India's Indigenous Medical Systems

A CROSS-DISCIPLINARY APPROACH

India's Indigenous Medical Systems

A CROSS-DISCIPLINARY APPROACH

edited by

SYED EJAZ HUSSAIN
MOHIT SAHA

PRIMUS BOOKS

PRIMUS BOOKS

An imprint of Ratna Sagar P. Ltd.
Virat Bhavan
Mukherjee Nagar Commercial Complex
Delhi 110 009

Offices at
CHENNAI LUCKNOW
AGRA AHMEDABAD BANGALORE COIMBATORE
DEHRADUN GUWAHATI HYDERABAD JAIPUR
JALANDHAR KANPUR KOCHI KOLKATA MADURAI
MUMBAI PATNA RANCHI VARANASI

First published 2015

ISBN: 978-93-80607-62-7

PUBLISHED BY PRIMUS BOOKS

Lasertypeset by Guru Typograph Technology
Crossings Republic, Ghaziabad 201 009

Printed and bound in India by Replika Press Pvt. Ltd.

Contents

Acknowledgements

WE ARE GRATEFUL to the Indian Council of Historical Research (ICHR), New Delhi, for providing financial assistance, and the Vice-Chancellor of Visva-Bharati for the fund from Study Circle, that enabled us to conduct the seminar on 'India's Indigenous Medical Systems: Historical Perspective and Contemporary Relevance'. My esteemed colleague, Sandip Basu Sarbadhikary, has played an instrumental role in ensuring the release of the latter. I would also like to thank all the contributors who held their patience throughout the entire process of publication of this volume.

SYED EJAZ HUSSAIN
MOHIT SAHA

Introduction

Syed Ejaz Hussain & Mohit Saha

Today history is not what the elders wrote; stressed and interpreted in context of land revenue and fiscal systems, peasants' rebellion and workers' movements or political and administrative structure, etc. Other factors also acted as the motor of change in society: production, dissemination and adoption of knowledge in general, and scientific knowledge in particular, has been the water mark for the growth, survival and extinction of civilizations. Medical science and health systems—conventional and modern, oriental and occidental—have also played some definite role in shaping and reshaping the society from the remote past. Greek, Arab, Chinese and Indian heritage in the medical knowledge are being explored today in context of modern scientific interpretation.

Social character and cultural polity of India is reflected in the domain of scientific and medical development of the country. The fact that India is generally termed as a 'recipient' society, and considering the manner in which Western science and medicine was received and perceived, exhorted the modern scholarship to explore the field of medicine and public health to find out how it was used as a tool of dominance and control in a colonial set-up. David Arnold's *Science, Technology and Medicine in Colonial India* (1993) was a pioneering hunt in this line of enquiry. Since then the subject has been extensively and critically examined, and diverse facts and facets have been brought about in scores of works broadly covering the colonial phase. This framework of historical writings particularly appealed to the revisionists who worked on pre-colonial or more precisely medieval history of South Asia. They were encouraged to investigate and examine the status and dynamism of science and technology as also medicine in the precolonial period in India, and to trace the indigenous roots of scientific developments.

Ayurveda, Unani and Siddha have been the three major systems of indigenous medicine in India. India's earliest indigenous medical system, Ayurveda, thrived on the two classical medical compendiums, i.e. *Caraka Saṁhitā* and *Suśruta Saṁhitā*. Ayurveda establishes that disease is a natural process and that symptoms are the reactions of the body to the disease. It forms a holistic healing science dealing not only with treatment of some diseases but projecting the system as a complete way of life. The goal of Ayurveda is prevention of disease as well as promotion of the body's own capacity for maintenance and balance of *Tridosha* or the three humours. Unani moved from Greece and Rome to Alexandria, Iran and finally reached Baghdad where a new dialogue and discourse between civilizations became a hallmark in the process of historical developments. Learned Muslims, Christians, Hindus and others translated several scientific and philosophical works including medicinal texts into Arabic in the middle of the eighth century under the rule of the Abbasid Caliphs, Harun Al-Rashid (AD 786–809) and his son Ma'mun Al-Rashid (AD 813–33).

When Mongols ravaged Persian and Central Asian cities like Shiraz, Tabrez and Geelan, a large number of scholars and physicians of Unani medicine fled to India and got patronage under the Delhi Sultanate. The Delhi Sultans, the Khaljis, the Tughlaqs, the Lodis and later the Mughal Emperors took keen interest in the promotion of Unani-tibb and extended state patronage to the scholars and physicians. They also enrolled some accomplished medical practitioners as court physicians. Among them Abu Bakr bin Ali Usman Kashani, Sadruddin Damashqui, Mian Bhowa bin Khawas Khan, Ali Geelani, Akbar Arzani and Mohammad Hashim Alvi Khan were some of the leading physicians whose experimentations and contributions to Unani-tibb became the groundwork for the growth of the system in India. At the same time the spirit of dialogue and discourse between civilizations and institutions of knowledge was revived and rekindled in India. Ayurveda, Unani-tibb and Siddha practitioners benefited from the sharing and exchange of observations and knowledge with each other in an unbiased and cooperative manner and thus helped enrich India's indigenous medical systems.

During the British rule, indigenous medical systems suffered a setback and their development was hampered due to withdrawal of governmental patronage. European and British physicians like Manucci, François Bernier, John Fryer and John Ovington criticized the Indian physicians and surgeons for their ignorance of anatomy and surgical methods. Earlier, in the sixteenth-century Goa, the Christian medical practitioners who considered themselves the 'doctors of soul', initiated various works of mercy like running orphanages and educational institutions, simply as a means to achieve the ends of raison d' être or conversion of the entire world to Christianity. The members of the Society of Jesus and the Royal Hospital of Goa, at least, practically worked for it—as is evident from the narration of the Portuguese doctor, Garcia da Orta who stayed in Goa from 1534 to 1563. But the Ayurvedic and Unani practitioners during the Sultanate period never had any such agenda, nor did any such idea germinate in Mughal India.

In spite of the onslaught and attack by the Europeans, the indigenous medical systems enjoyed faith among the masses and continued to be practiced both in rural and urban areas, and in fact still cater to medical needs of a large chunk of the country's population. Though there is great respect for allopathic medicine, there is immense faith in the abilities of traditional medical healers and practitioners to treat some chronic and seasonal diseases. Ayurveda, Unani, Siddha and other conventional systems of healing have been undergoing several changes in the method of treatment, research and examination of drugs, control and standardization, preservation and promotion of herbal plants, mass production and supply of medicines and their advertisements through electronic and print media as well as the growing concerns for community or public health. Instead of traditional examinations of the patient's urine and stool, modern techniques of investigation such as microscopic examination, chemical analysis, radiography and electrocardiography, etc., are now encouragingly adopted and employed by the practitioners of Ayurveda and Unani.

The present volume is based on papers of a seminar on 'India's Indigenous Medical Systems: Historical Perspective and Contemporary Relevance' held in the Department of History, Visva-Bharati, Santiniketan. This Department offers an optional paper at the postgraduate level on History of Science and Technology which incorporates a good portion on India's Indigenous Medical Systems especially Ayurveda and Unani. Interestingly the seminar was attended by faculty from various streams, Allopath, Ayurveda, Unani, historians as well as faculty from science and humanities. They shared a common platform and exchanged their experiences and observations to best utilize for the society the knowledge and potentiality of the healing systems we have inherited. The volume incorporates a total of nineteen research papers contributed by the scholars and faculty of various streams like history, medicine and surgery, humanities, science and information technology to the achievement of this common goal.

Deepak Kumar has surveyed the history of medicine in South Asia and has raised certain pertinent questions relating to collaboration and conflicts between the indigenous and Western systems. He has stressed that both Ayurveda and Unani interacted with and borrowed from each other in India after the introduction of Galenic traditions in medieval period and the concept of *arka* had entered Ayurveda. He has argued that several Sanskrit medical texts were translated into Arabic and Persian but instances of Islamic works being translated into Sanskrit are very rare. He has also pointed out that when the Western medical system entered India, there was again a period of collaboration and conflicts; Western medicine emphasized the cause of disease using the tools of microbes and microscopes but the indigenous system laid stress on the power of resistance in human body. Still, a dialogue began between both systems—indigenous and Western, but this dialogue was not translated into real practice by the medical practitioners.

Ishrat Alam has harnessed upon the untapped Dutch sources to probe how the people of divergent societies across continents and civilizations tried to understand the disease processes and possible medicines or treatment procedures. The pre-modern society in Japan, Ceylon, China and India or anywhere else was always open and receptive to new concepts and ideas about diseases and medicines, and was always inclined to adopt and integrate new methods of curing or preventing and controlling diseases. During the sixteenth–seventeenth centuries, Europeans, especially the Portuguese, the Dutch and the English physicians and surgeons who visited India 'were understandably perturbed over relatively high mortality rate amongst them in comparison to the indigenous people in the territories they were trading'. The author has briefly surveyed the Ayurvedic and Unani biomedical knowledge and methods of treatment and then shifted to the observation of European medical practitioners in India. Introduction and use of *Chob-i chini* or China root in various Asian societies is interesting information brought to light by the author.

In his article 'Rise and Decline of Surgery in Indigenous Medicine with Emphasis on Unani-tibb', Syed Ejaz Hussain has discussed the various kinds of medical instruments and tools produced in India and the Islamic world on the basis of the descriptions in *Suśruta Saṁhita* and *Kitab Al-Tasrif.* Sterilization of the medical instruments, introduction of experimental surgery, dialogue of exchange and sharing of knowledge between Ayurveda and Unani are the chief points addressed by him. Hussain has posited that overstress on maintaining the balance of humours (or *tridosha* and *akhlat*) in Ayurveda and Unani-tibb might have played a role in the torpid growth and decline of surgery in India's indigenous medical systems.

Debraj Chakraborty has explored the development of medicine and public health at the time of Jahangir who extended support and patronage to medicine and public health. A number of hakims and vaidyas flourished, and several dispensaries/hospitals were started during this time. But when an epidemic-like plague broke out, the Emperor and his hakims were rendered helpless and unable to control it—as a result of which hundreds of people died of such epidemics.

Achintya Kumar Dutta has traced the trajectory of Ayurveda through the nineteenth and twentieth centuries, and has examined the efficacy/inefficacy of Ayurveda in combating and controlling epidemics and some fatal diseases. The individualistic and cultural framework of Ayurveda, the author argues, robbed this system of treatment and its potentiality, while there were some regional factors for its decline in Bengal particularly.

Sujata Mukherjee has examined the process of encounter between Ayurveda and Western medicine. She has identified the potentiality and dynamism of Ayurveda, and the response of Ayurveda practitioners to the challenges posed by the introduction of Western medicine, particularly in colonial Bengal.

Nupur Dasgupta has traced, in historical perspective, the birth of *dravya* (concept of drugs) and the emergence of Ayurveda Material Medica as a discipline in the nineteenth century. This was at a time when the British physicians, scientists and botanists took keen interest in both classical texts and indigenous medical practices, and documented the knowledge on medicine to expose it to the Western world.

Inoculation and the role of *tikadars* in the socio-cultural milieu of nineteenth and twentieth centuries Bengal has been the subject of investigation in the chapter of Arabinda Samanta. What social resistance and challenges grew especially after the introduction of vaccination for smallpox in Bengali society has also been probed by the author.

Chhanda Chatterjee has brought to light forgotten work of Dr Martin Honigberger who came to Punjab from Transylvania during the reign of Maharaja Ranjit Singh. She argues that Honigberger, who did not have a high opinion of indigenous methods of treatment in India, was equally well aware of the pitfalls of Western medicine. Honigberger discovered several medicinal herbs in Punjab and Kashmir and provided some meeting points between indigenous and Western medicine.

Arunangshu Ganguly and Anil Bharani have scientifically studied the Terminalia Arjuna bark extracts which are used in various forms for the treatment of a variety of cardiovascular disorders. On the basis of clinical trials and tests they have attempted to establish that Terminalia Arjuna has been used in India for heart disease from very ancient times and was prescribed by Vagbhatta and other physicians in early modern period and is, in fact, still found useful in the treatment of various heart disorders.

Growth and acceptance of Unani medicine in India and some neighbouring countries is the subject of Anis Ahmad Ansari. The government patronage, enactment of various acts and establishment of an institution like AYUSH, has given encouragement and support to the Unani medicine. Not only several dispensaries and hospitals but Unani-tibb medical colleges are flourishing at several places in India and abroad.

Ashhar Qadeer has evaluated some major works on Unani-tibb composed in India. These works have incorporated various aspects like terminology, diseases and methods of treatment of Ayurveda described in several works in Sanskrit. He has posited that Unani medicine—that owes its origin to Greece—has so profoundly transformed in Indian climate and temperament that its basic character has changed, and it looks foreign to Greece and more indigenous to India.

Concept, classification and comparison of treatment in Ayurveda, Unani and Siddha have been revisited by Parthasarathi Giri. He has rued that the lack of scientific research on Western lines acted as the bottleneck for the lagging behind of the Indian systems of treatment which were simply considered as art.

Mohit Saha has identified some Indian plants and herbs which have been traditionally used for the treatment of jaundice. Some of these plants are now patent and are being used for the treatment of Hepatitis B, as has been established by clinical trials by some allopathic practitioners. The author has advocated for cross-pathy practices among both qualified Allopathic and Ayurvedic practitioners, but the chief obstacle in this connection is the MCI clause which prohibits the allopathic practitioners to prescribe drugs from Ayurvedic system of medicine. He has argued that the benefit of the patient, in fact, lies in the optimal balance and evidence-based use of the two systems and this needs to be encouraged, especially in developing countries like India which has a very inadequate doctor-patient ratio.

Encounter with Western medicine and the disadvantageous position of surgery in indigenous systems are the chief points of contention of the paper of Jayanta Bhattacharya. He has emphasized that the growth of knowledge pertaining to human anatomy was the chief characteristic of Western medicine, while Ayurveda could not develop or even borrow this knowledge. Sushruta's *marman* theory enabled the traditional practitioners to perform even rhinoplasty, yet the knowledge of anatomy did not undergo any epistemological change. However, the excellent knowledge of chemistry and botany survived and sustained the Indian systems of medicine and this often inclined the natives to reject the Western medicine.

Nirmalya Banerjee and Madhumita Majumdar have concentrated on the biological evaluation and medicinal properties of orchids, a group of charming flower plants which has been largely used for preparing various drugs like 'Chyavanprash' and even 'Vanilla'. As botanists, they have also suggested methods and strategies for protection and preservation of the numerous varieties of orchids.

Habibur Rahaman has briefly traced the growth of organized documentation of ethno-botanical medicine in India. He has identified thirty-four plant species of Birbhum district of West Bengal, that have been used as mono-herbal and poly-herbal forms for the cure of twenty-six types of different diseases and ailments in the Santhal society of the district. He has also enumerated these plant species on the basis of their botanical names followed by local names, parts used, names of the diseases, mode of administration, distribution, and chemical constituents. But the Santhal tribes never came out of their magico-spiritual shell.

S.N. Ojha debates on the question of the introduction of ontology and bio-informatics into India's indigenous medical systems. The process for this, he argues, already began some twenty-five years ago. This has provided a foundation for crossing the cultural barriers such as religio-spiritual framework in case of Ayurveda, Unani and Siddha. The growth of ontology, thus, may support the need of the healthcare process in transmitting, re-using and sharing patient data.

Notion of health and masculinity formed a part of the discourse of nationalism in Bengal in the late nineteenth and early twentieth centuries. In this context, Amrit Sen has tried to focus on the *Khadya Bigyan* or *The Science of Food* (1936) of Acharya Prafulla Chandra Ray who prescribed certain indigenous dietary practices as source of preventive and curative medicine for Bengali people and rejected the colonial dietary practices for them.

Across-the-board presentations in the volume expect a wider audience including the postgraduate students and research scholars as well as those who are avid to know peripheries of historical inquiry.

1

History of Medicine in South Asia

Some Concerns, Some Questions

DEEPAK KUMAR

> Medical history, without any doubt, is first of all history, a historical discipline like the history of philosophy, the history of art, or the history of music. It, therefore, has the general methods of historical research in common with other historical disciplines. But it is a special history and therefore different from all others, with problems and methods of its own. . . . Medical history, therefore, will study health and disease through the ages, the conditions for health and disease, and the history of all human activities that tended to promote health, to prevent illness, and to restore the sick, no matter who the acting individuals were.
>
> —H.E. SIGERIST, *A History of Medicine*, vol. I, New York, 1977

THE DOYEN OF medical history thus explained the significance and scope of the discipline he so passionately promoted. Earlier, the approach to the past was basically medical. He was one of the early few to visualize history of medicine as 'a critical historical discipline in which historians, philologists, philosophers and physicians collaborated'. He asked new questions: What health conditions were in a given society at a given time? Were there very many illnesses or few? What diseases prevailed? How did the people live? The rich and the poor, the master and the slave; under what conditions did they produce food and commodities, what was their housing like, their nutrition, their recreations? What was done to promote health and to prevent illness? What were the tools—religion, education or both? To these he added the history of hygiene and public health.[1] He constructed a social history of medicine not only from the point of view of physicians but that of the patient. How did the patients view the ailment and the cure? How were they treated? At what cost? Sigerist presented medical history not only as the concern of history but as 'the

*This essay is based primarily on his introduction to *Disease and Medicine in India*, New Delhi, 2002. For some recent references he is grateful to Dr V.K. Yadavendu.

compass that guides us into the future', or rather as 'medicine' per se. His was a vision of medicine, not just what medicine has been, but what it is and should be.[2] In an age when science and art of medicine has become very complex with specialities and supra-specialities, history of medicine provides a vantage point from which medicine can be seen as a whole.[3]

Sigerist was a pioneer but not alone. He represented an era of great technological changes which had brought the world closer. Fielding Garrison, for example, showed concern for 'the medicine and sanitation of the whole world'.[4] The colonized world also received attention, thanks to its unique tropical environment and problems. In this genre come Harold Scott's *A History of Tropical Medicine* and Charles Wilson's *Ambassadors in White*.[5] These were supplemented by a number of medical memoirs and travelogues which brought hitherto less known areas and its diseases into focus.[6]

The Indian Weltanschauung

How does the above outline fit into the Indian landscape? How did the Indians create, promote and view their medical thought and practices? From time immemorial, the Indian medical men, inspite of their scripture-orientation, have insisted on the supreme importance of direct observation of natural phenomena and on the technique of a rational processing of empirical data. The *Caraka Saṁhitā*, an ancient medical text, says, 'To one who understand, knowledge of nature and love of humanity are not two things but one'.[7]

In the Indian world view, nature and culture, subject and object were never seen in an adversarial mould.[8] But it was definitely complex; different thought processes and views were expressed and these could coexist. So one has superstition and reason both together. Again, it is this trend which takes even *yukti-vyapashraya bhesaja* (rational medicine) to the mirth and mire of metaphysics.[9] From magico-religious beginnings to rationalistic therapeutics and then back to decadence, it must be a fascinating journey. What were the factors responsible for the ups and downs and frequent changes in assumptions? Was it because of the priestly class and the *varnasrama* hierarchy which controlled both knowledge generation and knowledge dissemination? The priests would naturally be interested in supernaturalism and mystification of nature. Why did the medical men bow to them?[10] Probably they had no other option.

Similarly, for the medieval times one needs to know how traditional or canonical knowledge always claimed superiority. For example, how the Mutailites (who based their arguments on reason but without contradicting the Koranic observations) were gradually replaced by the fatalistic Asharites who repudiated rational thought? Al-Hytham's ideas and experiments in optics later degenerated into metaphysical debates. Why could the experimental rigour of a Susruta or Al-Hytham not be institutionalized? As a perceptive scholar explains: 'A society oriented towards fatalism, or one in which an interventionist deity forms part of the matrix of causal connections, is bound to produce fewer individuals inclined to probe the unknown with the tools of science.'[11]

To this was added a highly divisive caste system very peculiar to the South Asian society. Caste led to the ruinous separation of theory from practice, of mental work from manual work.[12] Faith and caste were to prove a fatal combination. The whole society was obsessed with spiritual and social engineering. So India produced Nanak, Kabir and Meera but no Harvey or Vesalius. The political and social leadership was no less responsible. There, no doubt, was an enormous intellectual (or cultural?) failure on the part of the ruling class.[13] Abul Fazl, a reliable witness to the Mughal era, mourned: 'The blowing of the heavy wind of *taqlid* (tradition) and the dimming of the lamp of wisdom . . . the door of "how" and "why" has been closed, and questioning and enquiry have been deemed fruitless and tantamount to paganism.'[14]

It is not that the Asians did not value knowledge. Here, knowledge developed through commentaries which were both valid and useful. But these hardly held the possibilities of paradigm shifts. Traditions stood like rock. Very few could hope to transcend the limits of faith, culture and canonized knowledge (e.g. *Siddhantas* or *Saṁhitās*). People could still be creative and the society did advance from simple to complex, rural to urban, etc. In this context, what was the medical scenario in South Asia? A formidable medical tradition had evolved, no doubt, but were new questions asked? Changes did take place; new interactions were made, but was there any recognizable shift?

Certain questions appear which may be difficult to answer in terms of ancient and medieval Indian histories but which should nonetheless deserve some attention. How was healing practised and who practised it? How was disease perceived? Medical anthropologists have looked into the magico-religious rites, rituals and the shamans. Can these be contextualized historically? How can one chart the interaction between the great and little traditions in terms of folk medicine and ethnohistory?[15] How did the many distinct and competing practitioners relate to each other—for example, the Ayurveda, Unani and folk practitioners? This question is put in sharper focus when modern medicine entered new lands riding the colonial wave. Colonialism required bodies to travel from one place to another and this influenced the relations between the bodies and the pathogens. Moreover, the colonizers were naturally anxious about their fragility either in the face of larger natural and social environments or in relation to other bodies (indigenous or foreign) that constituted an implicit threat.[16] What were its epidemiological consequences? Sanitation and concerns for public health? Then, how much 'public' was public health?[17] Colonial expansion strengthened the alliance between science and State and the concept of state science/medicine emerged.[18] How did it function? What was its impact? Is there anything specifically colonial about colonial medicine?

Ayurveda as 'the science of (living to a ripe) age', sans mantras, appeared around Buddha's time. The concept of humours or *dosas* which has been central in Ayurveda is nowhere seen in the Vedic literature. Nor does it reflect Hippocratic or Galenic thinking. Ayurveda's emphasis on humoural 'balance', moderation, etc., seem rather closer to Buddha's 'Middle Path'. Disease causation in Ayurveda is not only because of humoural 'imbalance' (*vaisamya*) but for a variety of reasons like weather, food, emotional agitations, sins from past life and even 'sins against wisdom' (*prajna paradha*).[19] Its protagonists might have been inaccurate in their knowledge of human physiology, but they were extremely good at plant morphology, its medical functions and therapeutics.[20] Both Charak and Susruta put emphasis on direct observation which is extremely significant. In any case, ancient medicine or Ayurveda remains a living and fertile area of research and interpretations such as social history of medicine, non-Sanskritic medical practices, religious and folk healing, barber-surgeon traditions, history of healing places from epigraphic records and other narratives of disease and healing.[21]

The scenario becomes even more interesting when the Islamic medical men introduced the Galenic tradition. There gradually appeared a hybrid of Muslim-Hindu system known as the *Tibb.* They differed in theory, but in practice both traditions seem to have interacted and borrowed from each other. From the Islamic side the concept of *arka* entered Ayurveda. Several Sanskrit medical texts were translated into Arabic and Persian, but instances of Islamic works being translated into Sanskrit are rare.

To this one can add the travelogues and writings of a number of European travellers like Francois Bernier, Niocolao Manucci, Garcia da Orta, and John Ovington who wrote extensively on Indian medical practices. They looked at these practices with curiosity and disdain.[22] But in the use of drugs Europeans and Indians learned from each other, as the works of van Rheede, Sassetti, and da Orta would testify.[23] The Europeans introduced new plants in India that were gradually incorporated into the Indian pharmacopoeia. Indian diseases received graphic description in Ovington's travelogue.[24] The best account of smallpox and the Indian method of variolation was given by J.Z. Holwell in 1767. To him, this method although quasi-religious, still appeared 'rational enough and well-founded'.[25] The travellers depicted Indian medical practices more as a craft and one that was governed by caste rules and wrapped in superstition. Yet they could not help admiring the wonder called rhinoplasty (on which modern plastic surgery is founded), nor could they deny the efficacy of Indian drugs. The Indians for their part did not completely insulate themselves from the 'other' practices. As the interaction grew in the eighteenth century, the vaidyas even took to bleeding in a large number of cases. Yet while the European medical men were gradually moving, thanks to the works of Vesalius and Harvey, from a humoural to a chemical or mechanical view of the body, Indians remained faithful to their texts.[26]

The Colonial Interventions

Mark Harrison rightly argues that the development of public health in India has to be seen 'in terms of a dynamic matrix of motives and sectional interests within and between European and Indian communities'.[27] But he finds the scope and effectiveness of colonial medical intervention rather 'limited'. Widespread indigenous taboos and suspicions, and the reluctance of the Indian rentier class to pay, precluded the possibility of 'any vigorous programme of sanitary reform'.[28] In such explanations, the role of the State unfortunately gets marginalized. Modern medicine entered India riding the colonial wave and, as a recent critique puts it, colonial medicine did not mean altruism, it meant uncanny imperialism.[29] No wonder, it failed to make the transition from state medicine to public health.[30] And public health itself could never be defined in terms of 'human rights', in colonial conditions it was just the management of dangerous bodies. Notions about the 'danger of contact' grew stronger with the broad acceptance of microbial pathology at the end of the nineteenth century. Local people came to be seen as 'natural reservoirs' of germs. Medical theories that emerged thereupon exonerated the socio-economic conditions and the (ill) effects of imperialism and instead blamed the victims.[31]

In the given scenario of complete hegemonization, the possibilities of intercultural interactions were rather limited. The indigenous systems felt so marginalized that they sought survival more in resistance than in collaboration. Total acceptance of new knowledge sometimes did mean total rejection of the old. Under such pressure, some of the 'old' withdrew into their own shell. Yet the majority of Indians had favoured revival and synthesis. There were several areas in which the Western and indigenous systems could collaborate but did not. The former put emphasis on the cause of the disease, the latter on *nidana* (treatment). Microbes and microscopes constituted the new medical spectacle. But the vaidyas put emphasis on the power of resistance in the human body. The improvement of the *Kshetra* (body of the patient) is far more important than the microbe and its destruction.[32] The Westerners were forced to take cognisance of indigenous drugs and the vaidyas took to anatomy, ready delivery of medicines, quick relief and so forth. But the comparison ends here. As a recent critique argues, they were inclined to borrow but could not 'create a dialogue between the two epistemics'.[33] Borrowed knowledge seldom develops into organic knowledge. This was true also of the hundreds of doctors produced by the government medical colleges annually. In the melee, some really good opportunities were lost. All guns were targeted at the government: 'Let the government renounce its special care for English medicines. When fought on equal fields, we can see the valour of this unscientific system. Then only we can understand whether native medicine is relevant to science and how far the science of English medicine is magnificent.'[34]

Such criticisms were never taken seriously by the practitioners of Western medicine. Perhaps, they were too sure of their competence and superiority. They continued to ridicule the 'other'. As a professor of physiology at Lucknow wrote: 'The financing of Unani and Ayurvedic institutes by Government in the hope of finding some soul of goodness in them is precisely on a par with the same government financing archery clubs to find out the possibilities of the bow and arrow in modern warfare.'[35]

Unfortunately, the modern medical men were too sure of their competence and superiority.[36] The Bhore Committee on medicine in India (1944) reinforced these convictions of Western superiority.[37] Nevertheless, thanks to the new developments in medicine, health was poised to become a rallying point of unity and a centre of cooperative action.[38]

Health was to come on the political centre-stage in another sense also. A.V. Hill who in 1944 reported on the state of scientific research in India, talked of a quadrilateral dilemma, i.e. population, health, food and natural resources. To him, the fundamental problems of India were 'not really physical, chemical or technological, but a complex of biological ones referring to population, health nutrition and agriculture, all acting and reacting with another'.[39] Colonial India, no doubt, had its limitations. Could independent India meet the challenge?

Exploring New Subthemes

Canonical medical texts have so far been a favoured area of attention. In India, for example, the texts of Charaka, Susruta, Madhav and Vagbhatta have been commented upon by many scholars.[40] These need to be contextualized. It is possible to think of and attempt a balance between text and the context, between social constructivism and historical relativism. In the Indian context, it is even more important. To achieve this, a sound knowledge of the classical language in which a text is written is necessary. Then, this needs to be related to the numerous commentaries that have followed an established text.[41] After all, in India, knowledge advanced more through commentaries written in different periods than through a canonical text. Their critical assessment would require help from philologists and philosophers. It is a daunting task but nevertheless rewarding.

Coming closer to modern times, a critical study of the travelogues, missionary accounts and the despatches of the surgeon on board a ship or on distant shores, would be extremely relevant. These may bring to fore the nuances of civilizational encounter. As colonization set in, medicine acquired new dimensions. The colonial medical men, trained as they were in rudiments of botany, zoology, geology and other practical sciences, emerged as colonial scientists. Their works have received a great deal of attention in recent years. Yet a lot more remains to be done. These colonial scientists showed remarkable understanding of not only the topography, flora and fauna but the cultures they encountered. For example, long before Darwinism appeared or was accepted, a medico-botanist wrote: 'It is remarkable that the incarnations of their God Vishnu should be in conformity to the modern views respecting the gradation of animal forms, as displayed in ascending from the less to the more highly developed, so the incarnations proceed from the fish to the tortoise, thence to the pachydermatous boar, the carnivorous lion, dwarf and Ram, etc.'[42]

Others tried to convey to the Indians the message of William Harvey and the Age of Enlightenment that he represented:

> True philosophers who are only eager for truth and knowledge never regard themselves as already so thoroughly informed but that they welcome further information from whomsoever and from whensover it may come. Nor are they so narrow-minded as to imagine any of the Arts or Sciences transmitted to us by the Ancients in such a state of forwardness or completeness that nothing is left for the ingenuity and industry of others. . . . Neither do they think it unworthy of them to change their opinion if truth and undoubted demonstration require them to do so; nor do they esteem it discreditable to desert error though sanctioned by the highest authority.[43]

Could this message have been appreciated by the Indians, and if so, how and to what extent? This would be equally valid for other Asian societies and cultures as well. The Indians accepted British law without much fuss but not British medicine. The response was basically three-pronged: (1) conformism, (2) defiance, (3) quest for alternatives. Several questions emerged in the debates at both national and local forums. Was indigenous medicine to be patronized because it was found to be 'cheap' and 'popular'? What were the 'pressure groups'? Was there actually a protest against modernization of Indian medicine? Did the voice of 'defiance' end up being a voice on 'defence' of the indigenous system or was it also able to launch a critique of the Western medicine at a deeper level? In any case the West loomed large. It was difficult to oppose the West, even more difficult to ignore it.

Here, one may pause to reflect on how different colonized societies responded to the colonial medical interventions. For this purpose, in-depth comparative studies are required. The Dutch incursions in East Asia, for example, created a 'Dutch School' of physicians as opposed to the traditional 'Chinese School'.[44] Exchange in terms of medical ideas may not have been vigorous but the early colonial medical men did produce a number of medical-ethnographic, climatological and topographical descriptions. Some of these were of outstanding scientific value while some reinforced or even created myths about racial and physiological differences. The 'natives' had no means to defend themselves; there was (perhaps still is) no level field, much less level pegging.[45] In Shamanistic healing, the human body is thought of as a microcosm that is constantly influenced by the macrocosm. And what happens within the microcosm is believed to affect the macrocosm. Thus, breaches of *adat* (customary rules) may cause natural disasters or epidemics. This etiology raised doubts and invited derision. Yet some recognized the time-honoured curing devices of traditional Japanese and Indian health care. The meridians used in acupuncture are very real links in the nervous system and the main *chakra* (energy centres) along the *susumna* (spinal column) in yoga theory do correspond to the main glands of the body.[46]

Unlike in India, where there was huge distance between the colonizer and the colonized, in colonial Taiwan, the government was much more interventionist.

Here, the traditional *pao-chia* system was integrated with a modern police network and was also utilized as the lowest level of public health administration.[47] This system of collective responsibility was effective yet oppressive. Its chief proponent was Goto Shimpei whose concepts of society and state were basically 'biological'. Had A.V. Hill this example in mind when he referred to India's problems as basically 'biological'?[48] In all the East Asian societies, rapid post-war development has created sophisticated modern health care systems. Yet at the same time each society has maintained traditions of medical practice stretching back over centuries with a shared Confucian heritage, Daoist medical lore and useful folk wisdom resulting in linked forms of traditional Chinese medicine.[49] In China, modern nationalism rather helped. It offered 'license both to cultural iconoclasm and to cultural nationalism—the one to destroy the old culture as harmful to the nation, the other to cherish it as the hallmark of the national genius'.[50]

Apart from the forays into the dichotomies of cultural texts which has enormous relevance for public health debates, there are several other sub-themes which call for attention. How and to what extent medical pluralism is desirable?[51] Acceptance of differing views may on the whole be encouraged but can one tolerate certain particular approaches like witchcraft or the Nazi medical experiments?[52]

Long ago, Thomas McKeown had argued for a sociological approach instead of a linear one. He called for a medical history with 'public interest put in'.[53] In addition history of medicine must take cognisance of issues like gender and health, health and business, drug industry and bioethics, etc. Another area meriting attention is that of chronic diseases and disabilities. One needs to move away from excessive obsession with toxicology and pathology and think of occupational health hazards and environmental medicine.[54] Who can forget the Bhopal tragedy of 1984? Industrial technology has probably killed more people than military technology. There are new developments, for example, nanotechnology. These fine tools often play the lead role in the patient's treatment. Instead of the technology being just a tool in the physician's hands, the tool becomes the focus of the care and the physician becomes the mechanism by which the tool is applied. The questions of law, technology and ethics here get intertwined.[55] In fact, medicine itself emerges as techne, a concept that integrates theoretical, practical and evaluative aspects and bridges the conceptions of medicine as science and as art.[56] What a canvas and what a feast! I trust the historians would rise to the occasion.

Notes

1. H.E. Sigerist, 'The Philosophy of Hygiene', *Bulletin of the Institute of History of Medicine*, vol. I, 1933, pp. 323–1.
2. Owesei Temkin, 'Henry E. Sigerist and Aspects of Medical Historiography', *Bulletin of the History of Medicine*, vol. XXXII, no. 6, 1958, pp. 487–95.
3. D.V. Subba Reddy, 'Evolution of the Study and Writing of History of Medicine', *Indian Journal of History of Medicine*, vol. VI, 1961, pp. 21–39.

4. Fielding H. Garrison, 'Geomedicine: A Science in Gestation', *Bulletin of the Institute of History of Medicine*, vol. I, 1933, pp. 2–9, idem, *An Introduction to the History of Medicine*, Saunders, Philadelphia, 1929.
5. H.H. Scott, *A History of Tropical Medicine*, 2 vols., Baltimore: Williams & Wilkins, 1939–42; C.M. Wilson, *Ambassadors in White: The Story of American Tropical Medicine*, New York: Henry Holt & Co., 1942.
6. The examples can be seen in Ronald Ross, *Memoirs*, Murray, London, 1923; P. Manson-Bahr and A. Alcock, *The Life and Works of Sir Patrick Manson*, Cassel, London, 1927; Victor Heiser, *An American Doctor's Odyssey*, New York: Norton & Co., 1936; G.S. Seagrave, *Burma Surgeon*, New York: Norton & Co., 1943, etc.
7. Debiprasad Chattopadhyay, *Science and Society in Ancient India*, Calcutta: Research India, 1977, p. 7.
8. Ole Brunn and Arnae Kalland, eds., *Asian Perceptions of Nature*, London: Curzon Press, 1995.
9. R.C. Majumdar's enthusiastic account of Ayurveda is an example. See D.M. Bose et al., eds., *A Concise History of Science in India*, New Delhi: INSA Pub., 1971, pp. 213–62.
10. This question is relevant for present time as well. If a particular political dispensation imposes astro-medicine, should the medical institutions accept it?
11. Pervez Hoodbhoy, *Islam and Science: Religious Orthodoxy and the Battle for Rationality*, London: Zed Books, 1991, p. 120.
12. The intellectual portion of the community being thus withdrawn from active participation in the arts, and how and why of phenomena—the coordination of cause and effect—were lost sight of—the spirit of enquiry gradually died out. Her (India's) soil was rendered morally unfit for the birth of a Boyle, a Descartes, or a Newton. . . . P.C. Ray, *History of Hindu Chemistry*, vol. II, Calcutta, 1909, p. 195.
13. Athar Ali, 'The Eighteenth Century—An Interpretation', *Indian Historical Review*, vols. 1–2, 1979, pp. 175–86.
14. Quoted in Irfan Habib, 'Capacity of Technological Change in Mughal India', in *Technology in Ancient and Medieval India*, ed. A. Roy and S.K. Bagchi, Delhi, 1986, pp. 12–13.
15. D.V. Hart, *Filipino and Malayan Humoral Pathologies: Folk Medicine and Ethno-history in South-East Asia*, Data Paper no. 76, Ithaca: Cornell University, n.d.
16. Alan Bewell, *Romanticism and Colonial Disease*, Baltimore: John Hopkins University Press, 1999, p. 24.
17. C. Hamlin, *Public Health and Social Justice in the Age of Chadwick: Britain 1800–1854*, Cambridge: Cambridge University Press, 1998, pp. 1–14.
18 For details see, Deepak Kumar, *Science and the Raj*, 2nd edn., Delhi: Oxford University Press, 2006.
19. Dominik Wujastyk, *The Roots of Ayurveda*, New Delhi: Penguin, 1998, pp. 1–38.
20. G.P. Majumdar, 'Health and Hygiene', *Indian Culture*, vol. II, nos. 1–4, 1935–6, pp. 633–54.
21. Dominik Wujastyk, 'Indian Medical Thought on the Eve of Colonialism', *IIAS Newsletter*, 31 July 2003, p. 21.
22. A European traveller, Edward Ives (1755–7) thus writes of the Indian belief that 'man was divided into two or three hundred thousand part; ten thousand of which were made up of veins, ten thousand of nerves; seventeen thousand of blood, and a certain number of bones, choler, lymph, etc. and all this was laid down without form or order, either of history, disease or treatment.' Quoted in H.K. Kaul, *Travellers India: An Anthology*, Delhi, 1979, p. 299.
23. For details see John M. de Figueredo, 'Ayurvedic Medicine in Goa according to European Sources in the Sixteenth and Seventeenth Centuries', *Bulletin of History of Medicine*, vol. 58, no. 2, 1984, pp. 225–35.

24. A. Neelmeghan, 'Medical Notes in John Ovington's Travelogue', *Indian Journal of History of Medicine*, vol. VII, 1962, pp. 12–21.
25. J.Z. Holwell, *An Account of the Manner of Inoculating for the Smallpox in the East Indies*, London, 1767, p. 24.
26. M.N. Pearson, 'The Thin End of the Wedge: Medical Relativities as a Paradigm of Early Modern Indian-European Relations', *Modern Asian Studies*, vol. 29, no. 1, 1995, pp. 141–70.
27. Mark Harrison, *Public Health in British India*, Cambridge: Cambridge University Press, 1994, p. 228.
28. Ibid., p. 234.
29. Anil Kumar, *Medicine and the Raj*, New Delhi: Sage, 1998, p. 218.
30. David Arnold, *Colonizing the Body*, Delhi: Oxford University Press, 1993, p. 3.
31. Warwick Anderson, 'Where is the Postcolonial History of Medicine', *Bulletin of History of Medicine*, vol. 72, 1998, pp. 522–30. On the contrary, some scholars argue that there never was a colonial divide between colonizers and the colonized. Instead, within a generation of conquest, local collaborators had emerged who saw that their family's ways forward was through learning and imitating European ways. Sheldon, Watts, *Epidemics & History*, London: Yale University Press, 1997, p. 271.
32. *Dhanwantari* (Malayalam), 4 February 1925, pp. 133–5; see also G. Srinivasa Murti, *The Science and the Art of Indian Medicine*, Madras: Theosophical Pub., 1948, pp. 139–42.
33. K.N. Panikkar, 'Indigenous Medicine and Cultural Hegemony: A Study of the Revitalization Movement in Keralam', *Studies in History*, vol. 8, no. 2, 1992, pp. 283–307.
34. *Dhanwantari*, 18 October 1920, p. 146.
35. *Indian Medical Gazette*, vol. 62, 1927, p. 223.
36. 'The indigenous system of India has been a cause of disappointment to us not because they are successful rivals of modern medicine, but because we have been able to borrow or steal from them so little that is of real value'. J.W.D. Megaw, 'Confidential Note on the Working of the Punjab Medical Deptt.', 6 September 1928, IHD, 1.1, 464 India, Box 5, f. 34, Rockefeller Archive Centre (RAC).
37. A prominent member of this Committee was Sir Weldom Dalrymple Champneys (1892–1980). In a lighter vein he composed: 'My name is –er-Eustace, As you see, I'm fine specimen of the Master Race You may think my conversation inane, but to manage these dirty Indian does not need a brain!' Champneys Papers, GC/139/H. 2/10, London: Wellcome Institute.
38. It was argued that things like penicillin and the sulpha drugs could be 'the ingredients of a new synthesis. But indigenous drugs and methods had no place in it'. Diary of Raymond Fosdick (Director, RF. 1938–48). RG. 12.1, RAC.
39. A.V. Hill, *Scientific Research in India*, London: Royal Society, 1944; idem, *The Ethical Dilemma of Science and Other Essays*, New York: Rockefeller Institute Press, 1960, p. 375.
40. P.V. Sharma, *History of Medicine in India*, New Delhi: INSA, 1992.
41. Jan Meulenbeld's, gargantuan *History of Indian Medical Literature* is an example.
42. J.F. Royle, *An Essay on the Antiquity of Hindoo Medicine*, London: Allen & Co., 1837, p. 178.
43. G.R. McRobert, 'William Harvey's Message to India', *The Indian Medical Gazette*, April 1929, pp. 225–8.
44. Peter Boomgaard, 'Dutch Medicine in Asia, 1600–1900', ed. David Arnold, op. cit., 1996, pp. 42–6, note 44.
45. Deepak Kumar, 'Unequal Contenders, Uneven Ground: Medical Encounters in British India, 1820–1920', in *Western Medicine as Contested Knowledge*, ed. Cunningham and B. Andrews, Manchester: Manchester University Press, 1997, pp. 172–90.

46. Ina E. Slamet-Velsink, 'Some Reflections on the Sense and Nonsense of Traditional Health Care', in *Health Care in Java*, ed. P. Boomgaard et al., Leiden: KTLV, 1996, pp. 65–80.
47. One *chia* was made up of ten households, and one *pao* was composed of ten *chia*. The system was used to prevent epidemic diseases like plague. Kohei Wakimura, 'Mortality and Public Health under the Colonial Rule: India and Taiwan, *Osaka City University Economic Review*, vol. 34, no. 1, October 1998, pp. 1–16.
48. See Note 39.
49. Ian Holliday, 'Traditional Medicine in Modern Societies', *Journal of Medicine and Philosophy*, vol. 28, no. 3, 2003, pp. 379–89.
50. The first important patron of 'reformed' or 'scientificized' Chinese medicine was Yen Hsi-shan, the Governor of Shansi. In 1921, he set up a 'Research Society for the Reform of Chinese Medicine', which would try to combine the best features of the Chinese and Western medicine. R.C. Croizier, 'The Ideology of Medical Revivalism in Modern China', in *Asian Medical System*, ed. Charles Leslie, California: Cambridge University Press, 1977, pp. 343–4.
51. For critical appraisal see, S. Cant and U. Sharma, *A New Medical Pluralism?*, London: UCL Press, 1999; R. Porter, ed., *The Popularisation of Medicine, 1650–1850*, London: Routledge, 1992.
52. As Ernst argues, 'one has to steer between the Scylla of imposing the well-tried and supposedly superior scientific criteria of biomedicine and the Charybdis of leaving the public exposed to potentially unprofessional, unethical and fraudulent practices'. W. Ernst, *Plural Medicine: Tradition and Medicine*, London: Routledge, 2002, pp. 1–18.
53. Thomas McKeown, 'A Sociological Approach to the History of Medicine', *Medical History*, vol. XIV, 1970, pp. 342–51; Reiterated in D. Porter, 'The Mission of Social History of Medicine: A Historical View', *Social History of Medicine*, vol. 7, no. 3, 1995, pp. 345–59.
54. Paul Weindling, ed., *The Social History of Occupational Health*, London: Croom Helm, 1985, p. 6.
55. Lars Noah and Barbara Noah, *Law, Medicine and Medical Technology*, New York: Foundation Press, 2002.
56. Bjorn Hofmann, 'Medicine as Techne: A Perspective from Antiquity', *Journal of Medicine and Philosophy*, vol. 28, no. 4, 2003, pp. 403–25.

2

Diseases and Medicines in the Pre-Modern World

Divergent Societies' Assessments

Ishrat Alam

In the present essay, an attempt has been made to understand disease processes in different societies, which, needless to say, requires integration of biomedical and historical knowledge. Such an exercise will play a significant role in collaborative and multidisciplinary research in this field by exploring the history of disease processes and contemporary human interventions. During the sixteenth–seventeenth centuries, Europeans, especially of Portuguese, Dutch and English origins (since I am dealing with their accounts), were understandably perturbed over relatively high mortality rate amongst them in comparison with the indigenous people in the territories they were trading. The differential experiences of tropical people attracted the attention of curious individuals who tried to understand the distinctiveness of the knowledge system(s) of people they had come into contact with. The exercise in understanding of such systems, will, it is hoped, help in (1) focusing on large scale dynamics of disease transmission in specific historical contexts, (2) in reconstructing some disease process that affected Asian population, and (3) in understanding introduction of some Euro-Afro American diseases into South and South-East Asia along with north European companies' arrival on these lands and their deleterious consequences on the demography of receiving societies. Some remarkable studies have been done to understand transoceanic exchanges and their biological or cultural consequences. But they are mostly concerned with Africa.[1] Studies on the Indian Ocean have been relatively fewer, however, the Indian Ocean also attracted the attention of some scholars towards such an important but largely neglected area of enquiry.[2]

As a backdrop, it is required to have a preliminary knowledge about the prevailing systems of identification and treatment of diseases in Asian societies on the eve of the arrival of European trading companies. The Ayurvedic system was possibly the most known and documented ancient system. The art of selecting substances which could be assimilated by the human system with benefit, and their cooking and compounding to give the most nourishment and health, constituted integral components of the ancient medical science of India. The term Ayurveda itself was concerned mainly with the prolonging of healthy life and prevention of disease and senility and only secondarily with curing of disease.[3]

The Ayurveda essentially believed in the humoural theory which was geared to the three major branches of medical knowledge; physiology, pathology and treatment. The actual term used in the Ayurveda is *tridosa*. Unlike humours identified in Europe, there were glaring differences between the *tridosa* concept of the Ayurveda and the Greek humoural theory. *Vayu*, *pitta* and *kapha* were supposed to be present in all living creatures, diffused simultaneously in every minute portion of the organism and to activate and govern the entire biological process between conception and death.[4] R.C. Majumdar was of the opinion that the conventional equating of the three humours with air, bile and phlegm possibly had a Greek origin.[5] A disease was caused by any disturbance in the equilibrium or agitation and, therefore, the cure of the disease lay in restoring the desired equilibrium or by pacification, restitution or expulsion of the offending *dosas*. The curative measures were resorting to administration of *bhesajas* (substances having the desired potentiality of restitution, restoration or pacification) and by the processes of cleansing, evacuation or surgery.[6] To the ancient Indian system of therapeutics was added another system popularly known as Unani-tibb or Arabian medicine by European historians. The Unani-tibb is essentially based on the Greek system which was founded by Hippocrates (*c.*460 BC), born on the island of Kos.[7] It is known as Unani owing to its Greek origin where it was established by Hippocrates and developed by Aristotle, Galen, and other Greek practitioners of medicine. Borrowed from the Greeks, the Arabs developed it further from the last quarters of the seventh century in conjunction with the Persian medical traditions.[8] According to Hippocrates, all living organism consisted of four humours—blood, phlegm, black bile and yellow bile.[9] Each of these consisted of four elements, viz., fire, water, air and earth—each of which in turn possessed some particular quality—heat, coolness, dryness and humidity. The essential factor in life is the natural heat, the seat of which is the left heart, and it pervades the entire organism. Any unsettlement due to internal or external causes, in the humours and their elements, led to disease, the natural heat tries to combat it. It is the responsibility of the physician to boost the natural healing power of the organism by suitable medicine when required, and not to supersede or impede it. However, the therapeutics of Hippocrates was not bound by any fixed rule. It was essentially individualistic. Under this system, the physician should treat the sick and not the sickness.[10]

In the Islamic world, the earliest independent Arab medical treatise, *Firdaus-ul Hikmat* (AD 850) was composed by Ali b. Rabban who summarized the whole system of Greek medicine as well as the Indian system of medicine on the basis of four important Indian medical works of Charaka, Susruta, Nidana, and Astangahridya. Following him, his student, Abu Bakr Muhammald b. Zakariyya al-Razi (Rhazes of medieval Europe) (d. first quarer of tenth century AD), made a thorough study of both the systems, was in charge of many hospitals, introduced the system of maintenance of records of every patient admitted into hospitals, and imparted practical training to the students.[11] He studied both the systems and emphasized both the maintenance of records relating to particular patients afflicted with particular disease(s), as also the method of practical training, a method which was adopted by the physicians as well.[12] But Abu Ali Husain b. Abdallah b. Sina (Avicenna AD 980–1036) and his *Qanun* (Canon) occupied the central place and dominated the world of medicine for subsequent centuries till the seventeenth century.[13] What is still more interesting is the fact that practitioners of medicine scattered in various parts of Islamic world continued to produce in Arabic and Persian, a whole series of books based on the Greek system of therapy, and in the course, anticipated the 'so-called modern theory of the circulation of blood as well as the germ theory'.[14] Similarly, they made contributions in the field of symptomatology, special pathology, epidemiology, ophthalmology, dietetics, toxicology and midwifery.[15] They were successful in pointing out the connection between exophthalmoses and goitize, introduced the process of bleeding for the treatment of cerebral haemorrhage and apoplexy, performed gastric lavage, used opotherapy and could keep a patient unconscious for seven days.[16] They were instrumental in evolving delicate surgical instruments, performing the amputation of the ovula, and exicisioning of the whole tongue, and removing the diseased bone from the skull and replacing it by that of a dog.[17] They contributed enormously to therapeutics, pharmacy and pharmaceutical techniques, and used many drugs and chemicals which were entirely unknown to the Greeks.[18] This Greco-Arabic medical knowledge system was ostensibly enriched further when it came into contact with the indigenous Ayurvedic system.[19]

In the context of medieval India, the first interaction with the outside world could be traced from the establishment of the Delhi Sultanate during which an interface took place between the indigenous Ayurvedic and *'Ilm-ul Tib* systems which had a reciprocal and pragmatic impact on both the divergent traditions.[20] In the sixteenth–seventeenth centuries, with the advent of the Europeans, another system was introduced into the Asiatic world.

To begin with, I will refer to Babur's observations about diseases and medicines which he encountered.

On 4 June 1505, Babur reports that his mother had fever.[21] He writes 'Blood was let without effect and a Khurasani doctor, known as Sajjid Tabib, in accordance with the Khurasani practice, gave her watermelon, but her time to die must have come, for on the Saturday after six days illness, she went to God's mercy'. Babur reports (29–30 April 1519) that he had burning fever: 'I got myself let blood. I had fever with sometimes two, sometimes three days between the attacks. In no attack did it cease till there had been sweat after sweat. After 10 or 12 days illness, Mulla Khwaja gave me narcissus mixed with wine; I drank it once or twice; even that did no good.'[22]

At another place talking about the therapeutic quality of lime (*B. Umu, C. acida*), Babur observes, 'If a person poisoned drink the water in which its fibres have been boiled, danger is averted'.[23]

Once Babur ate poisoned food and fell extremely sick. He reports further, 'on Saturday I drank a bowl of milk, on Sunday *'araq* in which stamped-clay and the best theriac *tiriaq-i-faruq* (an antidote), a strong purge. As on the first day, Saturday, something very dark, like parched bile was voided.'[24] He considered opium good enough for curing ear-ache.[25] Once during his march from Piag, he reported about the sudden appearance of boils on his body and he was treated by an Ottoman Turk (Rumi) who 'used a remedy which had been recently discovered in Rum. He boiled pepper in a pipkin; I held the sores in the steam, and, after steaming ceased, laved with hot water; the treatment lasted sidereal hours.'[26]

This is a clear attestation of the fact of transmission of medical knowledge from Europe to India.[27]

Babur writes about the use of pepper remedy, '. . . it must have been somewhat hotter than before, for it blistered (*qapardi*) my body, giving me much pain'.[28]

The Mughal court could attract possibly the most skilled physicians from other empires especially Iran, and the examples are galore. Interestingly in *Ain-i Akbari*, one comes across a list of no less than sixty-nine physicians.[29] Of them Hakim Misri occupied possibly the most important position.[30] At another place his name appears in the list of 'XVIII Commanders of Four Hundred'. According to Badauni, he was a very learned man and a clever doctor.[31] Next one hears about Hakim u'l Mulk whose real name was Shamsuddin, and like several other doctors, he had come from Gilan on the Caspian to Akbar's court.[32] Mulla Mir, also known as Mulla Mir Tabib Hairat, grandson of Mulla Abdul Hay Tazdi was another important physician.[33] Hakim Abul Fath was the son of Mulla Abdur Razzaq of Gilan. His name was Masihuddin Abul Fath. His two brothers, Hakim Humam and Hakim Nuruddin, also left Gilan and came to India.[34] He was a commander of 1,000, but according to Abul Fazl, he enjoyed the power of a vakil.[35] Hakim Zanbil Beg was, according to Badauni, a *muqarrib* or personal attendant on the emperor.[36] Hakim Ali of Gilan had migrated to Akbar's court. Once Akbar tried to test his acumen as a physician by giving him several bottles of urine of sick and healthy people and even of animals to distinguish their origin.[37] Hakim Ali correctly distinguished the different sources of urine.[38] In the 40th year, Hakim Ali was commander of 700 and earned the title of *Jālīnus-uz Zamani*, 'The Galenus of the age'. Subsequently, Jahangir made him a commander of 2,000.[39] His son Hakim Abdul Wahhab was given a rank of commander of 500, fifty horses.[40] Hakim Hasan had also come from Gilan,[41] as also Hakim Fathullah, the latter was greatly admired for his knowledge of medical literature.[42] In the first year of Jahangir's reign, he was a commander of 1,000, 300 horses.[43] His son Fathullah was later a doctor of Shahjahan.[44] Hakim Masihul Mulk had originally migrated from Shiraz and reached Akbar's court via the Deccan. He was appointed physician to Sultan Murad.[45] Hakim Jalaluddin Muzaffar of Ardistan was initially a doctor of Shah Tahmasp and later migrated to Akbar's court,[46] where he was liked by both Akbar and Jahangir. Jahangir had made him a commander of 3,000, 1000 horses. He suffered from *qarha-i Shush* (ulceration) or disease of the lungs for twenty years prior to his death for, he had been accidentally poisoned by his compounder.[47] Hakim Lutfullah, son of Mulla Abdur Razzaq of Gilan, was considered an able doctor by Badauni. Badauni says of him: 'He has read very many works on medicine, and his knowledge of astronomy is great. He has now gone to Kabul to treat Qilij Khan'.[48] Hakim Saiful Mulk Lang was given the nickname of '*Saiful Hukama*' 'the sword of the doctors' by his contemporaries and according to Badauni the popular perception was that, 'he killed his patients'.[49] He hailed from Damawand near Tehran and had great knowledge of medicine.[50] Badauni writes, 'As ill luck would have it, whenever this physician undertook the cure of a sick man, the unfortunate patient surrendered his life to the messenger of death, for which reason the wits gave him the nickname of was that, "*Saif-ul Hukama*" "sword of physicians"'.[51] Hakim Humam's real name was Humayun,[52] and though he was commander of 600 only, he was liked by Akbar.[53] Hakim Ain-ul Mulk was another important physician[54] as was Hakim Shifai, who was born at Isfahan, was a friend of Shah Abbas-i Safavi and later served under Akbar.[55] After him Abul Fazl gives a list of forty-six physicians who were of indigenous origin.[56] Of them, Shaikh Hasan of Panipat and his son Saikh Bina were renowned physicians. Shaikh Bina's son Shaikh Hasan or Hassu became very famous under Jahangir, and the emperor conferred the title of Muqarrab Khan on him.[57] He was hailed by his contemporaries as a good reputed surgeon. Abul Fazl also refers to Mahadev, Bhim Nath, Narayan, and Shivaji as important physicians of Akbar's reign.[58] But what is lamentable is the fact that one does not come across any narrative wherein the instruments, or methods used by them are discussed.

Jahangir provides us information about diseases and related issues during his time. His description of what was apparently the first advent of plague does deserve the attention. He writes: 'In this year, or rather in the 10th year after my accession, a great pestilence appeared in some places in Hindustan. The commencement of this calamity was in the parganahs of Panjab, and by degrees the contagion spread to the city of Lahore. Many of the people, Musulmans and Hindus, died through this. After this, it spread to Sirhind and the Duab, until it reached Delhi and its surrounding parganahs and villages, and desolated them. At this day, it had greatly diminished. It became known from men of great age and from old histories that this disease had never shown itself in this country before. Physicians and learned men were questioned as to its cause. Some said that it came because there had been draught for two years in succession and little rain fell, others said it was on account of the air which occurred through the draught and scarcity. Some attributed it to other causes. 'Wisdom is of Allah, and we must submit to Allah's decrees'! 'What does a slave who bows not his neck to the order'.[59] This is a surprising piece of evidence because much before Jahangir, Ibn Battuta in his travels undertaken between AD 1325–54, refers to occurrence of 'the Great Plague' at Damascus in July 1348.[60] Therefore, evidence provided by Jahangir assumes great significance. It seems plague was a late comer in the history of diseases in India. Did this disease reach India from Europe, West Asia or South-East Asia? It needs to be investigated.

Jahangir also tells about dog bite and its consequences. He writes that he was familiar with the fact that if any animal was bitten by a mad dog, the animal was sure to die. He cites the examples of two elephants which died because they were bitten by a mad dog.[61] Though the people were familiar with the impact, they obviously had neither identified the cause of death nor its remedy. As to rabies, later Niccolao Manucci refers (between the seventeenth and eighteenth centuries) to a newly married man who on his wedding night cut his bride to pieces. It was reported that he had been bitten by a mad dog three months before. The remedy for rabies was to cauterize the wound at once. Alternatively, if the bitten person went on a sea voyage, it was believed he would recover immediately.[62]

Jahangir reports about severe headache followed by fever for few days during which he had lost appetite. He writes,

> On Tuesday, 15th, I found I had a severe headache, which at last ended in fever. At night I did not drink my usual number of cups, and after midnight crop-sickness [increased crapulousness] was added to my fever, and till informing I rolled about in my couch. On Wednesday, the 16th, at the end of the day, the fever diminished, and after asking the advice of my doctors, I took my usual number of cups on the third night. Although they urged me to take some broth of pulse and rice, I could not make up my mind to do so. Since I arrived at the age of discretion, I never remember having taken *bughan* broth, and hope that I may not want it in future. When they food for me this day, I had no inclination for it. In short, for three days and two nights I remained fasting. Though I had fever for a day and a night, and my weakness was such that it appeared as if I had been confined to bed for a long time, I had no appetite left, and had no inclination towards food.[63]

Jahangir's description of one of his intimate attendants, Inayat Khan's death also provides some reference to a case of irresistible addiction to opium consumption. That along with the consumption of wine had resulted in a fatal combination leading to the inevitable death of Inayat Khan. Jahangir had ordered Hakim Rukna to attend on him, give Inayat Khan re-medial medicines, but all his efforts failed, for against the advice of Hakim Rukna, Inayat Khan insisted on more doses of opium and wine. Jahangir got his painters to draw a portrait of Inayat Khan and allowed him to proceed to Agra. But, as Jahangir writes, 'Next day he travelled the road of non-existence'.[64]

During the sixteenth and seventeenth centuries, certain developments took place in the history of medicine in India which did not take place in the two concurrent systems of medicine namely Ayurveda and Unani (possibly owing to its origin in Iona, Greece, '*Graeco-Arab*').

Around this time, an interesting interaction was taking place between Europeans and Indians at Goa, which had been conquered by Afonso Albuquerque for the Portuguese king in 1510 and which remained their mainstay till the whole of the sixteenth and seventeenth centuries under discussion.

In early seventeenth century, Edward Terry noticed:

> The common diseases of the countrey are blaudie fluxes, hot fevers and calentures [calentures, that is a tropical delirium]; in all which they prescribe fasting as a principall remedie. That filthy disease, the consequence of incontinencie, is common among them. *The people in generall live about our ages; but they have more old men.*[65]

John Fryer (1670s) noted: 'Notwithstanding this Mortality to the *English*, the Country people and naturalized *Portugals* live to a good Old Age, supposed to be the reward of their Temperance; indulging themselves neither in Strong Drinks, nor devouring Flesh as we do'.[66] Though he was generally critical of Asian surgery, he praised mangoes of Goa as having medicinal properties: 'they make them break out, and cleanse the blood, and Salivate to the height of Mercurial Arcanaes; and afterwards fatten as much as Antimony, or acorns to dogs'.[67]

Similarly, Francois Bernier (who remained in India between 1659 and 1967) observed:

> I have no doubt that the happy ignorance which prevails of many distempers is fairly ascribable to the general habits of sobriety among the people, and to the profuse perspiration to which they are perpetually subject. The gout, the stone, complaints in the kidneys, catarrhs and quartan agues [recurrent malaria] are nearly unknown; and persons who arrive in the country afflicted with any of these disorders, as was the case with me, soon experience a complete cure. Even the venereal disease, common as it is in *Hindoustan*, is not of so virulent a character, or attended with such injurious consequences, as in other parts of the world. But although there is a greater enjoyment of health, yet there is less vigour among the people than in our colder climates; and the feebleness and languor both of body and mind, consequent upon excessive heat, may be considered a species of unremitting malady, which attacks all persons indiscriminately, and among the rest Europeans not yet inured to the heat.[68]

Later, he wrote more generally on Indian healing techniques:

> On physic they have a great number of small books, which are rather collections of recipes than regular treatises. The most ancient and most esteemed is written in verse. I shall observe, by the way, that their practice differs essentially from ours, and that it is grounded on the following acknowledged principles: a patient with a fever requires no great nourishment; the sovereign remedy for sickness is abstinence; nothing is worse for a sick body than meat broth, for it soon corrupts in the stomach of one afflicted with fever; a patient should be bled only on extraordinary occasions, and where the necessity is most obvious—as when there is reason to apprehend a brain fever, or when an inflammation of the chest, liver, or kidneys, has taken place.

Whether these modes of treatment be judicious, I leave to our learned physicians to decide; I shall only remark that they are successful in *Hindoustan*, and that the *Mogul* and *Mahometan* physicians, who follow the rules of *Avicenna* and *Averroes*, adopt them no less than do those of the *Gentiles*, especially in regard to abstinence from meat broth. The *Moguls*, it is true, are rather more given to the practice of bleeding than the *Gentiles*; for where they apprehend the inflammations just mentioned, they generally bleed once or twice, not in the trifling manner of the modern practitioners of *Goa* and *Paris*, but copiously, like the ancients, taking eighteen or twenty ounces of blood, sometimes even to fainting; thus frequently subduing the disease at the commencement, according to the advice of *Galen*, and as I have witnessed in several cases.[69]

M.N. Pearson rightly stated that:

Bernier was writing as an expert commenting on his peers, in other words in his case the Unani practitioners, often Persians, who ministered at court, where he lived. But as in Europe, folk remedies and supernatural notions coexisted more or less easily in India with this relatively academic medical knowledge. Several European visitors reflected the state of folk medical knowledge in Europe when they commented on popular practice in India. Cholera was probably the most feared disease, especially on the west coast and in the south. The British in India thought it was caused by eating fish and meat together. They treated it by applying a hot iron to the ball of the patient's foot. If the patient winced, he would soon recover, but if no pain was felt the patient would soon die. Ovington, an educated man and a clergyman, noted that cholera [mordechine] is 'violent Vomiting and Looseness, and which is caused most frequently by an Excess of Eating particularly of Fish and Flesh together. It has been Cur'd by a Red-hot Iron clapt to the Heal of him that is sick, so close that it renders him uneasie by its nearness, whereby it leaves a Scar behind it'.[70] For fevers in general the remedy was to 'Take an iron ring about an inch and a half in diameter and thick in proportion. Then heating it red hot in the fire, extend the patient on his back, and apply the ring to his navel, in such a manner that the navel may be as a centre to the ring. As soon as the patient feels the heat take away the ring as quick as possible when a sudden revolution will be wrought in his intestines'.[71]

Pearson also cites Niccoalo Manucci to argue how little difference there was between the latter's knowledge and folk medicine. For instance, in Bassein, Manucci refers to a woman of good station who produced a girl after a pregnancy of three years.

Similarly, M.N. Pearson pointed out that till eighteenth–nineteenth centuries, people were not familiar with the notion of anatomy and continued with traditional herbal medicines and long abstinence from food. He refers to an instance:

How to write a charm to cure fevers: Take some olive leaves and on a Saturday, being yourself in a state of purity, write on one of the leaves, 'Hell is hungry', on another, 'Hell is refreshed', and on the third, 'Hell is thirsty'. Put these in a rag and bind them on the left arm of the patient. Make two intersecting triangles on a sheet of paper with one continuous motion of the hand, sew this up in a sheet of cloth and tie it round the patient's neck. When the fever has left, throw the cloth into a well or river.[72]

All such superficial practices were possibly owing to severe shortage of qualified doctors throughout India. Commenting on this aspect, Tavernier wrote:

It should be remarked that in all the countries we have just passed through, both in the Kingdom of Carnatic and the Kingdoms of Golkonda and Bijapur, there are hardly physicians except those in the service of the Kings and Princes. As for the commonalty, when the rains have fallen and it is the season for collecting plants, mothers of families may be seen going in the mornings from the towns and villages to collect the samples which they know to be specifics for domestic diseases. It is true that in good towns there are generally one or two men who have some knowledge of medicine, who seat themselves each morning in the market-place or at a corner of the street and administer remedies, ether potions or plasters, to those who come to ask for them. They first feel the pulse, and when giving the medicine, for which they take only the value of two farthings, they mumble some words between their teeth.[73]

Similarly, when Abbe Carre fell sick, he was advised by a Persian noble 'as to providing someone who can give you remedies and treat your illness, you are aware that there is no doctor or surgeon amongst us; we hardly know what such a man is, and Europeans are only consulted when one of them happens to be passing in this country'.[74]

Peter Mundy (19 May 1633) reported that on the request of Sayyid Shikam, son-in-law of Dalis Khan—late Governor of Baroda by the chirurgeon's mate Richard Barber—the chirurgeon's Mate cured to foot of a Moore [a Muslim], a friend of his 'which had been a long time score and almost grown to a Canker'.[75]

Abbe Carre (1672) reports about M. Deslong (Dellon) who was an employee of the French East India Company, how he left the Company and settled at Daman where he was 'considered to be the cleverest doctor in India, though all his science consisted of knowing how to bleed'.[76]

Tegenapatnam was under the rule of Khan-i Khanan. Khan-i Khanan fell sick at Vellore and the Dutch chirurgeon cured him of the ailment.[77]

Next one hears about upper chirurgeon Simon de Wolff in 1654. He was lent to Khan-i Khanan and he personally visited Bijapur to remain with the King who had been suffering from a disease for the last 12 years and could not be treated with opium. The King Mohammad Adil Shah died on 4 November 1656 and Simon de Wolff returned to Paliacatte.[78]

The Mughal emperor Shahjahan had asked for two painters and one chirurgeon in the Mughal court in 1656. In 1662, the Nawab Musemchan [Muazzam Khan] was trying to conquer Assam. It was reported that chirurgeon Gelmer Vosburgh stood separated due to high tide;[79] it is also said that Gelmer Vosburg fought against a force of 15,000–20,000 persons.[80] In 1685, it appears that the Verenigde Ooostindische Compagnie (VOC) sent a junior chirurgeon (onderchirurgijn) to serve the Mughals.[81]

There is also news of Jan Baptista Potvliet, a chirurgeon who was sent to serve Prince Azim Terra.[82]

Thus, one finds that the factors of various East India Companies were constantly in search of medicines in Asia. Among them it is found that the VOC was following a conscious policy of engaging doctors of medicine, the chirurgeons, at Amsterdam Chamber by selecting them in the presence of the directors (Bewindhebberen). They were classified into three categories.[83] They were provided medicine chests to treat the Company servants on the sea if they suffered unclean diseases or wounds during the voyage.[84] After a long discussion, it was resolved by the VOC officials that the instruments and tools, the chirurgeons estimated to be supplied, should be included in the Bill of Lading in order to deliver these to them on reaching the destination in order to avoid holding the chirurgeons responsible for some shortcomings to be detected in the latter.[85]

The medicine chests contained varieties of medicines. The chirurgeons believed that some of those medicines used to lose their potency once they entered into the tropical climate.[86]

All chambers of the VOC had decided to have a consolidated list of medicines to be sent to the East Indies (1676).[87] The VOC, particularly perturbed on account of the sealing of medicines from the medicine chests, wanted to take remedial steps against the same by the 1670s.[88] A series of steps were, in fact, adopted like provision of medicines on the ship were to be had only at earmarked ports like Texel or Goeree, etc., assigning particular quota of wine for chirugeons, etc.[89] Jacobus Bontius, by a resolution of the Gentlemen Seventeen ('Heeren Zeventien') on 24 August 1626, was appointed as 'Doctor, Pharmacist, and Superintendent of Surgeons (Chirurgijns) in (the Dutch East) Indies.[90] He sailed for the Indies on the ship the *Vianeh*, on 16 March 1627 in the fleet of Jan Pietersz, Coen[91] and reached Batavia on 13 September 1627.[92] Equipped with knowledge of anatomy through his acquisition of a doctorate in medicine in 1614 at Leiden and with the assistance of two resident surgeons—Andrew Durie, surgeon of the hospital and Adam, surgeon of the Dutch garrison—he conducted at least nine post-mortem dissections to ascertain impact of various diseases on different parts of the body.[93]

Bontius had identified nineteen major diseases of the belly, chest and skin prevalent in the East Indies that were not known in the Netherlands.[94] He treated them with the locally available remedial herbs.[95] Harold J. Cook cites treatment of 'papy' (locally called beriberi). First, its symptoms, humoural pathology, causes were diagnosed[96] and then cure was conceived. Bontius prescribed 'moderate exercise when possible and strong rubdowns—a method practised by the Bengali slaves and Malayam women although, like bathing, not by the Dutch themselves—which should be accompanied by fomentations and baths made from the 'noble' herb called 'lagondi' (or eastern privet), white the feet and hands are anointed with oil of cloves and mace mixed with oil of roses'.[97] When Bontius himself suffered from the disease, he tried 'lagondi' for sometime but soon switched over to China root (of which much will be said later)—a medicine much used by all the Indians, and particularly the Chinese.

Bontius felt that he 'could not move his legs or arms but with difficulty'.[98] However, compared to China root, lagondi was considered a better herb, a divine remedy by the people of the Indies, 'who used it in the form of fomentations, baths, and poultices to treat almost all diseases, promote menstruation, ease childbirth, cure all ills of the uterus, promote urination, relieve complaints of the bladder and kidneys, and ease the pains of colic. 'In a word, the panacea of the ancients was nothing to this of ours'.[99]

Possibly, he quickly went to the Moluccas (islands) and Timor soon after his arrival at Batavia.[100] During the commencement of the twin sieges by the Sultan Ageng, the Prince of Mataram (first from 22 August 1628 to 3 December 1628 and the second from 21 August 1629 to 2 November 1629), Bontius was in Batavia.[101] During the four-month interval between the two sieges, Bontius had suffered from malaria, beriberi and dysentery. After his recovery, his second wife Sara Gerardi died on 8 June 1630 and their two sons succumbed to presumably any of these ailments.[102] Around this time, he became a member of the Council of Justice and eventually succeeded Antonius van den Heuvel as 'advocate fiscal' on 1 May 1630. It is suggested that possibly owing to his deteriorating relationship with Governor General Specx, he left Batavia in 1631.[103] He died on 29 November 1631 at Batavia.[104] Bontius was not particularly pleased with the publication of his work. One of his four volume books was ready for publication by 1631 of which the first volume 'Notae in Garciam ab Orta', which was the most important of the series, was ready for press by 1631 but could finally be printed only in 1642.[105] Thus, Bontius stayed in South-East Asia for more than four years, utilizing this time to write his two works namely, *Historia Aninralivm* and *Historia Plantarum*.[106]

He could not finish both the works due to his death. It has been pointed out that Willem Piso published Bontius' unfinished works. He published *De Conservanda valetudine*, a work about prevention of diseases based on Bontius' information.[107] He also borrowed liberally from Bontius, already famous work *Notae in Garciam ab Orta*, where he had dealt with betelnut, tamarind, and Circuma wortel [a herb (the *curcuma longa*), also called Crocus from which a yellow stuff was obtained, used in the preparation of curry and ointment].[108] Bontius also wrote about an edible bird's nest (a name given to several plants from their appearance especially Monotropa and Neottia (bird's nest orchis),[109] bat (flying fox), extinct Dodaers or Dronte (little grebe, dabchic), Moluccen crawfish, tea, slimeapples, etc.[110]

It has been argued that Zacharias Janssen was the first to make the magnifying glass, but it was Cornelis Jacobszoon Drebbel who actually had manufactured the instrument called microscope.

Zacharias Janssen could enlarge the object from 3 to 9 times—Drebbel in 1621 and 1622 could enlarge the object 30 times in length and breadth, and by 1625 he improved it by 150 times.[111] Fifty years later, Antony van Leeuwenhock could enlarge the object 270 times.[112]

During the 1660s, Harold J. Cook observed that new initiatives were taken by the VOC in this sphere. He gives full credit to Robert Padtbrugge, born in 1637, a physician for transformation of VOC's general isolate observations about local medicines into a policy of gradual substitution of European medicines by locally available indigenous ones in the treatment of both European as well as local people.[113] He had left the Netherlands in February 1664 and reached Batavia in July and from there went to Ceylon in September 1664.[114] Padtbrugge served as merchant in the Western quarter of the VOC and was a member of the Council of Justice.[115] Despite such engagements, he continued to take an interest in medicine and natural history and presumably was responsible for provoking 'the Gentlemen (Heren) XVII into action'.[116] In 1668, he submitted his reports about minerals, herbs, medicines, etc. One of such reports has survived which contains a study made for the Gentlemen XVII (Heren XVII) as well as for the High Government at Batavia.[117] He referred to varieties of medicinal (*hulpmiddelen*) herbs, and selected a list of thirty of the best medicinal plants and herbs of Ceylon. Apart from such a change in policy about substitution of European imports of drugs to increasing reliance on Asian herbal treatment, another important step taken by the VOC was the establishment of a medical shop (*medicinal winkel*) in 1663 at Batavia. The VOC was also trying around this time to press for the development of Batavia and its environs independent of home finance.[118] The Gentlemen XVII presumably inspired by Padtbrugge's incessant invocations, sent a letter on 9 May 1669 to the Council of Indies at Batavia.[119] In turn, the Council at Batavia instructed Padtbrugge, the surgeons of the VOC and others to investigate such things and report back to them.[120]

Following Padtbrugge's report, Andreas Cleyer, new head of the medical shop and entrusted with the task of distilling chemical medicines, seized the additional opportunity.[121] Along with the charge of medical shop at Batavia, he was given the title of the physician.[122]

On 24 April 1669, the High Government at Batavia wrote to the Government of Ceylon that Cleyer had the knowledge about some medicinal plants which grew in Ceylon 'in particular colocynth apples in the Jaffnapatnam region and sarsaparilla near Calelure in the neighbourhood of Colombo'.[123] The High Government at Batavia had sought the help of Doctor Robertus Padtbrugge in this regard. Unfortunately, this coincided with Padtbrugge's departure to the Netherlands.[124]

Important steps were taken under new head of the medical shop, (May 1667) Andreas Cleyer, though he himself was not a physician. He was posted as rector at Batavia.[125] He had already requested drugs from the Cape of Good Hope.[126] At Table Bay (VOC established its factory there in 1652), by the mid 1660s local plants of botanical and medicinal significance were cultivated.[127] It gained reputation for being the chief place where acclimatization of plants from the entire Dutch East Indies took place. It was at Cleyer's initiative that the Governor and the Council in Batavia wrote to the Commander in Cape to send 'garden seeds, artichoke plants, and medicinals' for the medical shop at Batavia. He also took interest in the medicinal plants of Ceylon.[128] Ryckloff van Goens, the Governor of Ceylon, requested the Council at Batavia to send few chemists to identify and collect drugs and accordingly two chemists like Abraham Goetjens and Willem de Witte were sent to Ceylon.[129] Along with the chemists, Van Goens also succeeded in receiving a physician Paulus Hermann in 1672.[130]

It is suggested that Cleyer was also instrumental in prompting botanical work elsewhere. The Council at Batavia, presumably at Cleyer's initiative, wrote to the governor and Council of Coromandel to send 'colocynth apples, nux vomica ['vonut nuts', from which strychnine would be extracted 150 years (?) later (question mark mine)], and dried myrabolans, 'in which Mr Joachim Fijbeco (also being a good herbalist) is to be recommended to add such medicinal herbs, which grow on the coast'.[131] Similarly, a letter was sent to the Directorate of Bengal: 'Since Mr Jacob Frederik Strick Berts, first surgeon in Bengal (since he had long resided in the land of the Mogul and has roamed through it) must necessarily have obtained great experience and knowledge of many medicinal drugs and herbs in those lands',[132] Jacob Frederick Strick Berts was entrusted with the task of composing a list of such herbs and send them to Batavia in order to reduce the demands made on the home country.[133]

During the sixteenth to seventeenth centuries, the Portuguese, first the Jesuits and with them others, came into contact with the people of Japan. Luis de Almeida was possibly one of the first Portuguese to reach Japan to practice medicine in 1555.[134] He started practising medicine with the permission of the daimyo (lord) at Funai (mod. Oita) in the principality of Bungo, east of Kyushu.[135] He could establish his reputation for treating gunshot wounds with 'cander', a Japanese system of diagnosis which showed a swelling or carbuncle.[136] Almeida started training medical practitioners which, by 1558, had transformed into a school where Europeans along with Japanese were receiving both theoretical and practical education.[137] It is reported that the Franciscans also set up hospitals after their arrival in Kyoto.[138] Paul de Tonomine, a converted bonze and a student of Almeida, took charge of medicine at the Jesuit foundation in Funai.[139] Another person known as Keyu, was a Portuguese surgeon at Osaka.[140] Kurisaki Doki (who had remained with the Portuguese since 1590 when he was eight years old) became a very famous surgeon at Nagasaki.[141] But this trend was short-circuited by Hideyoshi who unlike his predecessor, Nobunaga, destroyed churches and also got a few Christians, executed.[142] His successor, Ieyasu, the first Tokugawa shogun, at the initial stage had no problem with the Christians, but soon started distrusting them. The subsequent period under his successors witnessed an extremely hostile policy of the state towards Christians.[143] Harold J. Cook's study of Chuan, Kichibei and Gensho is indicative of the fact that the Dutch surgeons/physicians could impart Dutch knowledge about medicine/surgery to their Japanese counterparts.[144] The curiosity of Japanese practitioners of medicine about Chinese or European systems led them to obtain books written in Dutch and get them translated into Japanese.[145] Caspar Schamberger accompanied the special envoy Andries Frisius to the shogun,[146] for the shogun Ietsuna was ill at Edo and his officials had requested

Schamberger's assistance in his treatment. As a consequence, Schamberger was allowed to stay for another six months to impart his knowledge of surgery which eventually led to the establishment of a 'Caspar-style surgery' (*Kasuparu-ryu geka*).[147] Inomata Dembei, an associate of Schamberger, wrote two books, namely *Kaspor-ryu-i-sho* (Medical Book of the Caspar School) and *Oranda-geka-sho* (Book of Dutch Surgery).[148] Kawaguchi Ryoan, a disciple of Dembei, further ensured the spread of the so-called Caspar system to other parts of Japan like Kyoto, northern Honshu and Shikoku within twenty years and published a book on Caspar's methods (*Caspar dempo*) in 1661.[149] Apart from the king, even the Japanese aristocracy expressed its interest in European surgery and medicine. For example, Inoue Chikugo-no-Kami, Governor of Nagasaki, asked the VOC to supply him works on anatomy in Portuguese and received Rembert Dodoen's *Herbarius oft cruidt-boeck*, and in 1654 he also got several works on anatomy translated from Dutch into Portuguese. In the same year, Gensho was instructed to compile a work on the surgical methods of the Dutch.[150] The VOC surgeon Hans Jonson had already written *Komo-ryu-geka-homo* (Secret Outlines of red-haired school surgery), and by 1669, Gensho wrote a thirteen volume treatise on medical botany.[151] Schamberger's diagnosis and prescriptions had received considerable acceptance, for later on personal physicians of daimyos tried to learn about Dutch medicine and surgery.[152] Hatano Gento, for example, in 1650 sought a certificate to prove that he was associated with the Dutch system of medicine and surgery on Deshima.[153]

Certificates were further obtained by Arashiyama Hoan, physician of daimyo of Hirado and his student Kasturagawa Hochiku, following which they started a medical tradition known as Kasturagawa school which was based on Dutch methods.[154] Not only that, one noted surgeon Daniel Busch who was one of the signatories of Hoan's certificate was officially allowed to treat patients in Nagasaki.[155] Similarly, Kichibei, the famous translator, obtained a certificate on Deshima in 1668 which enabled him to practice medicine and surgery at Edo[156] and he established a school known as 'Nishi-method' (*Nishi ryu*) which was a combination of the Chinese, Portuguese, and Dutch systems.[157] It is interesting to note that such an interaction between the Japanese and the Dutch resulted in production of certain texts dealing with both the systems of medicine and surgery. Narabayashi Chinzan (also known as Shingohei) was a student of Willem Hoffman (chief surgeon on Deshima from 1671 to 1675) and later practised and taught Western medicine and became the precursor of the 'most famous families of physician-translators'.[158] He published a six volume treatise called *Koi-geka soden* (An explanation of Dutch surgery).[159]

In the 1660s, according to Harold J. Cook, the Japanese elite evinced keen interest in the Dutch medicine. He cites the example of successful treatment with Dutch medicine of Inaba Masanori, daimyo of Odawara, Lord of Mino. And *rojyu* (a senior councillor or 'elder' in the Shogun's government), who was suffering from gout was treated by Schamberger at Edo. One finds a mention about Inaba's interest in the *dagh register* (daily account) of 1668 where it says that he had ordered for number of books on medicine in Dutch including an anatomical work *Spiegel der anathomie* and *Hortus Eystettensis*.[160] Before him, in November 1667, the *bugyo* of Nagasaki had requested the VOC for a physician, not merely a surgeon.[161] This request was reiterated in 1668 during the annual visit of by the Dutch station chief to Edo.[162] Another request was made subsequently.[163] The Japanese translator Sinosie, in fact, left the Dutch with the impression that the shogun wanted them to send him a personal physician, although that might not have been intended.[164] Cook suggests that daimyo Inaba, who wanted a Dutch physician, might have been the author of this request.[165] The Dutch reaction to such requests was extremely slow. It was only in 1672 that the Dutch attended to shogun's requests. The VOC considered five physicians for their posting in Japan between October 1672 and February 1673,[166] of which two were presumably more competent by virtue of having acquired doctorates in medicine. One was Adriaan van der Poel (b.1642) and the other was Willem ten Rhijne (b.1649). Of the two, the latter was enrolled with Sylvius who was busy developing his theory about acids and alkalis in the cause and treatment of diseases.[167] Ten Rhijne found value in both chemical and Hippocratic medicine.[168] In June 1673, he sailed for Batavia aboard the ship *Ternate* and reached Batavia at the end of January 1674 with a month long layover at the Cape.[169] He suffered from a pestilential fever during the second part of his voyage and treated himself with heavy doses of Monsiegneur Charras's 'Trochiscki de Viperis' (pastiles of viper-flesh).[170]

At Batavia, he met Hermann Busschoff who had observed the practice of moxibustion among the Chinese and Japanese to cure ill health.[171] Later, Busschoff wrote a book on moxibustion therapy and sent it to Utrecht where its publication generated a lot of curiosity about moxa, moxibustion and its efficacy as treatment.[172] Ten Rhijne reached Japan on 31 July 1674.[173] He had found it difficult to communicate with the Japanese; nevertheless, he found there Shodayu Motogi and Iwanaga Soko who could understand him, as also European astronomy, medicine and surgery.[174] Of the two, Iwanaga helped Ten Rhijne by translating Chinese texts on medicine and surgery which were already available on Deshima.[175] Ten Rhijne in turn tried his Japanese counterparts to know about four general causes of 'carbuncles',[176] an ailment caused mainly by (1) blood, (2) mental depression, (3) (disorder of) the liver, and (4) 'moisture'—or in other words, blood, passions, digestion, and environment, respectively.[177] With great difficulty, he could manage to get Iwanaga translate texts from Chinese into Japanese and Shodayu from the Japanese into Dutch which Ten Rhijne then turned into Latin.[178] The most appreciable aspect of the Chinese medicine which attracted Rhijne's attention, was various diagrams which were synthesized into four representations, two Japanese and two Chinese, each pair showing the back and front of the body they had earmarked points with green colour for inserting the needle, and points with red colour for intended moxibustion.[179] Ten Rhijne admired the accuracy of their knowledge about the practice of treating certain diseases through moxibustion and acupuncture. Both the Chinese and the Japanese systems did not approve of phlebotomy due to their common belief that such an exercise would shorten the life.[180] As an alternative to phlebotomy, therefore, the Chinese and the Japanese, according to Ten Rhijne, had developed the above two methods 'of venting impurities and "winds" (which caused the pains) from the blood'.[181] Ten Rhijne was apparently fascinated by these two methods which led him to write a treatise on them.[182] His efforts, accompanied by his insatiable desire to know more paid dividends. He was well received by the Shogun at Edo.[183] He also treated some patients with Dutch medicines.[184] On December 1675, one translator Tominaga Ichirobei borrowed a book on anatomy, the *Opera Spiegel* to show it to bugyo and then returned the same on 10 January 1676, which is indicative of the positive response from the Japanese state as well as practitioners. Throughout his stay in Japan, Ten Rhijne was continuously consulted by Japanese authorities of the state and medicine.[185]

Ten Rhijne left for Batavia from Japan on 27 October and reached Batavia on 13 December 1676.[186] The Governor General at Batavia, Joan Maetsuyker, noted in his missive of 13 February 1677, that despite Ten Rhijne's helpful nature and generous instructions to the Japanese (of course, in medicine and surgery), the Japanese did not show matching gratitude towards him.[187] At Batavia, he assisted Cleyer with his studies of Asian medicinal plants and practices, between 1677 and 1679.[188] Ten Rhijne's assistance to Cleyer, in fact, led to his fame because of Cleyer's publication of information about Chinese pulse doctrine.[189] The latter had gathered information about Chinese medical practices through Philippe Couplet;[190] through him, Cleyer managed to obtain materials compiled by Michael Boym about Chinese medicine and practices.[191] In fact, it was Boym, a Polish member of the China mission, who first introduced Europeans to Chinese medicine and the Chinese method of touching the pulse for diagnosis and prognosis.[192] Eventually, because of all this, Cleyer could publish the *Specimen medicine Sinicae, sive opuscula medica ad mentem Sinensium* (The Pattern of Chinese medicine, or medical, work according to Chinese thought).[193] The *Specimen* was divided into six parts (*opuscula*). Cleyer refers to Wang Shuhe which was supposedly a late medieval version of *Mo Chüeh*.[194] But it seems *Mo Chüeh* is possibly *Mo Ching* (Pulse Manual) compiled by Wang Hsi. The latter was identified by Cleyer as Wang Shuhe, though he was usually called Wang Shu-ho. The text itself was complied around AD 300 from the *Nei Ching*, *Shang han tsa ping lun* and other early classics.[195] By this time, Chinese medicine had drawn to its close. But this shows how determined Cleyer was in his pursuit! The third part of the text refers to a compilation of Michael Boym, which led to the publication of Boym's *Clavis medica* in 1686 as a reprint.[196] The *specimen* acquired the status of one of major texts that dealt with the Chinese system of medicine. John Floyer's studies of the pulse was based on this.[197] As a result of all this, Ten Rhijne could publish his work by May 1683 and it was well appreciated by his contemporaries in Europe.[198]

It was well known by 12 February 1685s letter that Ceylon had the privilege of having numerous kinds of medicinal herbs.[199] It was hoped that this would turn out into a viable business. There was also claimed to be a demand for sending a doctor, three to four pharmacists, and three to four good botanists to understand the herbs.[200]

Paulus Hermann, a botanist (herbalist) and doctor,[201] was sent to Ceylon on the Governor of Ceylon, Rijcklof van Goens' request, in November 1671 and reached Ceylon in 1672.[202] Hermann was appointed as doctor to the hospital in Colombo. According to Governor General Rijcklof van Goens and his team at Batavia, Paulus Hermann had collected 10,000 special plants, shrubs (Reesters) and herbs (kruijden)—so many of which, Van Goens asserted, were till then never known to any authority.[203] Van Goens considered Ceylon a blessed country, having as many varieties of worthy and delightful medicines as any country could have, and where everything was in such an abundance that it was hoped that very soon there would be no need to import medicine from the Netherlands.[204] He, in fact, goes to the extent of saying that the book *Hortus Malabaricus* which was sent by the Gentlemen XVII contained nothing that was not known in Ceylon and in fact was available in abundance, and therefore, there was no need to seek for them in the Malabar.[205] It was also asserted that Ceylonese medicines were better than those found in Malabar, like the Ceylonese cinnamon which had overtaken the wild cinnamon found in Malabar.[206] It was at this time that Paul Hermann was busy writing his book on medicine.[207] Once he was back in Europe in 1680, Hermann had built up the botanical collections and there was a considerable growth in cultivation of such curious plants.[208] Despite his various acts of commissions and omissions in Ceylon, Hermann was appointed Professor in the medical faculty at Leiden in recognition of his fundamental work.[209]

Another interesting name one hears is that of Engelbert Kaempfer who had joined the VOC in 1685 and visited Bandar Abbas, Persia (1685–8) and Deshima (Japan) (1690–2) and collected information about various diseases and medicine. He had obtained a medical degree from Leiden in 1893 on ten exotic facts that he had observed (Decadem observationum exoticarum), such as—a worm from which people of and around Hormuz and much of the Persian Gulf suffered which was identified as *dracunculus*, the *mumia* of Persia called *Mouminahi*, and acupuncture and moxibustion.[210] He identified acupuncture as 'a Japanese cure for colic' (Senki' in Japanese) and according to him, it arose from a gas of the intestines, mesentry, omentum, peritoneum and muscles of the abdomen which was expelled by the use of needles on certain loci.[211] He confirmed that moxa was a Chinese and Japanese substance used in cantery. Kaempfer gained fame and reputation after the publication of his book *Amoenitatum exoticarum politico-physico-medicarum faciculi* V ('Exotic politico-physico-medical pleasantries in five sections') in 1712.[212]

Hendrik Adriaan van Rheede tot Drakenstein (1636–91) had an interesting career in the VOC.[213] He along with Heer van Mydrecht, had established a 'montsterweverye' (sample workshop with looms) and decided to engage the best artisans and weavers to weave cloths from silk, tusser, Mogta and cotton.[214] But this experiment apparently failed. His calculation was that the VOC had lost approximately 38 tons worth of gold (i.e. 380 million guilders) in private trade.[215] On 21 February 1687, he wrote in length against the practice, purchase of silk,[216] sericulture,[217] indigo cultivation and its preparation,[218] printing/painting of chirtz,[219] assaying of gold,[220] and pearl fishery.[221] During his tenure at Malabar, Van Rheede had launched his large collaborative study which eventually came to be known as *Hortus Malabaricus*.[222] Van Rheede had established a chemical laboratory in Cochin in 1674.[223] He engaged the chemist Paulus Meysner to prepare 'Waters, oils and salts' from the 'famous medicinal herbs, fruits and roots' of Malabar, 'and to examine in what respect they are equal to or excel the European ones, in order to provide the Company's medical shop therewith and to avoid the annual expense of many ineffective leaves, roots, seeds and ointments [being sent] from Batavia to Ceylon'.[224] Van Rheede mentions in the preface to the third volume of the *Hortus Malabaricus* that he was trying to save expenditure on import of medicine from the Netherlands by attempting to substitute this with the expanding knowledge about local drugs.[225] He was particularly delighted to know about distillation of oil from the roots of local cinnamon, which was used at the hospital of Cochin with good result.[226] But the High Government at Batavia (letter dated 22 October 1675) prohibited Van Rheede's further work, on the pretext that distilled cinnamon oil of Malabar would damage Ceylonese cultivated cinnamon's market in Europe. Van Rheede had argued (letter dated 10 February 1676) that the Singalese of Ceylon were familiar with cinnamon oil since they had been using it in betel-chewing for long, and in effect ignored the directive from Batavia.[227] Rheede was assisted by Mathew of Saint Joseph, originally called Pretro Foglia, a keen medical botanist.[228] Mathew had earlier examined the plants of Lebanon and Basra.[229] He went on to narrate his experiences of flora and fauna in his book *Viridarium Orientale* ('Garden of the Orient'), 1675.[230] Van Rheede was also ably assisted by a good team, comprising of Paulus Hermann who had advised him to revise Mathew's organization of the information which he was collecting; Antoni Jacobsz Goetkint, an artist who could make accurate drawings of the plants; Marcelus Splinter, a fine draftsman; Johannes Casearius also helped him by 'putting the results of their studies into proper Latin; Christian Herman van Donep who translated from Portuguese into Dutch and Manuel Carneiro who translated from local languages into Portuguese.[231] Apart from them, Paulus Meysner, chemist and head of the local hospital; local surgeons from Karapuram (south Cochin), Itti Achudem, belonging to the caste of Chogans, whose main occupation was coconut industy and who was generally familiar with local botany; Ranga Botto, Vinaique Pandito and Apu Botto who were scholars and had fled from Goa "because of the increasingly intolerant Counter—Reformation there" were also engaged in his work.[232] The impact of such a large number of Indians participating in collection of material for *Hortus Malabaricus* is reflected in the following of the Ezhava system of classification.[233] In 1677, Van Goens, due to obvious reasons, got Casaerius and Van Rheede at Batavia from Malabar.[234] While in Batavia, Van Rheede continued to work on *Hortus Malabaricus* in association with other botanists like Willem Ten Rhijne, Louys de Keyser, and Hermann Grim. Van Rheede made startling observations in his *Hortus Malabaricus.* He claimed, for example, that true calumba root, which was used widely in Europe, actually grew in Malabar and not in Ceylon; it was infact only imported into Europe through Colombo and therefore it was called "Colombo" root associated with Ceylon'.[235]

Georgius Rumphius also known as 'Pliny of the Indies, the blind seer of Ambon', is best known for his works *D'Amboinsche rariteitkamer* ('The Ambonese curiosity cabinet'), 1705 and *Het Amboinsche kruid-book* (*Ambonese Herbal Book* in 6 volumes), 1741–50—both of which were based on his work done in the 1660s and 1670s. Rumphius (b.1627) had joined the VOC in 1652. It is suggested that he was inspired by Bontius.[236] Rumphius had sent, six chests of rarities—plants, etc., to Pieter Blaeu (1627–1706), Secretary of Amsterdam Chamber.[237] He was also a mathematician.[238]

Thus, due to such concerted efforts on the part of the VOC, its officials from Ceylon started reporting from 12 February 1679 that there was no need to import drugs and medicines from Europe.[239] Wouter Schouten (1676) observed presence of arts and sciences among Muslims and Hindus (Heydenen lit. heathens, pagans) in Bengal, but few were trained in practice.[240] Doctors and itinerant healers [? *Wandtheelders*] were in huge abundance. However, the Dutch surgeon who was *schrander* (shrewd) was esteemed above all those persons who were *geleerde* (learned).[241] He especially speaks about one such friend and fellow brother (Medebroeder) Sr. Johannes Thadema, who was stationed at Hughly and was held in high esteem by all those Muslims and Hindus who were distinguished in their crafts[242] and had become very prosperous.[243] Wouter Schouten's next observation is still more interesting. With regard to Bengali *medecijnmeesters* (medicine masters), i.e. surgeons, Schouten found that they did not practice the 'art of Anatomy' or the dissection of human body, but instead supported such *ongefondeerd* (unestablished), science founded upon pure (*loutere, louteze?*), *ondervindingh* (experience), which they annotated, regularly in their *geschred en Boecken* (manuscripts), and thus rendered them more accessible for future, readers.[244] He further states that they (Hindu?) (which included) women and men, young and old, weak and strong all alike, protected themselves with a herbal drink, although the Muslims kept away from such treatments. The Hindus also practised smearing their bodies with sandal/saffron or purifying their bodies with the burnt ash of cow dung among other things. The heathens would sometimes offer paddy which had rice as food for the cows; the cow dung produced as a result of manuring this paddy was regarded highly by the heathens and was much sought after. They used to pick all the whole grains which being dried was considered not only as good medicine for sick persons and invigorating (en tot een hertsterckingh), but was considered auspicious.[245]

Schouten further observed that the *Chirurgijns* (Bengali surgeons), had definitely none or surely very little knowledge about 'Mamiale operatie' (dissection of human body) and suggested that the art of anatomical surgery could be exported.[246]

Schouten found that the Mughal army, when pitted against the hostile army, requested for the hakims (Mooren) usually or one or more surgeons from the VOC according to their capacity who were fully trusted by the Great Moors (muslims).[247] He further informs about the caste group of *baertscheerders* (barbers), just like they were on the Coromandel Coast and Arakan, who were to be found in great abundance in Bengal.[248] These barbers had no shops but would be found along the streets and ways, and were present everywhere.[249] They did not serve only the Muslims or the Hindus, the Dutch or the English or the Portuguese exclusively. Rather, they spoke to the people on the streets and did not interfere with their faiths. The barbers would sit on a stone or some other thing, and other than their usual task, would also perform manicures and pedicures, and clean ears.[250] They were paid poorly, about 20–30 caucus and little bit of corn.[251] Their tools were also poor; they carried one *spigeltje* (small mirror), *wetsteentje* (small sharpening stone), and one small cup in place of a saving basin. These tools would be carried in their girdles or in a *riem* (strap). They mostly visited the people in their houses.[252]

But if one turns his attention to other sources one finds that the situation was not so dismal after all. There were some areas where manual treatment of injuries or disorders of the body were treated by surgeons very completely. In 1528, the stepmother of the Mughal Princess Gulbadan had accidentlly pulled the latter's hand in such a manner that it had caused dislocation.[253] It was set and bound up not by a surgeon but by a *kamangar* (bow-maker).[254] There were specialized persons called *jarrahs* who treated wounds and practised bloodletting.[255] During Jahangir's reign (1605–27), Muqarrab Khan rose to *jarrahs*, a very high status and was appointed Governor of Gujarat.[256] However, it was Hakim Momena who performed bloodletting in Jahangir's case in 1619.[257] The *jarrahs* were regarded 'as little more than *hajjams*' (glorified barbers) as is clear from the use of the term 'the hajjam's glass' (*shisha-i hajjam*).[258] The two dictionaries Sirajuddin Ali Arzu's *Chiragh-i Hidayat*,[259] and Tek Chand Bahar's *Bahar-i Ajam* (1740)[260] refer to the glass (tube) that the bloodletter used, to suck out blood.[261] It seems that the professional *jarrahs* of some status would have had forsaken their old profession of barbers. It has been argued that owing to the grip of the caste system over contemporary society the two professions/crafts of physician and surgeon remained separate—which, in fact, could be the reason behind the absence of textual evidence for India's remarkable achievement in plastic surgery. It seems the practitioners of this art were illiterate who, therefore, could not write about what they were doing.[262]

Venitian Niccolao Manucci was possibly the first to report about the practice of nose-restoration. In 1686, he found in Deccan:

> At the commencement of the war when the men of Bijapur caught any unhappy persons belonging to the Moguls who had gone out to cut grass or collect straw or do some

other service, they did not kill them but cut off their noses. Thus they came back into the camp all bleeding. The surgeons belonging to the country cut the skin of the forehead above the eyebrows, and made it fall down over the wounds on the nose. Then, giving it a twist so that the live flesh might meet the other live surface, by healing applications they fashioned for them other imperfect noses. There is left above, between the eyebrows, a small hole, caused by the twist given to the skin to bring the two live surfaces together. In a short time the wounds heal up, some obstacle being placed beneath to allow of respiration. I saw many persons with such noses, and they were not so disfigured as they would have been without any nose at all, but they bore between their eyebrows the mark of the incision.[263]

Later, Honigberger, himself a physician, reported from Lahore in 1852 that an 'Akalee or Nahung' had his nose cut off by Ranjit Singh. But, according to Honigberger, his nose was so well restored in the mountains that he thought nothing better could be performed in Europe.[264] Honigberger refers to the European method under which such operation was usually performed with 'the cuticle of the arm'.[265]

G.T. Vigne (1839) found that Kangra (Himachal Pradesh) had acquired a unique reputation 'for a very different reason—that performance by its inhabitants of the operation of nasotomy, if such a term may be applied where a new feature is given'.[266] G.T. Vigne informs that he extracted information about this practice from two reluctant practitioners. He writes:

. . . that they first give the patient a sufficient quantity of opium, bang or wine, to render him senseless: they then, so I was informed, tap the skin on the forehead, above the nose, until a sort of blister arises, from which a piece of skin, of the proper shape, is then cut, and immediately applied as a nose, *sewed on* [emphasis mine], and supported by pieces of cotton. The wound is then dressed with an ointment,[267] in which blue vitriol is one ingredient. . . . G.T. Vigne refers to a superstition which had rendered Kot Kangra as an exclusive place where only such a surgical operation could be conducted.[268] We hear about several persons who had been operated upon, and were returning homeward, looking proud of their acquisition, but a sorry substitute for the old feature.[269]

Apparently this precursor of the current 'plastic surgery' method had received considerable fame and could attract patients from as far as Iran.[270]

This practice, according to the local people, could be dated back to Akbar's time (1556–1605).[271] It is reported:

The Emperor Akbar ordered that of some miscreant to be cut off, and the sentence was carried into execution. Sometime afterwards he made his appearance with a new nose; and the astonished monarch asked how he had acquired it. He was informed that Budjn, a surgeon of his own, had given the man his new nose; and he rewarded his skill by putting him in possession of a Jaghir at Kangra, and gave him the necessary writing, which is still (1839) in possession of his descendants at Kangra, the Sikhs, of course, having taken possession of the Jaghir.[272]

John Martin Honigberger, a physician in the court of Ranjit Singh, narrated an interesting event about the restoration of the nose of an Akale or Nahung, whose nose, ears and hands had been cut off by order of Ranjeet Singh (he had even deserved the gallows), and whose nose had been so well restored in the mountains that we were all surprised, and confessed it could not have been better done in Europe. As we know, from history, this operation was even in the remotest antiquity, practiced by the Hindoos, and they formed the nose out of the cuticle of the forehead, which proceeding is now, and always will be the same.[273]

Honigberger, then, distinguishes the Indian practice from that of Europe. He writes:

In Europe, where cutting off of nose is only in use, in exceptional cases—as when ulceration or other circumstances make it requisite—this operation is usually performed with the cuticle of the arm, and judiciously too, as according to our custom, the head mostly is uncovered, and a scar on one's forehead, with a new nose on the face, makes rather an ugly appearance, whilst, in the East, the scar remains hidden beneath the turban.[274]

By the sixteenth century, according to Needham and his associates, the China root was liberally used as a panacea against syphilis, possibly because it had acquired the reputation of being an efficient drug against the urino-genital diseases.[275] Its popularity in the contemporary European (possibly American too) society is attested by the publication of Ahdreas Vesalius' *Epistola rationem modumque propinaudi Racinis Chynae decocti . . . petractans six editions soon after its publication.*[276]

Within India it acquired popularity among the vaids and hakims alike[277] from its appearance in the sixteenth century till late nineteenth century. It started losing ground owing to the discovery and use of arsenic, mercury and bismuth,[278] and its popularity not only waned but lost all its glamour with the discovery of the wonder drug penicillin in the early twentieth century. [In later part of the present essay, there is more information about this.]

Thus, with the help of the above survey, one may say that all societies, irrespective of their continental association and solidarity, reflected a genuine interest on the part of the researchers to discover new botanical support for advancing their knowledge of medicines and the tryst with medicine still continuing.

Of all diseases, cholera was a major killer. There were serious outbreaks of it in Goa in the 1543, 1563, 1570, 1580, 1588, 1610, 1635, 1639, 1670 and 1680.[279] The Italian merchant Sassetti reported about its occurrence in Cochin in the 1580s.[280] The Venetian doctor Manucci (late seventeenth century) reported that *mort-de-Chien* (cholera) was the main killer. He reports that the cure for the disease was found in burning the heel of the patient with a red hot iron until the heat was felt.[281]

Smallpox, another scourge, makes its appearance in the medical literature of India from the seventh century onwards—nearly coincidering with its occurrence in the west and possibly a little after China.[282]

Before its control by vaccination, smallpox was an all-too familiar and dreaded epidemic in India. It was responsible for a high rate of mortality and was a major source of blindness besides other disabilities. There has naturally been some interest in the history of the disease and of the fight against it, and this has produced some valuable studies.[283] There were two viruses of the genus *Orthopoxvirus* which used to cause smallpox amongst humans. One was known as *variola minor poxvirus* which caused a mild form of the disease. It was also called alastrim and the fatality rate was low; it was possibly rare in India. The other was *variola major poxvirus*, in which the rate of mortality was exceptionally high.[284] Ralph W. Nicholas has suggested that references to the postural disease smallpox as *masurika* is found in Sanskrit texts dating back to over 2,000 years, showing that it was an ancient affliction in India. But his earliest references are actually from the medical treatises of Charaka and Sushruta, whose floruit period can be anywhere between fourth to sixth centuries BC and fourth century AD.[285] In the medieval period, the earliest reference that can be traced dates back to the eleventh century; Alberuni (AD 1030) refers to smallpox. In a very brief but interesting passage, he wrote:

> The Hindus who are the neighbours of those regions (of Lanka) believe that the smallpox is a wind blowing from the Island of Lanka towards the continent to carry off souls. According to one report, some men warn people beforehand of the blowing of this wind, and can exactly tell at what times it will reach the different parts of the country.[286]

By Alberuni's time, people had become familiar with both the viral strains. He writes, 'After the smallpox has broken out, they recognize from certain signs whether it is virulent or not'.[287] The familiarity with the disease and its devastating consequences also prompted attempts at medical control. Alberuni writes of both surgery and medicine: 'Against the virulent smallpox they use a method of treatment by which they destroy only one single limb of the body, but do not kill. They use as medicine cloves, which they have to the patient to drink, together with gold dust.'[288] This dreaded disease, in the absence of proper knowledge, also prompted use of ritual. Alberuni refers to the use of cloves as amulets. He writes, 'And besides, the males tie the cloves, which are similar to date kernels, to their necks'.[289] Alberuni's confident observation was that if those precautions were taken, 'perhaps nine people out of ten' had the chance to survive![290]

It is interesting to note the absence of any reference in Alberuni to the Goddess Sitala. It seems that the worship of Sitala as the goddess of the disease started much later. This argument gains strength also from the fact that it was only in the late fifteenth and early sixteenth centuries that a *parisista* (appendix) on 'The Pathology of Sitala' was added to the text *Madhavanidanam* by Madhavakara (composed in the early eighth century).[291] By the twelfth century, in Dalhana's commentary on Sushruta, one can find *Sitalika* as a popular designation for *masurika*. By the sixteenth century, the *Bhavaprakasa* written by Bhava Misra had an elaborate section on smallpox and appropriate therapy for different types of pustules.[292]

By the seventeenth century smallpox seems to have become still more widespread, and had transformed from a disease into a calamity. In 1644, Antonio van Diemen reported that 600 slaves (male and female) had reached Batavia from Masulipatam, and 135 had died during the journey due to smallpox.[293] In the Mathura region, there are references to twenty-five villagers as witnesses in sale deeds. Their personal descriptions were recorded before the Qazis (1653–1717). Of them, as many as ten had suffered from smallpox because their faces had pock-marks.[294] In the Cambay documents too there are references to the incidence of smallpox; in a document dated 20 Rabi I, 1104, or 29 November 1692, there is mention of a witness named Paswir, son of Rup Karan, who had smallpox marks on his face.[295] In another Cambay document, of 24 February 1716, once again the description of the face of the witness notes smallpox marks.[296] In 1718, the Dutch factors complained that 'due to the prevalence of smallpox one cannot get indigenous brick-layers to repair and restore the walls of Cochin (first)'.[297] On 21 October 1726, De Haan reported the prevalence of 'strong smallpox' in Malabar.[298] Similarly, it also affected the people of Punjab. For example, in a sale, deed of 1160/1748, both mortgagers, Gur Sahai and Karam Chand, have pock-marked faces.[299] Four years later, in 1752, another document from the same town has the description of a mortgager, Godaria, who bore pock-marks.[300] A careful scrutiny of these limited number of documents shows that from the middle of the seventeenth century the frequency and spread of the disease had increased considerably. The evidence of smallpox from Punjab assumes more significance in the light of its coinciding with the disease's occurrence in Bengal.[301]

It is in this context that the lengthy account about the goddess of smallpox in the Malabar region by a former Dutch reform missionary to Ceylon, should be analysed. This account was considered so important by its writer Philippus Baldaeus, that he wrote minute details of the disease.[302] The very title of the chapter on it is quite interesting. It reads, 'Handling of the daughter of Ixora (i.e. Ishwara) and the Origin of Smallpox. Fear and Service of the Malabaris for this, robbing of their temple at Madiri by the King of Cochin, their arrival at Koilang'.[303] Philippus Baldaeus provides information about the representation of smallpox in religious belief and ritual.[304]

According to this Dutch account, there was a devil named Darida who, through his devotion to Brahma, got the blessing that he could not be killed by anyone.[305] Darida was overwhelmed by the powers given to him by Brahma and, consumed with the thought of fighting Ishwara, reached Calaya, where Ishwara resided. Since Darida was protected by the blessing that no man could kill him, Ishwara sent a lady called Sorga to fight him who cut off his head. Yet Darida had his head restored by the blessing of Brahma. Then Ishwara sent five holy ladies, who was known as Chamundiga to the Malabaris. They too chopped off Darida's head, despite which he once again reappeared the next day. Ishwara finally consulted Vishnu, and that was how Patragali (identified as Bhadrakali) was born. Baldaeus describes the physical features and other paraphernalia of Patragali. One is told of how Goddess Patragali was infuriated and how she caused smallpox on the face of Ishwara. According to this version, it was thus that smallpox was born. Though this text is not free from anthropomorphism, it still considers that the disease had some natural causes.[306] Baldaeus is here narrating the history of smallpox in India as being interrelated with the goddess of smallpox, although both are obviously quite different things. This reflects the common practice of seeking and then interpreting a relationship between disease and divinities. However, it is clear from Baldaeus' account that the religious interpretation which the people of Malabar associated with the infectious disease did not exclude a naturalistic comprehension. Baldaeus refers to Greek and Jewish perceptions of the disease and compares them with the Indian perception:

> The diseases under which smallpox should be reckoned, were sent by God to punish the sin of the humans, but she has natural causes, she can originate from within or from outside, as air, food, drink, sleep, waking, rest and movement of the body, hunger, forcing and holding of excrement, fashions and times of the year . . . winds and venomous vapour of the air, as from the same scalding fever and pestilence.[307]

Baldaeus refers to the traditionally accumulated knowledge about the disease:

> Brahmins also known well, how, according to the size of the winds, each period of the year produces various diseases, so we found fault within Ceylon island,[308] and specially in the kingdom of Jafnapatan, in the province of Pachirapalli, how there in the Winter severe fevers and swelling up of bodies are caused by the saline and nitreous water, [and] how the mortality prevails among their cattle, is not unknown to them, how the aching eyes especially in Malabar tease the people, occurring from a spoiled air, how very often the fish (created by a stench in the water) like mad and silly ones proceed to the beach, and die in thousands, as few years ago happened in Ambonia, and earlier in Ceylon, and other places, where more has happened.[309]

Baldaeus also describes the seasonal pattern of the epidemic's visitation. He writes:

> So sees one in spiring that the Malabaris are attacked by smallpox, which without doubt originate from the heat and contaminated blood, and from other vicious humidity and fruits, which the common people mostly partake, who also are attacked by smallpox, for this season is also considered deadly or remediable, after that dampness was found venomous, so that some poxes are cured lightly, while others die in 12 or 18 days.[310]

This passage suggests that during the spring season, the transmission of the smallpox virus was greater, and shows a great resemblance with the seasonal pattern of its occurrence in Bengal.[311] It is now a known fact that the smallpox virus was more active and transmissible in dry weather conditions.[312] However,

Baldaeus' account suggests that a season in which there was dampness was more vulnerable to smallpox.[313]

As far as the medical treatment of the afflicted person was concerned, Baldaeus informs that, 'Some poxes were cured lightly, as against others that kill in 12 or 18 days (both) men and children, like the doctors and Comaras[314] abandon these in the country from their experience, or they are mortal or capable of cure'.[315] He adds:

> The Pagans, thinking that Patragali sends this disease, leave the patient at once. This can be the reason why the image of a woman is [there] among the Pagans, there a child strikes the poor on the neck, as seeking help from this idol, being deserted by men. Because they judge the disease is infectious and sticking: they give the patient over to one of the Comaras, being the devotees of Patragali pagod. Believing that Patragali causes the smallpox, they do then many oblations and ceremonies for the sick; to please this idol, cut off the heads of one or two hens, whose blood falling on the earth, was licked up by dogs.[316]

Elsewhere too, he speaks about the worship and rituals associated with treatment of the disease.[317] Curiously enough, he speaks about *Basuri*[318] as the daughter of Ishwara. This was why:

> the Malabaris gave this name to the smallpox, which they also hold to be the ulcer and the dagger of Patragali, therefore, when they see a patient with smallpox, they will worship him, because they think that Patragali is in his middle; so they do also to dead-body, calling it Pandara [Bhandara?], that is a royal treasure, they know well also that God is good and does harm to none: but that Patragali, because he produces this evil, must be reconciled with offerings.[319]

Interestingly, an iconoclastic attitude was developing amongst the people. Philippus Baldaeus also refers to some kind of counter-ideology prevailing in Malabar about the disease—they had started rationalizing the cause of its eruption. The entire passage on this is so unique as to deserve quotation. People believe:

> that also this disease is not caused by Patragali, because people have not sinned especially against her, it appears, because many *Brahmans* and devout *Comaras* die of this disease, though they are in friendship with this idol. Many have according to their own admission sinned greatly against Patragali and nevertheless do not die of this disease. Many dying of this disease, are known openly, they have certainly not sinned against Patragali.[320]

Despite such a sceptical attitude towards smallpox, Baldaeus does not refer to any medical treatment of the patient. However, he does refer to the diet that was prescribed. The patients were given *kanji*, i.e. well-cooked rice.[321] But they were not forced to drink it.[322] They were also treated with bleeding, purgation and taking of cold food.[323]

The mortality rate was possibly pushed up because of a corrupt practice among the people of Malabar. Baldaeus reports: 'And some die well by infirmity, and are also killed by the Comaras, as they see that with their removal, their profits can come to them, because they inherit all the household goods.[324]

The people in Malabar had a special temple for Patragali at Cranganore. It was also called the Temple of Pilgrimage 'because of the great influx of the people'. Since it had possibly acquired the status of a major shrine, popular religious fairs were held. Baldaeus writes about the day of the feast when thousands of Sanams(?) were sacrificed. It had become a very rich temple. The king of Cochin wished to take away part of this wealth so much so that he stationed his people at strategic places near the rivers and roads in order to rob the travelling pilgrims.[325]

While fear of the disease led to a religious ritual invented to protect people from the wrath of the goddess on the one hand, it also encouraged a rational effort to discover the causes of the disease. In the eighteenth century, they considered controlling it with the help of medical treatment. It has been suggested that the practice of variolation or smallpox inoculation may have had many independent sources of origin. It possibly developed independently in different parts of Eurasia and Africa.[326]

In 1654, one hears about Indick, a nephew of the deceased Chinese king, suffering from Morbum (morbus gallicus), i.e. syphilis and had requested the Governor-General to send a Dutch chirurgeon to treat him.[327] It is interesting to note that he requested for all Dutch medicine for his treatment despite knowledge of China roots usage in such afflictions. The VOC officials at Batavia instructed opperchirugijn Christiaen Beyer to proceed to China for treating Indick.[328] He tried all Dutch medicine but failed in his efforts and eventually returned to Batavia.[329]

In 1655, one hears about Khankhana (?) who had fallen sick at Veloer (Vellore) and was cured satisfactorily by the Dutch chirurgeon,[330] possibly, Simon de Wolff.[331]

The Mughal emperor Shahjahan had asked for two Dutch painters and one chirurgeon in 1657.[332]

The marmalade of the bark of nutmeg was considered useful in treating the sick persons.[333]

The nawab Muazzam Khan (Mosem Khan) continued his operations in Bengal and Assam and according to letter of 9 September 1662, he was assisted by the Dutch chiruageon Gelmer Vosburgh.[334]

According to Linschoten:

> The root came to India, and was there first knowne in Anno 1535,[335] for before that time they knew it not, for that as then cured the Poxe, (which in India is a common disease), with the woode called Guaiacum, that is brought out of the Spanish Indies, and was at that time in a manner weighed against gold: and as the land of China, is much subject to the disease of the Pore, it seemeth that God hath given them this roote to cure and help the same, and since it was knoune (and found out) in India they would never use any other remedy, because there is great store of it, and the best in all the world, whereby men in those countries doe not once make any account of the Poxe (or feare the healing thereof), for that it is more earlier healed then any other disease, also it

is no shame with them, although they have had it at ye least 3 or 4 times; this root is now with them in so great abundance, and common use, that it is very good cheape, for that it is not worth at the most above halfe a Pardaw the pound, which in Porting all money is a Teston and a halfe.[336]

Next Linschoten informs about the use of the drug. He writes:

The sicke persons doe use it in this manner following they [of the roote, and cut in small peeces or slices, the wayght of an ounce, which they seeth in foure pottes or quartes of water, letting it seeth till it be halfe consumed, whereof they seeth fresh every day: this water they must drink alone, and eat bisket with nothing els but small rosted Chickens, without any Butter, suet, salt, or any [other] sauce, but onely drie with the Bisket, and this must bee their dinner, at night some Reasons, and tosted breade with Hony and nothing els: every day twice they must lie [on their beddes] we covered to make them sweat, every time an hower, or an hower and a halfe, which they must continue for the space of thirtie days, always keeping themselves out of the ayre, and from the wind, and lapping their heads and their ears very close, staying continually within the house, and above all things abstayning from the carnell company of women.[337]

This process was to be followed for 15–25 days from 25th day onwards of usage in the above prescribed manner, the pain would start diminishing first, and by the 30th day pain along with other symptoms of the disease would disappear.[338] For the next 30 days the patient was expected to continue drinking China root water in the manner prescribed above.[339] Besides, the patient was also ordained to abstain from consuming:

fish, or any goose or heavie meates, as Oxe, Cow, or Hogges flesh, and such like, as also they must keepe themselves from [much] aire or sinde, whereby their bodies [being healed] may returne to their perfect healthes againe, and after these twenty or thirty days are [full] expired, then they must begin to use all kinde of meates and drinkes, although when the first thirtie days are out, they may well goe abroad. . . .[340]

In terms of price and availability in India, it was noted for its cost compared to other alternative drug and at the same time it was available in large quantity. Therefore, the usage of this democratic drug called China root had cured 'many thousandes' in India'.[341] The China root was considered equally efficacious in the treatment of the smallpox, piles and cramps '[palsies]', all kinds of cold, and gout.[342] Linschoten asserts that Emperor Charles was cured of gout by the use of China root.[343] He cautions people about the ill consequences due to its indiscriminate use[344] and advises that such medication should be practised in consultation with an expert physician only.[345] He points out also that the dosage of the drug varies according to climate, by comparing India and China's contrasting climatic conditions.[346] It was noticed that its consumption was found to be:

likwise good against all scabbes and swellings of the said Morbo Neapolitano, or ye French pockes, the best rootes are the blackest (Dutch original heaviest) with few knots and white within: for the reddish are not so good; the wood or tree whereof it growth is like a Haw—thorne, straight and about three or four spannes high, and the roote thereof is called the wood of China, or Pockewood; when they are greene they eate them raw, and being sodden they taste almost like sugar canes but not so sweet. The tree hath but few leaves, but they are almost like the leaves of a young Orange tree. These plants or trees in China are called Lampaton, as the Chinos themselves doe say. This shall suffice for this root of China called, because it is found in no place but in China. . . .[347]

Soon after Linschoten, Garcia da Orta reports about the curing of a person suffering from smallpox, with the use of China root, in Goa in the same year, i.e. 1535. The efficacy of China root became gradually famous in Europe, for 'soon afterwards in 1546 Andreas *Vesalius* published his important book on it from Basle'.[348]

China root (*Smalx China*) the famous *Radix Chinae* is a climber. Its lilaceous root contained the saponins and sapotoxins which were admittedly nothing more than mild nauseants.[349] The China root's medicinal properties were known by the time of Thas Hung-Ching who wrote his *Pen Tshab Ching Chi Chu* around AD 512.[350]

Jan Huygen van Linschoten visited Goa the late in sixteenth century, where he found that the main diseases to be *mordexijn* (cholera), the bloody flux or dysentery and fevers, especially malarial ones.[351] Syphilis (meaning not the American derived virulent strain, but the local version), which was treated with China root, had become a common disease. Some people reportedly contracted it three or four times.[352]

One knows of the time that Asad Beg Qazwini, a Mughal officer, had introduced tobacco along with hookah for the emperor's consideration in 1604.[353] Akbar's physician Hakim Ali had argued:

In fact, this [tobacco] is an untried drug, None of the old medical authorites (*hukama*) have written about it. How can we suggest that His Majesty take such a thing whose real essence is unknown. It is not proper for his Majesty to take it. . . . It is not necessary to follow the Europeans and to adopt a thing not known to our sages, and without experiment.[354]

To this, Asad Beg reacted in the following manner:

It is a wonderful thing that all customs of the world have come about [at one time or another], and from the time of Adam to this day everything has come by and by. Whenever anything new appears among one people, it gets to be known all over the World, and all people adopt it. Scholars and physicians need to apply themselves to learn of its usefulness or ill-effect and to experiment (with it). Maybe, [of now] they just do not know its (tobacco's) benefits. Thus China root (*Chob-i-Chini*) was not present in old times, and has appeared recently and is yet found beneficial in so many diseases.[355]

Thus, Asad Beg's argument in favour of adoption of a new drug or plant soon after its introduction dispels any notion about cultural inertia or wholesale rejection by the receiving culture.

Irfan Habib has discussed in detail the origin and the course of diffusion of China root.[356]

Pyrard de Laval who visited Goa (1608–10) in the early seventeenth century observed that burning fevers, presumably enteric fevers (typhoid) and dysentery were common, as was venereal disease.[357] So far the latter was concerned, there presumably was a milder Asian version already prevalent. Pyrard de Laval, however, was referring to a new, more virulent form which was probably introduced from America. He found the people of Maldives calling it 'farangui baescour' (farangi basur), i.e. European piles.[358] The Portuguese introduced the disease into China when the farmer seized the island of Tunmen in Guangdeng province. Li Shizhen noted in 1578, that syphilis, not mentioned in the ancient recipes, had arisen in Guangdong and then spread to all parts of China'.[359] The Persian term for this was *chob chini* which was adopted not only in Hindustani, Bengali, Punjabi, Marathi and Gujarati, but also in Sanskrit as *Chobachini*.[360] According to Linschoten, it was a god gifted remedy which became immediately popular soon after its arrival in 1535.[361] Linschoten's opinion finds support from Garcia da Orta (1563), in the sense that Garcia da Orta also considers 1535 as the year when a cure was first accomplished (presumably in India) through the use of China root.[362] The appreciation for the drug in Europe is reported by Andreas Vesalius in 1546.[363]

Linschoten (1583–8), praising medicinal qualities of China root observed:

> But returning to our matter of sicknesse, pockes and piles (lempten), with other secret diseases, they are [in those countries] very common and [not hidden] concealed, for [they thinke it] no shame, more then to have any other disease. They heal them with

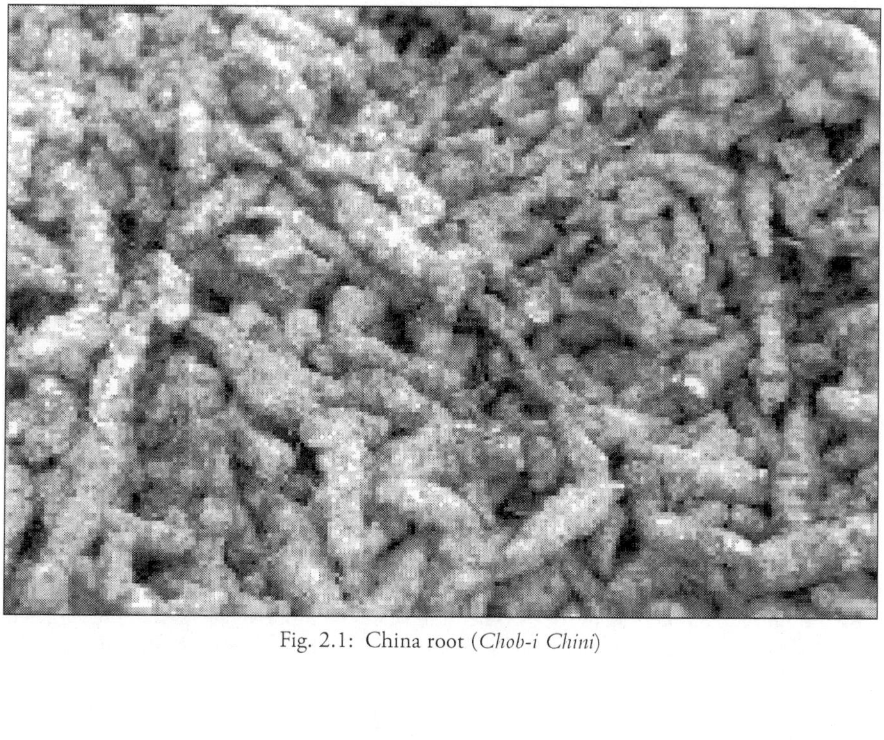

Fig. 2.1: China root (*Chob-i Chini*)

China root [wortel China]: there are [some] that have had them [at least] three or four times, and are not [anything at all] shunned or disliked for the same, but tore [both boast and] bragge thereof.[364] It is not anything perilous for the body, insomuch that they rather have them, and feare them lesse than any of the aforesaid disease.[365]

Therefore, according to Asad Beg, China root, though a novelty, was readily appreciated by all systems of medicine. It was also appreciated by the Ayurveda because in Bhava Misra's *Bhavaprakasha* (sixteenth century) it finds mentioned as a remedy against syphilis.[366]

Similarly, it entered the Unani System. Nurullah' Ata in his treatise *Risala-i-Chob-i Chini* (AH 944 /AD 1537–8) says that he had stayed nearly twenty years in India where he came to know about China root (*bikh-i-Chini*, *bikh* meaning root). He writes that the Portuguese were guarding its knowledge as a sedutously guarded secret and deliberately denying access to Muslims. Eventually, he obtained the knowledge as also a supply of drugs from Portuguese notables and started curing patients.[367]

Thus, on the basis of this brief survey above, I may suggest that the people across continents and civilizations were trying to understand the disease processes and were attempting to search for adequate medicines. None of the societies surveyed above was found averse to new concepts about diseases and medicines. In fact, they were in favour of adoption of adequate methods to cure or prevent diseases which the humanity across the globe was grappling with. It is an endeavour which still continues.

Notes

1. Cf. James L.A. Webb, Jr., 'Historical Epidemiology and Infectious Disease Process in Africa', *The Jornal of African History*, vol. 54, no. 1, 2013, pp. 3–10, especially for its encapsulation of major works and their arguments put in an extremely lucid and concise manner.
2. David Arnold, 'The Indian Ocean as a Disease Zone, 1500–1950', *South Asia*, vol. XIV, no. 2, 1991, pp. 1–21; M.N. Pearson, 'The Thin End of the Wedge, Medical Relativities as a Paradigm of Early Modern Indian-European Relations', *Modern Asian Studies*, vol. 29, no. 1, 1995, pp. 141–70; M.N. Pearson, *Towards Superiority: European and Indian Medicine 1500–1700*, James Ford Bell Library, Minnesota, 1989, pp. 1–44. Biswamoy Pati and Mark Harrison, *Health, Medicine and Empire, Perspectives on Colonial India*, Hyderabad, 2001; repr. 2006; see especially 'Introduction', pp. 1–36 for references to recent works. But these works deal mostly with the colonial phase of Indian history, Harold J. Cook, *Matters of Exchange, Commerce, Medicine and Science in the Age of Empire*, 1st pub. 2007, Yale University Press; repr., Hyderabad and Delhi, 2008, a work which is remarkable for the period it has covered.
3. R.C. Majumdar, 'Medicine', in *A Concise History of Science in India*, ed. D.M. Bose, S.N. Sen and B.V. Subbarayappa, New Delhi, 1971, p. 213.
4. Ibid., p. 240.
5. Ibid.
6. The use of 'humours' in Ayurveda, however, could not be equated with the meaning assigned to humours in the case of Greek or medieval European medicine, for the different and comprehension understanding of the term, please see, R.C. Majumdar, op. cit., p. 240.

7. See Una McGovern, *Chambers Biographical Dictionary*, Edinburg, 1st pub. 1987; repr. 2003, p. 730, S.V. *Hippocrates*.
8. M.Z. Siddiqui, 'The Unani Tibb (Greek Medicine) in India', in *A Concise History of Science in India*, ed. D.M. Bose, S.N. Sen and B.V. Subbarayappa, Delhi, 1971, p. 268.
9. Ibid.
10. Ibid.
11. Ibid., p. 269.
12. Ibid.
13. Ibid.
14. Ibid.
15. Ibid.
16. Ibid.
17. Ibid.
18. Ibid.
19. Ibid., pp. 270–3.
20. Iqtidar Husain Siddiqui, 'Science of Medicine and Hospitals in India during the Sultanate Period', *Indian Historical Review*, vol. 39, no. 1, June 2012, pp. 11–18.
21. Zahiruddin Muhammad Babur, *Babur-Nama* (Memoirs of Babur), tr. & ed. A.S. Beveridge, Delhi, 1989, vol. 1, p. 82.
22. Ibid., p. 399.
23. Ibid., p. 511.
24. Ibid., p. 543.
25. Ibid., p. 608.
26. Ibid., p. 657.
27. M.N. Pearson, op. cit., p. 9.
28. Babur, op. cit., vol. II, p. 660.
29. Abul Fazl, *Ain-i Akbari*, vol. I, tr. & ed. H. Blochmann, repr. 1927, rev. & ed. D.C. Phillott, Ori. repr., Delhi, 1977, pp. 611–13.
30. Ibid., pp. 550, 611; see also Abdul Qadir Badauni, *Muntakhab-ut Tawarikh*, vol. II, tr. & ed. Wolseley Haig, rev. & ed. B.P. Ambashthya, Patna, 1973, pp. 230–1.
31. Badauni, op. cit., pp. 230–1.
32. Fazl, op. cit., pp. 611–12.
33. Ibid., p. 612.
34. Ibid.
35. Ibid., pp. 468–9, 612.
36. Ibid., pp. 490, 612; Badauni, op. cit., p. 228.
37. Ibid.
38. Fazl, op. cit., pp. 519–20, 612.
39. Ibid.
40. Ibid., p. 521. Under Akbar, *manṣab* (numerical rank) signified paired ranks, the first designating *zāt* (setting personal rank and salary) and the second *sawār* (setting size of cavalry contingent and payment himself).
41. Ibid., p. 612; Badauni, op. cit., vol. II, p. 167, 'He was noted for his natural quickness of wit, but he had not learning in proportion . . .'.
42. Ibid., p. 612. Therefore, the assertion that the physician were not regarded as part of the Mughal ruling aristocracy requires some qualification (see Syed Ali Nadeem Rezavi's 'An Physician of the Aristocratic Mughal Empire: Muqarrab Khan', in *Medieval India 1*, ed. Irfan Habib, 1992, p. 154.
43. Fazl, op. cit., vol. I, p. 612.
44. Ibid.
45. Ibid.
46. Ibid., pp. 582, 612.

47. Ibid.
48. Ibid.
49. Ibid., p. 582.
50. Ibid.
51. Ibid.
52. Badauni, op. cit., vol. II, p. 237.
53. Badauni, op. cit., vol. III, pp. 226–8.
54. Ibid.
55. Ibid.
56. Fazl, op. cit., p. 529.
57. Ibid.
58. Ibid.
59. Jahangir, *Tuzuk-i Jahangiri*, tr. A. Rogers, ed. Henry Beveridge, 1st pub. 1909–14, 1989, vol. I, Delhi, p. 330.
60. Ibn Battuta, *The Travels of Ibn Battuta AD 1325–54*, tr. and notes from the Arabic text ed. C. Defremery and B.R. Sanguinetti, ed. H.A.R. Gibb, vol. I, Delhi, p. 143.
61. *Tuzuk-i Jahangiri*, pp. 242–3.
62. Niccolao Manucci, *Storia do Mogor or Mogul India*, Calcutta, 1966–7, vol. III, pp. 114, 117.
63. *Tuzuk-i Jahangiri*, vol. II, pp. 12–13.
64. Ibid., pp. 43–4.
65. Edward Terry (1616–89), in *Early Travels in India 1583–1619*, 1st pub. London, 1921, 1st Indian edn. 1985, p. 310.
66. John Fryer, *A New Account of the East India and Persia*, vol. I, p. 180 and see also vol. II, pp. 83–4.
67. Ibid., vol. II, p. 84.
68. Francois Bernier, *Travels in the Mogul Empire, 1656–1668*, tr. & ed. A Constable and V. Smith, London, 1914, pp. 253–4, see also M.N. Pearson, *Towards Superiority: European and Indian Medicine 1500–1700*, p. 12 especially for identification of 'quartan agues' with recurrent malaria.
69. Ibid., pp. 338–9, see also M.N. Pearson, *Towards Superiority: European and Indian Medicine 1500–1700*, pp. 12–13.
70. J. Ovington, pp. 204–5.
71. Dennis Kincaid, *British Social Life in India 1608–1937*, London, 1973, p. 7, cited by M.N. Pearson, *Towards Superiority: European and Indian Medicine 1500–1700*, p. 13.
72. Pearson, *Towards Superiority*, p. 14.
73. Jean Baptiste Travernier, *Travels in India of Jean Baptiste Tavernier*, vol. I, tr. V. Ball and W. Crooke, New Delhi, 1977, p. 271.
74. Abbe Carre, *The Travels of Abbe Carre in India and the Near East, 1672–74*, London: Hakluyt Society, Pearson, *Towards Superiority: European and Indian Medicine 1500–1700*, p. 271.
75. Peter Mundy, *The Travels of Peter Mundy in Europe and Asia, 1608–1667*, ed. R.C. Temple, London, 1914, pp. xlvi, 270–1.
76. Pearson, *The Travels of Abbe Carre in India and the Near East, 1672–1674*, tr. Lady Fawcett, ed. Charles Fawcett with assistance of Richard Burn, repr., Delhi, 1990, p. 680.
77. Coolhaas, *Generale Missiven Deel III: 1655–1674*, p. 27.
78. Ibid., p. 99.
79. Ibid.
80. Coolhaas, *Generale Missiven Deel IV: 1675–1685*, pp. 294–5.
81. Ibid., p. 814.
82. Coolhaas, *Generale Missiven Deel VI: 1698–1713*, p. 258.

83. Pieter van Dam, *Beschryvinge van de Oostindische Compagine*, vol. 1, ed. Dr F.W. Stapel, 's-Gravenhage, 1927, pp. 397, 614.
84. Ibid., p. 614.
85. Ibid., p. 615.
86. Ibid.
87. Ibid.
88. Ibid.
89. Ibid., pp. 615–18.
90. Cf. M.J. Sirks, *Indisch Natuuronderzoek-Een beknopte geschiedenis van de beoefening der natuur Wetenschappen in de Nederlandsche Kolonien*, Amsterdam, 1915, pp. 6–7.
91. Ibid., p. 7; Harold J. Cook, *Matters of Exchange, Commerce, Medicine and Science in the Age of Empire*, 1st pub. Yale University Press, 2007; 1st pub. in India, Hyderabad, 2007, p. 191, says that it was on 19 March 1627 on the basis of his reliance on M.A. van Andel, *Chirurgijns, vrije meesters, beunhazen kwalkzalvers: de Chirurgijns-gilden en de praktijk der heelkunde* (*1400–1800*), The Hague, 1941, Martinus Nijhoff, 1981.
92. Ibid.
93. Cook, op. cit., pp. 191–5.
94. Ibid., p. 196.
95. Ibid.
96. Ibid.
97. Ibid.
98. Ibid.
99. Ibid.
100. Ibid.
101. Ibid.
102. Ibid., p. 8.
103. Ibid., p. 9.
104. Ibid.
105. Ibid., p. 10.
106. Ibid.
107. Ibid., p. 11.
108. Pieter van Dam, *Beschryvinge van de Oostindische Compagnie*, ed. F.W. Stapel, vol. II, ed. 's-Gravenhage, 1939; repr. 1976, p. 604, S.V. Curcuma.
109. See *Chambers Twentieth Century Dictionary*, ed. A.M. Macdonald, New Delhi, revd edn. 1976, S.V. Bird.
110. Ibid., p. 11.
111. Cf. L.S.A.M. von Romer, *Historische Schetsen, Even inleeding tot het Vierde Congress der Far Eastern Association of Tropical Medicine*, 6–13 August 1921, p. 2.
112. Ibid., p. 4. It will be interesting to note here that people were aware of the extreme preciousness of the vision as one of the most important human senses and hence it would be logical to expect that the alleviation of weak eyesight and extension of the power of normal vision would have been one of the priorities in scientific endeavours. Magnification of an object so that it appeared larger to the eye than it really was, was known to the ancient Greeks and Romans from fourth BC onwards. But neither the name of the discoverer nor the date of the discoverer nor the date of the discovery are known. But optical magnification was one step forward towards developing microscope. See David Bardell, 'The Invention of the Microscope', *BIOS*, vol. 75, no. 2, May 2004, pp. 78–84 (Stable URL:http:/www.jstor.org/stable/4608700). Ibn al Haytham (*c.* AD 965–1039) also known as Alhazen had investigated magnification of an object by a piece of glass having plano-convex shape. But like Europeans, he saw no practical use for optical magnification (ibid., p. 79). Next one hears about Roger

Bacon (*c.* AD 12–92) who experimented with lenses and like al Haytham argued about its use as an aid for correcting vision. After the advent of the eyeglasses, there was an interregnum of nearly three centuries when another invention of equal significance took place as an optical aid to vision. The invention of the telescope and that of microscope are interwoven (ibid., p. 80). Both appeared about AD 1600 (the exact date is not known). The alignment of two lenses one behind the other to give greater magnification than that observed with just one lens is generally believed to be a chance discovery. The three Dutch spectacles Hans Jansen or his sons Zacharias or Hans Lippershey are given credit for this discovery. Jacob Metuis, a Dutch instrument maker, is also claimed to be the discoverer. However, the earliest record of the existence of a microscope is contained in a letter written by Constantijn Huygens in London on 30 March 1622 to his parents in the Netherlands. He informed his parents that he had purchased a 'lunette de Drebbel' (his term for the microscope). It is generally believed that he had made the microscope (ibid., p. 81). But there is no evidence to prove that. The earliest datable evidence of use of microscope comes from 1625 and 1630, when microscopic investigations were made of a bee and a weevil by Federico Cesi and Fransesco Stelluti (see, D. Bardell, 'The first record of microscopic observations', *Bio Science*, vol. 33, 1983, pp. 36–8). It has been suggested that the microscopes used for these observations were probably made by Galileo since it is known that in 1624 Galileo sent a microscope to Cesi in Rome. (see David Bardell, 'The Invention of Microscope', p. 81).

113. Cook, op. cit., p. 305.
114. Ibid.
115. Ibid.
116. Ibid.
117. Ibid.
118. Ibid.
119. Ibid.
120. Ibid.
121. Ibid., p. 308.
122. Ibid., p. 307.
123. Ibid., p. 308.
124. Ibid., p. 309.
125. W. Ph. Coolhaas, ed., *Generale Missiven van Gouverneurs-Generaal en Raden aan Heren XVII der Verenigde Oost indische compagnie, Deel III: 1655–1674*, ed. s-Gravenhage, 1968, p. 576.
126. Cook, op. cit., p. 308.
127. Ibid.
128. Ibid.
129. Ibid.
130. Ibid.
131. Ibid.
132. Ibid.
133. Ibid.
134. Ibid.
135. Ibid.
136. Ibid.
137. Ibid.
138. Ibid., p. 341.
139. Ibid.
140. Ibid.
141. Ibid.

142. Ibid., p. 342.
143. Ibid., pp. 342–3.
144. Ibid., pp. 346–7.
145. Ibid.
146. Ibid., p. 347.
147. Ibid. Cook refers to an anonymous work *Komo Geka* (Red Hair Survery) which described his methods of applying ointments, plasters, and poultices (ibid.).
148. Ibid.
149. Ibid.
150. Ibid., pp. 347–8.
151. Ibid., p. 348.
152. Ibid.
153. Ibid.
154. Ibid.
155. Ibid.
156. Ibid.
157. Ibid.
158. Ibid.
159. Ibid. Harold J. Cook has discussed the details of the book.
160. Ibid.
161. Ibid.
162. Ibid.
163. Ibid.
164. Ibid., p. 349.
165. Ibid.
166. Ibid.
167. Ibid.
168. Ibid.
169. Ibid.
170. Ibid.
171. Ibid., pp. 350–1.
172. Ibid., p. 351.
173. Ibid.
174. Ibid., p. 352.
175. Ibid., pp. 352–5.
176. Ibid., p. 354.
177. Ibid.
178. Ibid., pp. 354–5.
179. Ibid., p. 355.
180. Ibid., p. 356.
181. Ibid.
182. Ibid.
183. Ibid., pp. 356–7.
184. Ibid., p. 358.
185. Ibid., pp. 358–61.
186. Ibid., p. 361.
187. W. Ph. Coolhaas, ed., *Generale Missiven van Gouverneurs-Generaal en Raden aan Heren XVII der Vexenigde Oostindische Compagnie*, Deel IV: 1675–1685, 's-Gravenhage, 1971, pp. 159–60.
188. Cook, op. cit., p. 362.
189. Ibid.

190. Ibid., pp. 363–4.
191. Ibid., p. 365.
192. Ibid., p. 366.
193. Ibid.
194. Ibid., p. 366. Harold J. Cook has based his identification on Lu Gwei-Djen and Joseph Needham, *Celestial Lancets: A History and Rationale of Acupuncture and Moxa*, 1980, London, 2002, p. 277.
195. Joseph Needham and Lu Gwei-Djen, *Science and Civilization in China, Biology and and Biological Technology*, vol. 6, *Medicine*, edited with an introduction by Nathan Sivin, Cambridge, 2000, p. 52.
196. Cook, op. cit., p. 367.
197. Ibid.
198. Ibid., pp. 367–77.
199. Pieter van Dam, *Beschryvinge van de Oostindische Compagine*, ed. F.W. Stapel, vol. II (2), 's-Gravenhage, 1932, repr. 1976, p. 315.
200. Ibid., see also Valentijn, *Ceylon*, p. 53 where he speaks about 'delightful medicinal herbs' cited by F.W. Stapel, op. cit., p. 315.
201. W. Ph. Coolhaas, ed., *Generale Missiven van Gonverneurs-Generaal en Raden aan Heren XVII der verenigde oostindische compagnie, Deel IV: 1675–1685*, 's-Gravenhage, 1971, p. 295.
202. Cook, op. cit., p. 309.
203. *Generale Missiven, Deel IV: 1675–1685*, p. 295.
204. Ibid.
205. Ibid.
206. Ibid.
207. Ibid.
208. Cook, op. cit., p. 320.
209. Ibid., p. 16.
210. Ibid., p. 374.
211. Ibid., Cook uses the term points. I preferred to call it loci instead of points on the basis of Joseph Needham, Lu Gwei-Djen, op. cit., p. 61.
212. Ibid., pp. 374–5.
213. Johannes Heniger, *Hendrik Adriaan van Reede tot Drakenstein (1636–1691) and Hortus Malabaricus: A Contribution to the History of Dutch Colonial Botany*, Rotterdam, 1956, cited by Cook, op. cit., pp. 310–11.
214. Pieter van Dam, *Beschryvinge van de Oostindische Compagnie*, vol. I, ed. F.W. Stapel, 's-Gravenhage, 1932; repr. 1976, p. 23.
215. Ibid., p. 57.
216. Ibid., pp. 60–6.
217. Ibid., pp. 67–80.
218. Ibid., pp. 192–205.
219. Ibid.
220. Ibid.
221. Ibid., pp. 329, 412–33.
222. Cook, op. cit., p. 311.
223. Ibid.
224. Ibid., p. 311.
225. Ibid.
226. Ibid.
227. Ibid., pp. 311–12.
228. Ibid., p. 312.

229. Ibid.
230. Ibid.
231. Ibid., p. 313.
232. Harold J. Cook cites (p. 313). John M.de. Figueiredo, 'Ayurvedic Medicine in Goa according to European Sources in the Sixteenth and Seventeenth Centuries', *Bulletin of the History of Medicine*, vol. 58, 1984, pp. 225–35.
233. Ibid., pp. 313–14.
234. Ibid., p. 315.
235. Cf. C.G. Uragoda, *A History of Medicine in Sri Lanka from the earliest times to 1948*, Colombo, 1987, p. 68.
236. Cook, op. cit., pp. 329–30.
237. *Generale Missiven Deel IV: 1675–1685*, pp. 501–2, 603.
238. Ibid., p. 653.
239. Ibid., p. 295.
240. Wouter Schouten, *Oost-indische Voyagie*, vol. III, Amsterdam, 1676, pp. 112–13.
241. Ibid.
242. Ibid.
243. Ibid.
244. Ibid.
245. Ibid.
246. Ibid.
247. Ibid.
248. Ibid.
249. Ibid.
250. Ibid.
251. Ibid.
252. Ibid.
253. Gulbadan Begum, Memoirs (*Humayun Nama*), ed. & tr. A.S. Beveridge, London, 1902, text, p. 19, trans. p. 13, cited by Irfan Habib, 'Inside and Outside the Systems, Change and Innovation in Medical and Surgical Practice in Mughal India', in *Disease and Medicine in India, A Historical Overview*, ed. Deepak Kumar, Delhi, 2001, p. 79.
254. Ibid.
255. Irfan Habib, op. cit., p. 79.
256. Ibid.
257. Ibid.
258. Ibid.
259. Cited by Irfan Habib, p. 79. *Sirajuddin Ali Arzu's Chiragh-i Hidayat*, printed on the margins of *Ghiyasul Lughat*, Kanpur, 1899, p. 604.
260. Cf. Donald Butter, *Outlines of... Southern Districts of Oudh*, pp. 174–6, cited by Irfan Habib, pp. 80, 84.
261. Tek Chand Bahar, *Bahar-i Ajam*, vol. II, Lucknow, 1916, p. 186.
262. Habib, op. cit., p. 80.
263. Nicolao Manuchy (Manucci), *Storia do Mogor, 1656–1712*, tr. W. Irvine, vol. II, London, 1907–8, p. 301, cited by Irfan Habib, op. cit., pp. 8, 84.
264. John Martin Honigberger, *Thirty Five Years in the East*, repr. Calcutta, 1905, pp. 49–50, cited by Irfan Habib, op. cit., pp. 80, 84.
265. Ibid.
266. G.T. Vigne, *Travels in Kashmir, Ladak, Iskardu and C*, 2nd edn., 1884; repr., Karachi, 1987, pp. 140–1.
267. Ibid., p. 141.
268. Ibid.

269. Ibid.
270. Ibid., p. 140.
271. Ibid.
272. G.T. Vigne, op. cit., pp. 140–1.
273. John Martin Honigberger, *Thirty-Five Years in the East, Adventures, Discoveries, Experiments, and Historical Sketches relating to the Punjab and Cashmere, in connection with Medicine, Botany, Pharmacy &c.*, Calcutta, 1905, pp. 49–50.
274. Ibid., p. 50.
275. Ibid.
276. Ibid.
277. Habib, op. cit., pp. 73–4.
278. Ibid.
279. M.N. Pearson, *Towards Superiority: European and Indian Medicine 1500–1700*, p. 16.
280. Ibid.
281. Ibid.
282. Ibid. The other details are available in Irfan Habib's paper.
283. Ralph W. Nicholas, 'The Goddess Sitala and Epidemic Smallpox in Bengal', *The Journal of Asian Studies*, vol. XLI, no. 1, November 1981, pp. 21–44; David Arnold, *Imperial Medicine and Indigenous Societies*, Delhi, 1989, pp. 45–65; Dharampal, *Indian Science and Technology in the Eighteenth Century*, Delhi, 1971, pp. 141–63; Mridula Ramanna, 'Indian Response to Western Medicine: Vaccination in the City of Bombay in the Nineteenth Century', in *Art and Culture, Endeavours in Inter-pretation*, ed. A.J. Qaiser and S.P. Verma, Delhi, 1996, pp. 67–8.
284. Ralph W. Nicholas, 'T Goddess Sitala', p. 24.
285. Debiprasad Chattopadhyaya, *Science and Society in Ancient India*, Calcutta, 1977, pp. 24–32.
286. Edward C. Sachau, tr., *Alberuni's India*, vol. I, London, 1910, p. 309.
287. Ibid.
288. Ibid.
289. Ibid.
290. Ibid.
291. Ralph W. Nicholas, 'The Goddess Sitala', p. 26. Madhava Kara has given an extensive and comprehensive chapter on *masurika*, or smallpox. Nicholas is of the opinion that by the seventh century, smallpox had become so widespread in India that it demanded careful attention from experts dealing with medicine. In the same century, it was established in the countries around the Mediterranean.
292. Cf. ibid., p. 27.
293. Dr W. Ph. Coolhaas, *Generale Missiven Van Gouverneurs—Generaal en Raden aan Heren XVII der Verenigde Oostindische Compagnie, Deel II: 1639–1655*, Martinus Nijhoff, Gravenhage, 1964, p. 223.
294. Irfan Habib, *The Agrarian System of Mughal India*, 2nd revd edn., Delhi, 1999, p. 111. The first edition did not have this information.
295. NAI, 2702/4. I am grateful to my friend and colleague, S. Ali Nadeem Rizvi, for giving me information from the Cambay Documents, preserved in the National Archives of India, New Delhi.
296. NAI, 2695/16.
297. Coolhaas, *Generale Missiven, Deel VII: 1713–1925*, p. 374.
298. Coolhaas, *Generale Missiven, Deel VIII: 1775–1929*, p. 64.
299. J.S. Grewal, *In the By-Lanes of History, Some Persian Documents from a Punjab Town*, Shimla, 1975, pp. 175–6, 178.
300. Ibid., pp. 182, 184.

301. Cf. Nicholas, 'The Goddess Sitala', p. 33.
302. Philippus Baldaeus, *Nauwkeurige en Waarachtige Ontedekking en weder-legginge van Afgoderye der Oost-Indische Heydenen, Malabaren, Benjanen, Gentiven, Bramines*, Janssonius van Waasberge en Van Someren, Amsterdam, 1672, pp. 28–34.
303. Ibid., p. 28.
304. In some of the earlier literature on smallpox we find much information about the divine origin of smallpox. Compare accouts given by Nicholas, 'The Goddess Sitala', pp. 29–33.
305. Baldaeus, *Nauwkeurige en Waarachtige*, p. 28.
306. Ibid., p. 31.
307. Ibid. This important passage is deleted in the printed version by A.J. de Jongh. It is possibly because of this and some other omission of passages that Ralph W. Nicholas could not have access to this information.
308. Cf. Alberuni's account, and it appears that the eleventh century perception of holding Ceylon responsible for smallpox continued.
309. Baldaeus, p. 31.
310. Ibid.
311. Nicholas, 'The Goddess Sitala', pp. 38–9.
312. David Arnold, *Imperial Medicine and Indigenous Societies*, p. 46.
313. The dampness was because of the winter monsoon in India which causes rainfall in north-western India and the Tamil Nadu-Kerala costal areas. It is to be noted that since the winter monsoon blows from land to oceans, it is by and large less humid than the summer monsoon, and the consequent rainfall is also smaller. Nevertheless, it creates sufficient dampness.
314. Comaras could be indentified with the people called *Coramas*, who were low-caste illiterate people engaged in making baskets, and trading in salt and grain. See Francis Buchanan, *A Journey from Madras through the Countries of Mysore, Canara and Malabar*, vol. I, London 1807, pp. 249–50.
315. Baldaeus, op. cit., p. 32.
316. Ibid.
317. Ibid., pp. 32–3.
318. The term *basuri* was possibly used for the Sanskrit equivalent, *masuri*, which was the ancient term for smallpox. But *basuri* could be from the Arabic *basur*, 'piles, ulcers', etc.
319. Baldaeus, op. cit., p. 33.
320. Ibid.
321. Ibid., p. 32.
322. Ibid.
323. Ibid.
324. Ibid.
325. Ibid., p. 33.
326. David Arnold, *Imperial Medicine and Indigenous Societies*, p. 49.
327. W. Ph. Coolhaas, ed., *Generale Missiven van Gouverneurs-Generaal en Raden an Heren XVII der Verenigde Oost Indische Compagnie, Vol. II, 1639–1655*, 's-Gravenhage, 1964, pp. 783–4.
328. Ibid.
329. Ibid.
330. Coolhaas, *Generale Missiven, Vol. III: 1655–1674*, 1968, pp. 27–8.
331. Ibid., p. 99.
332. Ibid., p. 171.
333. Coolhaas, *Generale Missiven, Vol. III: 1655–1674*, 16 December 1660, p. 315.
334. Ibid., p. 445.

335. H. Kern, ed., *Itinerario, Voyage ofte Schipvaert van Jan Huygen van Linschoten near oost ofte Portugaels Indien*, vol. I, 's-Gravenhage, 1910, p. 160; see also, Arthur Cook Burnell, ed., *The Voyage of John Huyghen van Linschoten to the East Indies*, vol. I, 1st pub., London, 1885, repr. Delhi, 1988, p. 239; P.A. Tiele, ed., *The Voyage of John Huyghen van Linschoten to the East Indies*, vol. II, 1st pub., London, 1885, 1988, p. 107. According to P.A. Tiele, Garcia da Orlex in his *Colloquios* f. 177b, gave credit to the Chinese for introducing the drug into India, see, ibid., p. 107, fn 4.
336. Ibid., pp. 107–8.
337. Ibid.
338. Ibid., p. 108.
339. Ibid.
340. Ibid., p. 109.
341. Ibid.
342. Ibid., p. 110.
343. Ibid.
344. Ibid., pp. 110–11.
345. Ibid., p. 110.
346. Ibid.
347. Ibid., pp. 111–12.
348. Irfan Habib, p. 73. See also, J. Needham, Lu Gwei-Djen and Huang Hsing-Tsung, *Science and Civilization in China, vol. 6, Biology and Biological Technology, Part I, Botany*, Cambridge, 1986, p. 106.
349. Needham et al., op. cit., vol. 6 (1), p. 106.
350. Ibid., p. 226.
351. M.N. Pearson, p. 15.
352. Ibid.
353. See Irfan Habib, 'Inside and Outside the Systems Change and Innovation in Medical and Surgical Practice in Mughal India', in *Disease and Medicine in India: A Historical Overview*, ed. Deepak Kumar, Delhi, 2001, pp. 71–2.
354. Ibid.
355. Tr. and qtd. Irfan Habib, 'Inside and Outside the Systems . . .', p. 72.
356. Ibid., pp. 72–3.
357. M.N. Pearson, op. cit., p. 15.
358. Irfan Habib, 'Inside and Outside the Systems . . .', p. 72.
359. Ibid.
360. Ibid.
361. Ibid.
362. Ibid., p. 73.
363. Ibid.
364. Kern, op. cit.; see also, Burnell, op. cit.
365. Ibid.
366. Ibid.
367. Ibid. The other details are available in Irfan Habib's paper.

3

Rise and Decline of Surgery in Indigenous Medicine with Emphasis on Unani-Tibb

SYED EJAZ HUSSAIN

INDIA HAS BEEN a land of wisdom. It is a nation where civilizations congregate and merge. India's contribution to the production and dissemination of scientific knowledge, specifically in the fields of classic mathematics, astronomy and medicine has been widely acclaimed and acknowledged in the academic and scientific horizons. Its skill, knowledge and vibrant tradition of healing backed by rich natural and botanical resources—especially medicinal flora—captivated not only the Arabs and the Chinese but the Europeans too. Ayurveda, the oldest way of treatment, along with other systems like Siddha and Unani which developed later, have together provided a less expensive and efficacious health care to its vast populations both in urban and rural segments over centuries. Besides, the Indian traditions of health care systems also incorporate several non-drug therapies like yoga. All these systems are, infact, deep-rooted in the scientific and cultural traditions of the country.

The Indian medical system was well received in the Arab world. The Abbasid Caliphs and the contemporary Arab scholars harboured a great love and respect for Indian sciences including medicine. A number of renowned Indian vaidyas were invited to Baghdad, and some major Ayurvedic treatises were translated into Arabic such as *Suśruta Saṁhitā* of which the Arabic name is *Al-Kitab shahsun al-Hindi*, also known as *Kitab-i-Susurud*.[1] None of these translations are now known to exist, except a rendering of a book on poisons, which was originally translated into Persian for Khalid-Al-Barmaki, the Abbasid wazir, and later was translated into Arabic.

Abul Hasan Ali bin Sahl Rabban Al-Tabari (AD 810–61) (hereafter Abul Hasan Tabari), a Christian convert, born at Merv in Khurasan (now in Iran), was the first Perso-Arabic author who has described in some detail the Ayurveda and Indian medical practitioners in his work *Firdaus al-Hikmah* (*Paradise of Wisdom*). Of this work, five manuscripts are known, out of which one is preserved in the British Library, London[2] while one copy is available in the Raza Library, Rampur.[3] His other famous work on medicine *Al-Kitab Hafzh al-Sihat* (*Book on Preservation of Health*) is preserved in the Bodleian Library, Oxford.[4]

Abul Hasan Tabari recorded the Indian works of Jarak (*Caraka Saṁhitā*), Susrud (*Suśruta Saṁhitā*), Nidan (*Nidana*, a work on Pathology by Madhavakara) and Ashtankar (*Ashtangahridaya* of Vagbhatta). He has also referred to *Kutubun Imr'at Hindiyah* or *Books of an Indian Lady Doctor* which is also identified with *Rusa al-Hindiyah*, a book of an Indian gynaecologist mentioned by Ibn Abi Usaybi'ah (d.1270). The Indian lady doctor, according to Tabari, also prescribed medicines for beauty and shining of a woman's face. Tabari has explained in his work, Ayurveda's theory of *Panchamahabhuta* or the five basic elements, and *tridosa* or the three humours. The five basic elements are *al-ard* (*pirthvi* or earth), *al-ma'* (*apas* or water), *an-nar* (*tejas* or fire), *al-rih* (*vayu* or air), and *al-hawa'* (*akasa* or ether), while the three humours are *balgham* (*kapha* or phlegm), *al-rih* (*vayu*/*vata* or air) and *al-murra* (*pitta* or bile).[5]

Another prominent Arab physician Ibn al-Nadīm (d. *c*.388/998), the author of *Kitab Al-Fihrist*, has mentioned the names of twelve Indian vaidyas whose names are so distorted in Arabic transcription that it is difficult to trace them in classical Ayurvedic texts. Ibn al-Nadīm has also mentioned that the Indian physician Manka was invited to Baghdad by Yahha bin Khalid-al-Barmaki, the Abbasid wazir, for the treatment of Harun al-Rashid (AD 786–809), the Abbasid Caliph. Manka's treatment was successful, and not only was he richly rewarded by the Caliph, but he was also entrusted with the translation of medical books from Sanskrit to Arabic with the help of Arab physicians; *Al-Kitab shahsun al-Hindi* or *Kitab-i Susurud* was translated by him. Ibn al-Nadīm also informs that Ashtankar or Ashtangahridaya was translated by Ibn Dhan, the Superintendent of the Baghdad hospital, while Jarak or the book of Charaka was translated from Persian into Arabic by Abdullah bin Ali who had earlier translated this work from Sanskrit into Persian.[6] In its description of *salajīt* it has also mentioned how the *bhasma* or powder of gold, silver and copper was prepared for pharmaceutical use.

But the exchange and collaboration was not one-sided; it was bilateral. Ayurveda also adopted several techniques and new ideas from Unani-tibb. The elaborate technique of pulse examination and therapeutic use of mercury and opium was borrowed in Ayurveda from Unani-tibb. Theoretical knowledge of nādi may have been derived from Tantrik literature but its practical use in various aspects of ailing body examination was borrowed from Unani-tibb after the thirteenth century. Pharmaceutical use of mercury after purification by heating and calcination or making its powder, is not found in any classical Ayurvedic work; it began in India only after the thirteenth century under the influence of Unani-tibb. But it may be noted that *bhasma* or powder of gold, silver and copper was already known to the Indian medical practitioners. Kushta or preparing metal powder in Persian was perhaps borrowed from Ayurveda. Opium production began in India from the sixteenth century. Medical properties of opium were known to the Ayurvedic practitioners in a very limited way and the drug was imported here from Arabia. But later on, its wider application began under the influence of Unani-tibb.[7] Several Indian names like *atrifal* (Sanskrit *tri-phala*: a combination of three fruits or a myrobalan-electuary), *sandal* (Sanskrit *chandan* or odoriferous wood), *zanjabil* (Sanskrit *sringgavera* or dry ginger) and *kafur* (Sanskrit *karpur/kapur* or camphor), found their way into Arab pharmacopoeia. It is notable that *zanjabil* and *kafur* as well as *misk* and *oud* have occurred in the Koran (verses 76: 18, 76: 5 and 83: 26) also, as has been claimed by Syed Sulayman Hasan Nadvi in his work *Arab-o Hind ke Ta'aluqat*.

Manufacture of Medical Instruments

Growth of surgery in medical treatment exhorted the medical practitioners to evolve devices and manufacture tools and instruments useful for the purpose of surgery. Initially, these tools were very simple and primitive. They were generally made of iron and wood, etc. In course of time, with the progress in surgical skill, various other types of new medical tools and instruments were produced and some old instruments were improved. Surgery was performed in all ancient civilizations except China and Japan where it was a taboo on account of certain conservative attitudes like reference for the dead, filial piety and avoidance of bloodletting. Enough references and evidences are

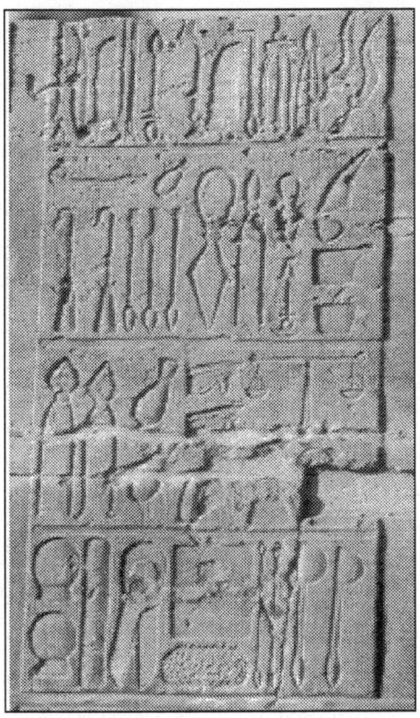

Fig. 3.1: Inscription of Ancient Medical Instruments
Found on the wall of an Ancient Temple in Kom Ombo City, Egypt
(Bone saws, suction cups, knives and scalpels, retractors, scales, lances, chisels and dental tools)

Source: Wikipedia, the free encyclopaedia
Accessed on 25 August 2013

found of the existence of surgery and practice of some surgical operations in Greco-Roman, Mesopotamian, Sumerian and Egyptian civilizations. Small surgical knife made of copper, scalpels and needles, spoon and some other types of simple surgical instruments have been found in archaeological discoveries, and references of some of the medical tools are found in classical historical literature also.[8] In November 2001, archeologists in Egypt discovered 30 surgical tools of bronze such as scalpels, needles and a type of spoon from the tomb of Skar, the oldest Pharaonic surgeon of one of Egypt's fifth dynasty rulers (Fig. 3.1) dating back more than 4,200 years.[9]

But the development of surgery achieved a landmark even in very ancient times in India. *Suśruta Saṁhitā* is the evidence of the growth and maturity of the Indian surgery in the classic age.[10] Apart from foreign body removal, suturing, cataract removal, fractured bone-setting and other techniques of surgical operations, *Suśruta Saṁhitā* also described the advanced technique of plastic surgery. Sushruta's contribution is far beyond the imagination of any other contempory surgeon in the world and he was undoubtedly far ahead of his time in this field. *Suśruta Saṁhitā* described in detail the various branches of surgery, surgical methods, and surgical instruments in one full chapter devoted to the subject of surgery. It has given detailed description of 121 types of surgical instruments of which 101 were blunt and 20 were sharp instruments. The blunt instruments were:

Svastika yantras	They were forceps of twenty-four types, each resembling the mouth of an animal or bird, and were used for extracting thorn or foreign bodies entrenched in bones.
Sandansha yantras	They were dissecting forceps or tongs in two styles used for extracting foreign bodies from skin, muscles, blood vessels and ligaments.
Tala yantras	They were spoon shaped instruments used for extracting foreign bodies from the ear, nose or a sinus.
Nadi yantras	They were tubular instruments of different diameters and lengths depending on the use, for inspection and treatment of diseased spots and also for removing foreign bodies.
Shalaka yantras	They were rod like instruments of twenty-eight types in specific lengths, circumferences and shapes used for specific operational procedure as for probing, retraction, separation, extraction, cauterization, cleaning wounds and applying drugs to a particular portion of the ailing body. Some instruments falling in this category were used for removing nasal polypi, cleaning urethra and applying collyrium.

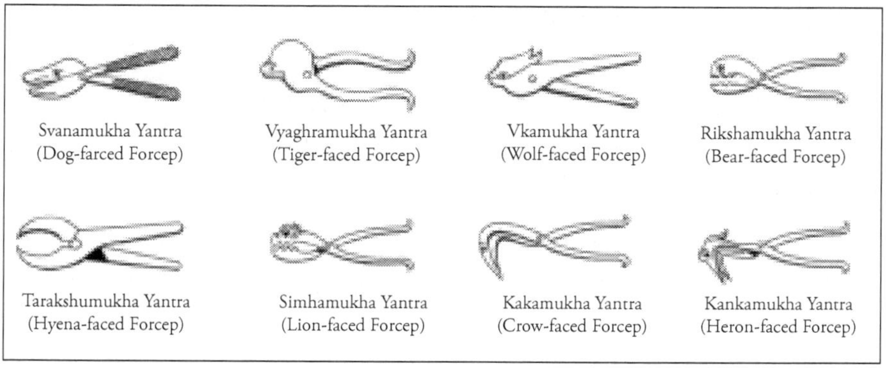

Fig. 3.2: Eight Kinds of Forceps Described by Sushruta

Apart from the above 101 blunt tools and instruments, *Suśruta Saṁhitā* has also described the details of 20 sharp instruments used for different categories of operations like *bhedya* (excision), *chhedya* (incision), *lekhya* (scarification), *vedhya* (puncture), *eshya* (probing), *aharya* (extraction), *visravya* (drainage), and *sivya* (suturing). The 20 sharp instruments were:

1. *Karapatra* (Bone saw or rongeur): An instrument for removing small rough portions of bone.
2. *Vriddhipatra* (Scalpel): A small straight knife with a thin sharp blade used in surgery and dissection.
3. *Mudrika* (Ring knife): A circular or oval ring with an internal cutting edge used to shave off tumors in the nasal and other cavities.
4. *Utpalapatra* (Lancet): A sharp-pointed surgical instrument, usually with two edges, for making small incisions.
5. *Suci sastra* (Suturing needle): Thread, gut, wire or needle used for sewing or joining a wound.
6. *Kusapatra* (Bistoury): Long surgical knife with a narrow blade.
7. *Vrihimukha* (Trocar): A sharp-pointed surgical instrument, used with a cannula to puncture a body cavity for fluid aspiration.
8. *Ara* (Awl): A pointed hand tool with a fluted blade used for piercing wood, leather, etc.
9. *Atimukha* (Hawk bill scissors)
10. *Sararimukha* (Scissors)
11. *Amtaramukha* (Curved bistoury)
12. *Trikurcaka* (Three edged knife)
13. *Kutharika* (Chisel)
14. *Vetasapatraka* (Scalpel of different type)
15. *Badisha* (Sharp hook)
16. *Dantasanku* (Tooth scaler/extractor forceps)
17. *Esani sastra* (Sharp probe)
18. *Mandalagra sastra* (Circular knife)
19. *Nakhasastra* (Nail parer)
20. *Ardhadhara* (Single-edged knife)

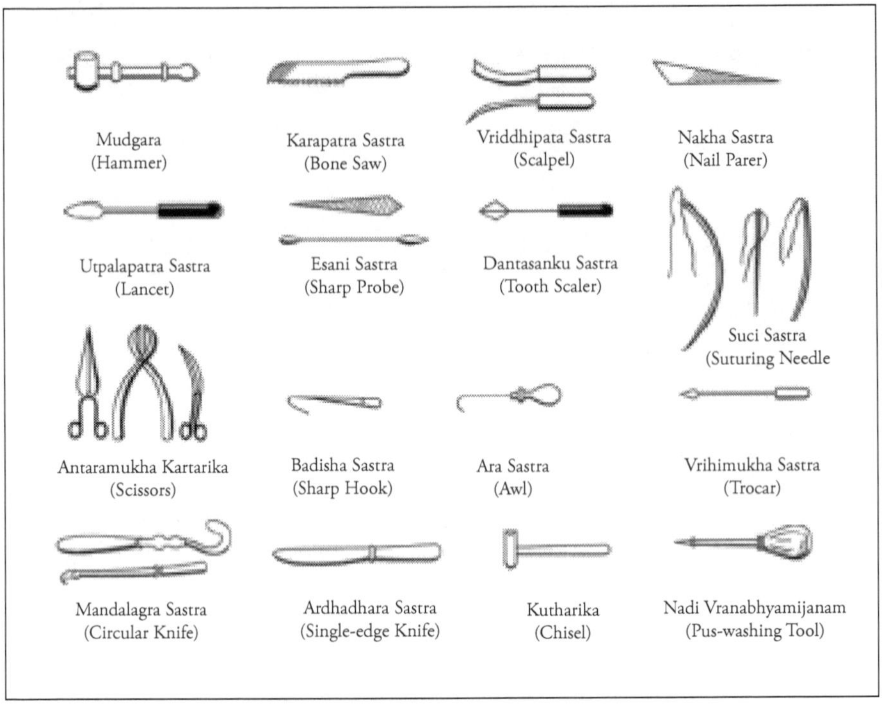

Fig. 3.3: Drawings of Some Other Tools Described by Sushruta

Based on these descriptions of various medical tools and instruments mentioned in *Suśruta Saṁhitā* and those used in rural India in the beginning of the twentieth century, Kaviraj Kunja Lal Bhishagratna in 1907 drew the sketches of some of the instruments in the first English translation of the legendary surgical work. Later commentators and other researchers on the subject reproduced these drawings. It may be noted that the operating portion or head of some of the instruments resemble the shape of a dog, tiger, wolf,

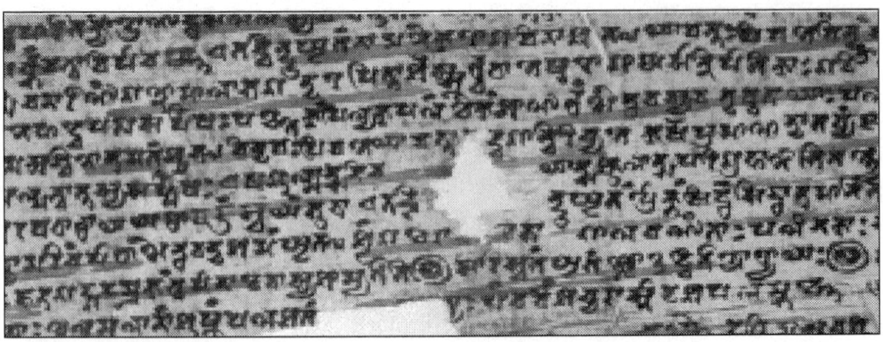

Plate 3.1: The Bower Mansucript (Bodleian Library, Oxford University)

Source: Wikipedia, the free encyclopaedia
Accessed on 25 August 2013

bear, lion, serpent hood or bird, etc., in order to make distinction for use and purpose of one instrument from the other. Sizes of the instruments are generally given in finger breadths.[11]

Arab Renaissance and the Growth of Medicine and Surgery

The period between eighth–tenth centuries is regarded as the Age of Arab Renaissance, when the Arabs and Persians began to study the Greek and Roman sciences in the university at Jundishpur of old Sassanid Persia. It was also the first school of Unani medicine where the Islamic scholars studied the works of Hippocrates, Galen, and other Greek physicians. Very soon these scholars familiarized themselves with the sciences and specifically the medical knowledge of Byzantium (modern Istanbul), Persia, India, and China. The Arabs' hunger for knowledge was especially aggravated when Abbasid Caliph Harun al-Rashid (AD 786–809) established the *Bayt al-Hikmah*, or House of Wisdom which served as a translation bureau in Baghdad. A massive translation movement now took place and scholars from Greece, India and other places were invited and leading works of science, philosophy, education, literature including medicine and surgery were translated into Arabic and Persian and later in turn into Turkish, Hebrew and Latin, in order to make them more widely available for further study and research. This brought about a revolution in the domain of knowledge. David W. Tschanz noted:

> The most important of the translators was Hunayn ibn Ishaq al-'Ibadi (AD 809–73), who was reputed to have been paid for his manuscripts by an equal weight of gold. He and his team of translators rendered the entire body of Greek medical texts, including all the works of Galen, Oribasius, Paul of Aegina, Hippocrates and the Materia Medica of Dioscorides, into Arabic by the end of the ninth century. These translations established the foundations of a uniquely Arab medicine.[12]

Translation of *Suśruta Saṁhitā* into Arabic, as noted above, was a part of this translation movement.

During the period of Arab enlightenment, three names reached the acme in the field of medicine and surgery, and their collective contribution not only heralded a new era in indigenous medicine, but their works also steered the growth of modern medicine in Europe. They were Abu Bakr Al-Razi (AD 850–932), Abu Ali Husain Abdullah bin Ibn Sina (AD 980–1037) and Abu Al-Qasim Khalf Ibn Abbas Al-Zahrawi (AD 936–1013). Al-Razi came to be known in Europe as Rhazes, Ibn Sina as Avicenna and Abu Al-Qasim as Abulcasis.

Al-Razi (Rhazes), born in the town of Rayy, near Tehran, was the most eminent physician of the ninth century and contributed 113 books on medicine including two encyclopedic works *Al-Kitab al-Hawi fi al-Tibb* (The Comprehensive Book of Medicine) and *Al-Kitab al Mansuri* (The Book for Mansur). *Al-Kitab al Mansuri*, presented to Mansur Ibn Ishaq, the ruler of Khorasan, carried a chapter on general surgery and bone fractures. Al-Razi dealt with hernia, tumours of the breast, skin and legs and the removal of leg varices. He used the previously known tools such as the scalpels (small light knife), hooks, retractors, pincers, scissors, needles and cautery tools that were made of iron or copper.

Al-Razi also invented some new instruments—for instance, for the removal of nasal polypi he used the knotted rope that passed from the nose to the mouth, and also employed different shapes of scalpels in surgery of the tumours. He was also the first to use the suture thread made of the intestine of animals—the catgut—and the first to use pure alcohol for wound cleaning and dressing. The use of the soporific sponge for inhalation anaesthesia was also one of his pioneering inventions. It was a sponge saturated with dissolved powder of opium, hyocyamus and mandragora (a short-stemmed European narcotic plant), placed on the nose and mouth before any operation to make the patient insensible to pain.[13] His treatise, *The Diseases of Children*, has led some historians to regard him as the father of pediatrics. He was the first to identify high fever and its cause. His work on kidney stones is considered archetypical.

Ibn Sina (or Avicenna) who was born in Bukhara (Persia) in today's Uzbekistan, was the most distinguished physician of Unani-tibb and composed over 107 books of which *Al-Qanun fil-Tibb*[14] or *The Canon of Medicine*, and *Kitab al-Shifa'* or *The Book of Healing* became most widely known. *The Canon of Medicine* is composed in five volumes. The third volume deals with all body diseases from head to foot while the fourth volume has discussed tumours, orthopaedic disorders and surgery. Ibn Sina also added some

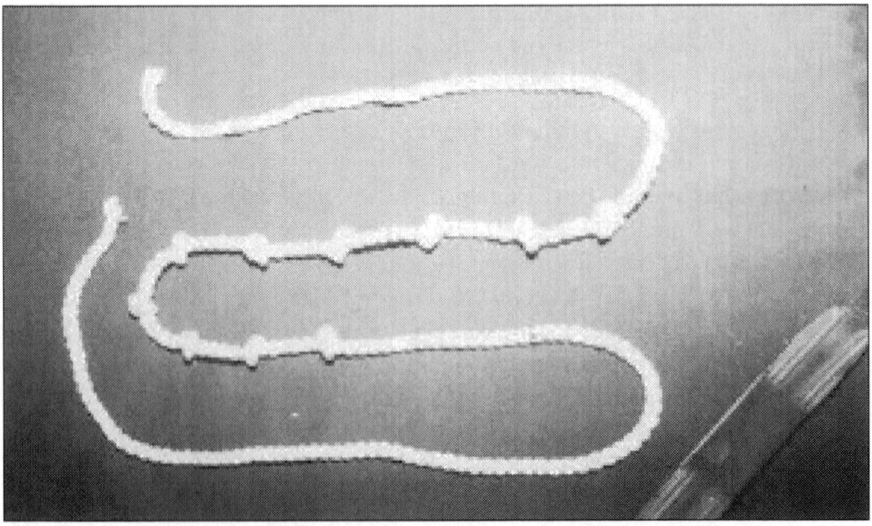

Plate 3.2: A Rope with Knots for Removal of Nasal Polypi by Rhazes
Source: Mostafa Shehata, 'Medical Instruments in Islamic Medicine'

new tools and improved some old tools used in surgery. He introduced the use of silver and gold in the manufacture of some instruments. David W. Tschanz has remarked, 'The Canon was used as a reference, a teaching guide and a medical textbook until well into the nineteenth century, longer than any other medical work.'[15]

In common surgery like tumour and pharyngeal operation, he used different sizes of scalpels, hooks, dilators, extractors, scrapers, needles and grasping forceps. In orthopaedic surgery, he used scalpel extractors, pincers, scissors and hand-saw, besides the wood splints to support fractures and dislocations. In thermo-cautery he used tools made of gold and presented a new innovation of a cautery tool enveloped by a tube, to be used inside the nose, mouth or rectum. He invented the first endotracheal tube, made of gold, to be introduced through the mouth to save suffocating patients.[16]

But the contribution of Abul Qasim Al-Zahrawi (or Abulcasis) was unparalleled so far as the growth of surgery was concerned. Born in Cardoba (Spain), his most outstanding work was *Kitab Al-Tasrif li-man 'ajaza'an al-ta'lif* or the arrangement of medical knowledge for one who is not able to compile a book for himself which contained thirty chapters, the last of

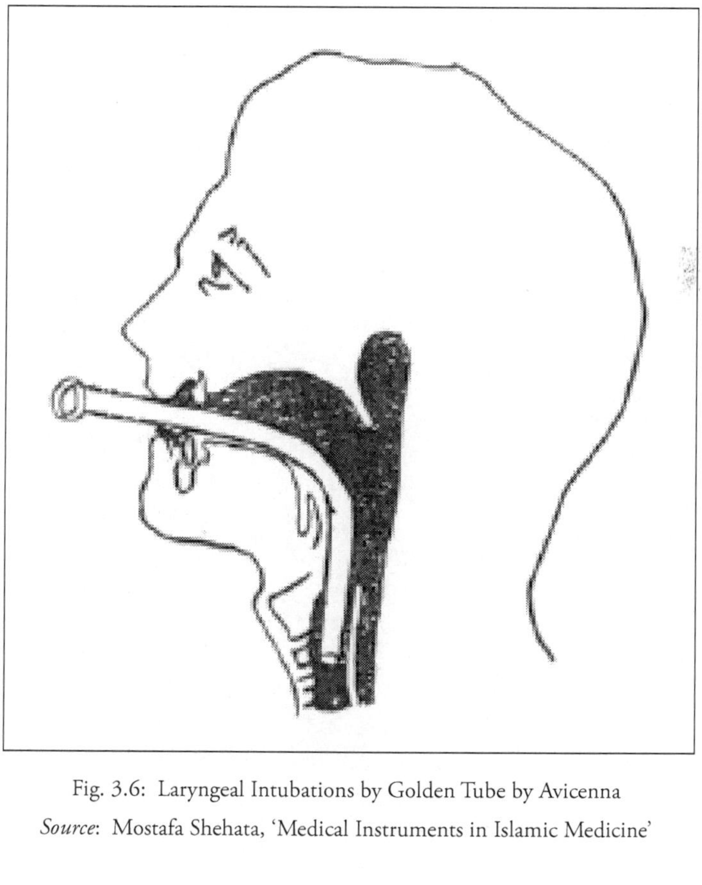

Fig. 3.6: Laryngeal Intubations by Golden Tube by Avicenna

Source: Mostafa Shehata, 'Medical Instruments in Islamic Medicine'

which, i.e. the thirtieth treatise dealt with surgery. Completed in AD 1000 *Kitab Al-Tasrif* was treated as a reference book in surgery even in Europe for long. Abulcasis was the first surgeon to describe and draw the pictures of more than 150 medical instruments like scalpels of different sizes and shapes, forceps, hooks, retractors, dilators, scrapers, cannulas, depressors, deceivers, crushers, extractors, pincers, scissors, tweezers and catheters, besides some tools for thermo-cautery. The cautery tools were of different shapes and sizes with single or double blades. Their tips were slender, punctuate, crescentic, rounded or lenticular. The scalpels were also of different shapes and sizes to suit the incisions at different parts of the body. The forceps were of the wide or pointed tip to be used for catching wound edges, palpation of the lesions and extraction of foreign object from the body. Hooks of various shapes and sizes with single, double or triple curved ends were also made and used in different locations of the body. Silver or gold wire was used for bridging loose teeth, small fine scalpels, pincers, scrapers, extractors were the other tools used for dental surgery. Trocars, made of iron or copper, with hollow cannulas were used to withdraw fluid from the abdomen, chest or cystic swellings. Pincers were used to crush urinary calculi and to extract a small diseased bone. Vaginal speculum made of metal or wood with a metal screw was used in obstetric surgery. On the other hand, hammers, hand saw and wood splints now began to be used in orthopaedic surgery. There are about 200 figures drawn on surgical instruments by Al-Zahrawi and about twenty-six of them were new ones mentioned by Al-Zahrawi for the first time.[17]

Abu Marwan Abdul Malik Ibn Zuhr, also known as Avenzoar (AD 1094–1162), and Abul Faraj Ibn Al-Quff (AD 1233–86) were two other prominent

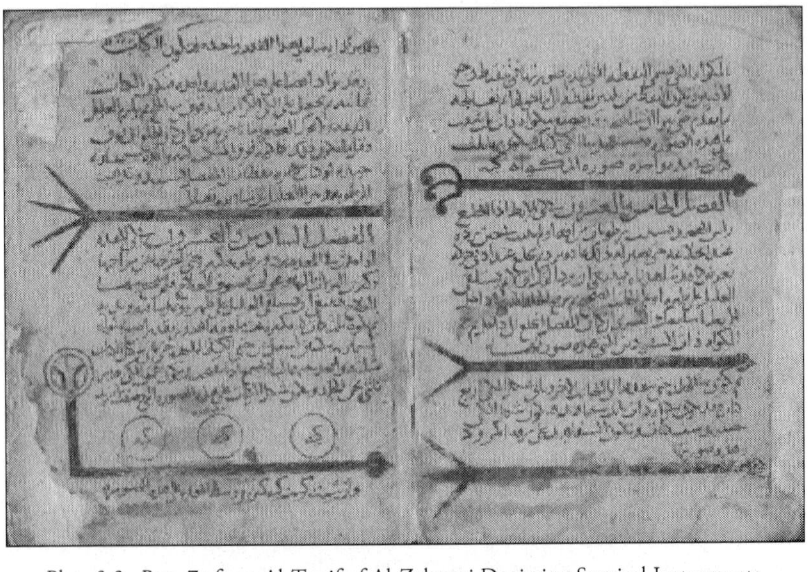

Plate 3.3: Page 7a from Al-Tasrif of Al-Zahrawi Depicting Surgical Instruments
Azerbaijan National Academy of Sciences, Baku

surgeons in medieval times. Ibn Zuhr was born in Seville, now south-western Spain. His work, *Kitab Al-Taisīr fil-Mudāwāt wal-Tadbīr* or *The Book of Simplification Concerning Therapeutics and Diet*, was well known for the progress of surgery. The work helped facilitate the growth of surgery. It was soon translated into Hebrew and Latin, and printed eight times in Latin between 1490 and 1554.

Though Ibn Zuhr used the surgical instruments invented by Abulcasis, he performed and perfected surgery of the kidney and urinary bladder by employing the technique for tracheostomy operation. He also designed the malleable catheter for oral feeding.[18] Ibn Al-Quff was a prominent surgeon who served in the army in Damascus and specialized in the surgery of wounds and tumours. In his reputed work, *Kitab Al-'umdah fi al-Jirahat* or *The Book on the Basics of Surgery*, he has given a detailed description of various types of surgical operations as also various tools and instruments used in these operations. His work was the most predominantly used in surgery during the entire medieval period. In this book he also explained the connections between arteries and veins which was the earliest description of what would be known as capillaries. He did this work before the invention of a microscope and also explained how valves worked and the direction in which they opened and closed. *Kitab Al-'umdah fi al-Jirahat* was published in Hyderabad, India in 1937.[19]

Most of the tools and instruments mentioned above were made of hard metals like iron or brass. However, lead, silver and gold were also used partially in some of the tools. In some cases, for instance, in the case of orthopaedic tools, wood was also used, while materials like glass, pottery or ceramic were used for making drug containers, mixers and droppers. Blacksmiths, goldsmiths and carpenters were involved in manufacturing these tools as per the requirements

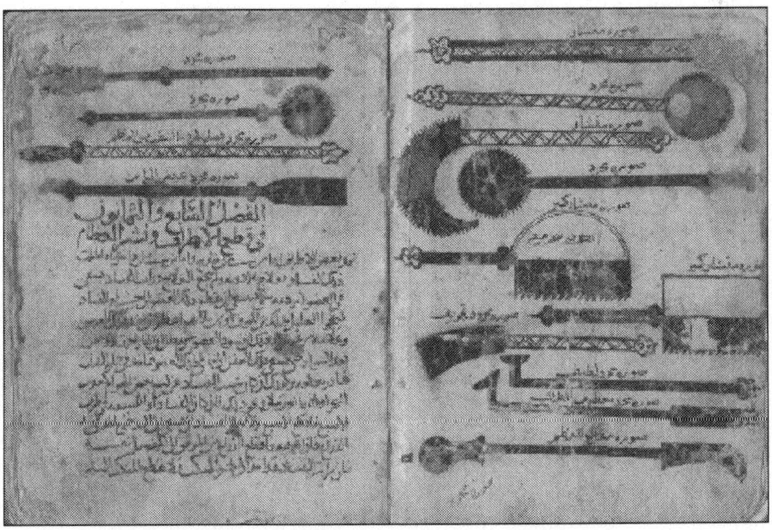

Plate 3.4: Page 7b from Al-Tasrif of Al-Zahrawi Depicting Surgical Instruments
Azerbaijan National Academy of Sciences, Baku

and directions of the physicians. Abulcasis was the first to use lead for making some of the instruments. Since lead was soft, it was easy to curve and bend an instrument made out of it, during surgical operation. Probes and hooks, therefore, were also especially made of lead for the purpose of extracting fishbone from the throat.

Sterilization of the Instruments

The discovery of microorganisms in 1675 by Antonie van Leeuwenhoek (AD 1632–1723), a Dutch merchant and scientist of Netherlands, who was known as the Father of Microbiology, brought a revolution in the field of medicine. But before the discovery of microorganisms, it was Ibn Sina who hypothesized that microbial disease (e.g. tuberculosis) and some other diseases could be contagious. He advised preservation of the medical instruments in fresh liquid bile as an effective antiseptic measure.[20] Fire heating of the instruments was the other method practised during the classical age of medicine for the purpose of controlling infections. Rhazes and Avicenna both recommended that surgical tools and cautery instruments be heated before their use as a safe antiseptic measure. They also used pure alcohol as an antiseptic agent for wound cleaning and operative dressings.

Introduction of Experimental Surgery

Animals have been used repeatedly throughout the history of biomedical research. Early Greek physician-scientists, such as Aristotle (384–322 BC), and Erasistratus (304–258 BC), performed experiments on living animals. Likewise, Galen (AD 129–199/217), a Greek physician who practised in Rome and was a giant in the history of medicine, conducted animal experiments to advance the understanding of anatomy, physiology, pathology, and pharmacology. However, experimentation on animals to test the toxicity of medicines first came about in the ninth century from Al-Razi. The latter is known to have given monkeys doses of mercury to test its safety for human use, as is recorded in a thirteenth century work, *Al-Jamie Limufradat Al-Adwiya Wal-Aghdiya* (Complete Book of Simple Medicaments and Nutritious Items) composed by Ibn Al-Baytar.[21] In Unani-tibb, Ibn Zuhr (Avenzoar) was the first to introduce a testing surgery on animals. Ibn Zuhr did animal testing as an experimental method for testing surgical procedures before applying them to human patients.[22] He performed the first experimental tracheotomy on a goat.[23] In his work, *Kitab Al-Taisir Fi Al-Mudawat Wa Al-Tadbeer*, he noted:

> Earlier on in my training when I read those opinions (controversies), I cut on the lung pipe (wind pipe, trachea) of a goat after incising the skin and the covering sheath underneath. Then I completely cut off the substance of the pipe an area just less than the size of a tirmisah (lupine seed). Then I kept washing the wound with water and honey till it healed and it (the animal) totally recovered and lived long time.[24]

Ibn Zuhr continued his experimentation on animals in his research on surgery. In the course of looking for a treatment for lung ulcerations he wrote:

. . . Thus remedies for lung ulcerations are there around in the universe but are yet unknown to us. That is because sheep when caught with a lung disease do leave the herd and wander about as if looking for something; shepherds say for a plant to eat and when they finish eating it their illness is relieved completely and are back to normal. I did inspect lungs of sheep with the evident effect of breach of continuity and with obvious evidence of healing and union. Up till now I did not know that medicine and I do think no one before me knew it either.[25]

In this way, right from the time of *Suśruta Saṁhitā* to the time of Abulcasis, indigenous medicine, especially surgery—both in Ayurveda and Unani-tibb— developed and reached an acme. *Caraka Saṁhitā*, *Suśruta Saṁhitā* and *Astangahridya* were already known to the Arab physicians and surgeons. These classical Indian works were also translated into Arabic. Hence it is natural that Arab physicians and surgeons must have benefited from the medical insights and surgical methods and instruments described by these works. An interesting fact, however, is noted. Al-Zahrawi (Abulcasis) and Ibn Zuhr (Avenzoar) were par excellence in the field of surgery and were credited to have introduced new innovations in surgical process and manufacture and use of several new medical instruments and tools. It is understood that though they belonged to medieval Al-Andalus or Spain, they must have heard and got access to the Arabic version of the Indian works especially *Suśruta Saṁhitā*; yet one does not find any reference to it in the works of these two surgeons.

Apart from manufacture of new surgical instruments and tools, some modern concepts like clinical trials, drug-potency studies, experimentation on animals and description of the true structure and function of the human body were set in motion during the golden era of ninth–twelfth centuries by the Islamic physicians and surgeons who worked in Egypt, Baghdad, Damascus, Tabriz, Isphahan, Rayy, and Cardoba, which were located in medieval Arabia, Persia and Spain. The Unani-tibb had, thus, reached a stage of maturity and become a well organized medical system before it was introduced into mainland India in the thirteenth century with the establishment of the Sultanate rule in Delhi.

Dialogue of Exchange and Share of Knowledge: Unani in India

A dialogue of exchange and share of knowledge in medicine had begun long before the establishment of the Sultanate rule in India when Indian physicians were invited to Baghdad and the translation of Indian medical works were rendered into Arabic in the eighth century at the great Islamic centre of learning and knowledge. It was perhaps due to this acquaintance that when Unani-tibb reached India, it was welcomed here and India's vast and varied medicinal flora was let open for Unani-tibb practitioners to utilize it in making medicines and conducting experiments and research. Expert Unani practitioners, hakims and tabibs began to visit, migrate and even permanently settle in India during the Sultanate as well as during the Mughal period. Scores of works and commentaries were composed and compiled by them.

Table 3.1: Prominent Physicians/Surgeons and their Works during the Delhi Sultanate

Sr. No.	*Name of Rulers*	*Famous Physicians*	*Famous Surgeons*	*Works composed (with year of composition)*
1.	Iltutmish, Razia, Balban	Abu Bakr bin Ali al-Kashani, Sadruddin Tabib, Alauddin, Badruddin Damishqi (famous during Khalji period also)		Al-Beruni's *Kitab-al Saidna* (was translated from Arabic to Persian)
2.	Alauddin Khalji	Maulana Hamid Mutriz, Maulana Sadruddin ibn Maulana Husamuddin Marikali, Yameni tabib Ilmuddin, Maulana A'izuddin Badayuni	Mah Chandra Tabib, Madrak Marzi Jaja Ilmuddin	
3.	Muhammad bin Tughluq	Zia Muhammad Masu'd Rashid Zangi		*Majmu'a-i Ziay'i* (1329)
4.	Firuz Shah Tughluq (himself a physician & bone-setter)	Ilyas bin Shahab alias Zia Anonymous		*Rahat-ul Insan* (1385) *Tibb-i Firuzshahi*
5.	Sikandar Lodi	Mian Bhowa Mian Taha Farmuli		*Ma'adan-ush Shifa-i-Sikandar Shahi* or *Tibb-i Sikandari* (1512)

Table 3.1 gives the names of the prominent physicians and surgeons during the rule of the Delhi Sultanate. Unani slowly reached even the remotest parts of the country and works on medicine began to be written in large parts of the country. Several hospitals were also started by the rulers.

When the Tughluq dynasty declined and independent provincial kingdoms came into existence in Bengal, Gujarat, Malwa, Deccan, Jaunpur and Kashmir, hakims and tabibs migrated to these places from Delhi as well as from Persia and some other countries. They flourished in these provincial kingdoms and under the patronage of the local rulers and governors contributed a lot of works. Names and works of some prominent Unani-tibb physicians are given in Table 3.2. It became a common practice to maintain Unani and Ayurvedic practitioners in the royal courts by the kings, sovereigns and governors. They provided treatment and medical suggestions to the royal house, harems, nobles and their family. Provincial rulers also established several hospitals.[26]

With establishment of the Mughal rule in the country, Unani got a new impetus along with Ayurveda. New hospitals came into existence and the number of physicians and surgeons swelled. Physicians emerged not only as a professional class but a certain hierarchy also developed. Besides, a variety of medical works were compiled. Patronage, grants and honours were also extensively bestowed upon the skilled and expert physicians, which in turn led to the growth of rivalry, competition and jealousy among the physicians and surgeons.[27] Besides, the provision of medical facility to the public became a state duty. Table 3.3 presents the names and works of prominent physicians and surgeons during the period of the great Mughals.

Table 3.2: Prominent Physicians and their Works under the Provincial Sultanates

Sr. No.	*Name of Rulers*	*Famous Physicians*	*Farmous Surgeons*	*Works composed (with year of composition)*
	SULTANS OF GUJARAT			
1.	Muzaffar Shah I	Shahab ibn Abdul Karim Nagori		(i) *Tibb-i Shahabi* (ii) *Tibb-i Shifa al-Khani* (1391)
2.	Mahmud Shah	Ali Muhammad ibn Isma'il Asawali Asili		*Shifa-i Mahmudi* (tr. of *Ashtangahridaya*)
	SULTANS OF MALWA			
3.	Mahmud Khalji I	Maulana Fazlullah (Chief Physician of Dar-ush-shifa, Mandu)		
	SULTANS OF KASHMIR			
4.	Sultan Zain-ul Abidin	Mansur bin Muhammad bin Yusuf Sri Bhatt	Physician & surgeon	(i) *Kifaya-i* (ii) *Mujahidia Tashrih-i Mansuri*
	ADIL SHAHI SULTANS OF BIJAPUR			
5.	Ibrahim Adil Shah II	Muhammad Qasim Farishta (historian)		*Dastur-ul Atibba* or *Ikhtiyarat-i Qasimi* (1590)
	NIZAM SHAHI SULTANS OF AHMADNAGAR			
6.	Burhan Nizam Shah	Hakim Wali Gilani		(i) *Taqwim-ul Abdan* (ii) *Risala-i Hifz-i Sihatt* (iii) *Taqwim-ul Amraz*
7.	Murtaza Nizam Shah	Zain-ud Din Samani (set up a Dispensary in Ahmadabad) Rustam Jurjani		*Zakhira Nizam Shahi* (1547)

(Contd.)

Table 3.2 (*contd.*)

Sr. No.	*Name of Rulers*	*Famous Physicians*	*Farmous Surgeons*	*Works composed (with year of composition)*
	QUTUB SHAHI SULTANS OF GOLCONDA			
8.	Muhammad Quli Qutub Shah	Mir Momin		*Ikhtiyarat-i Qutub Shahi*
		Shamsuddin Ali Husain al-Jurjani		*Tazkirat-i Kahhalin*
		Hakim Shamsuddin bin Nuruddin		*Zubdat-ul Hukama*
		Abdullah Tabib		*Tibb-i Farid*
		Taqiuddin Muhammad bin Sadruddin Ali		*Mizan-ul Tabai'*
		Nizamuddin Ahmad Gilani		*Majmu'a-i Hakim-ul mulk*
		Ismai'l bin Ibrahim Tabrezi		*Tazkirat-ul Hukama*

Table 3.3: Prominent Physicians and their Works during the Great Mughals

Sr. No.	*Name of Rulers*	*Famous Physicians*	*Famous Surgeons*	*Works composed (with year of composition)*
1.	Babur (and Humayun)	Khwaja Nizamuddin Ali Khalifa	Syed Tabib Khurasani, Atka Bakshi	
		Mir Abul Baqa Yusuf Herawi (flurished in Humayun's time also)		(i) *Jami-ul Fawa'id* (ii) *Fawa'id-ul Akhyar* (1507) (iii) *Qasida fi Hifz-ul Sihhat* (1530) (iv) *Riyaz-ul Adwiya* (1539) (v) *Tibb-i Yusufi* (vi) *'Ilaj-ul Amraz*
		Muhammad Baig		*Dastur-ul Fasd*
2.	Akbar	Ali Husain Gilani Abul Fath Gilani		(i) Commentary on Avicenna's Canon (ii) Mujarrabat-i Ali Gilani
		Shamsuddin Gilani	Shaikh Bina	*Khulasa-i Bina*
		Hakim Ain-ul Mulk		(i) *Fattahi* Commentary on Avicenna's Canon (ii) Sharh-i *Qanooncha*

(*Contd.*)

Table 3.3 (*contd.*)

Sr. No.	*Name of Rulers*	*Famous Physicians*	*Famous Surgeons*	*Works composed (with year of composition)*
		Humam bin Abul Fath (one of Akbar's nine jewels),		
		Muzaffar bin Muhammad al-Husaini al-Shifai, Shah Fathullah Shirazi, Ilmuddin, Maulana Jalaluddin Md. Ardistani, Mahadev, Bhim, Nath and Narayan		*Tibb-i-Shifai*
3.	Jahangir	Hakim Amanullah		(i) *Ganj-i Badaward* (ii) *Ummul 'Ilaj* (iii) *Dastur-ul Hunud* (tr. of Madan Vinod a Sanskrit work)
			Muqrrab Khan	*Anis-ul Kuhhal*
		Hakim Sadr		(i) *Hidayat-ul Hikmat* (ii) *Hifz-i Sihhat*
		Rukna Kashi Shaikh Momena Shaikh Hamiduddin Abd-ush Shakur Hakim Ruhullah		
4.	Shah Jahan		'Ain-ul Mulk Shirazi	(i) *Alfaz-ul Adwiya* (1628–9) (ii) *Tibb-i Dara Shikohi* (iii) *Qutas-ul Atibba* (iv) *Anis-ul Mu 'alijin*
		Mir Muhammad Hashim		*Hashia* (marginal notes) on (i) *Tafsir-i Baizawi* (ii) *Asbab-o 'Alamat*
		Taqrrub Khan, Fathullah Shirazi, Tabiba Satiunnisa Khanum (Gyneocologist)		
5.	Aurangzeb	Khair Andesh Khan (Etawah)		*Khair-ul Tajarib*
		Muhammad Akbar Arzani,		(i) *Tibb-i Akbari* (ii) *Mizan-i Tibb* (iii) *Tibb-i Nabvi*

(*Contd.*)

Table 3.3 (*contd.*)

Sr. No.	*Name of Rulers*	*Famous Physicians*	*Famous Surgeons*	*Works composed (with year of composition)*
				(iv) *Muffarih-ul Qutub* (v) *Qarabadin-i Qadri* (vi) *Mujarrabat-i Akbari* (vii) *Hudud-ul Amraz* (viii) *Tibb-i Hindi*
		Muhammad Mehdi Ardistani, Muhammad Raza Shirazi		(i) *Riyaz-i Alamgiri* (ii) *Riyaz-i Manazir*
			Alvi Khan Shirazi Shivji	

Growth and Decline of Surgery in Indigenous Medicine

The rulers in medieval India, both Sultanate and Mughal, maintained a large army and remained involved in frequent military engagements as they had to fight wars and battles for expansion, consolidation and security of their kingdoms and Empires. Hence, they also needed to maintain a good number of physicians and surgeons. Mah Chandra Tabib, Madrak Marzi, Jaja and Ilmuddin were prominent surgeons during the Khalji period. *Sirat-i-Firuz Shahi* notes that Firuz Shah Tughluq himself was a master bone-setter; he joined the fractured bone of a good number of his soldiers. Firuz Shah had established a large hospital known as Bimaristan in Delhi. *Sirat-i Firuz Shahi* informs that:

Amrāẓ har nau' dawai mufrad wa murakkab dar shafakhāna Firuz Shahi muhaiya mi dārand. Marīẓ wa saqīm wa waẓī' wa sharīf wa ahrarār wa 'abīd wa qarīb wa ba'īd ashfa' hāsil mi kardad wa aṯ'ima' wa aghziya muwafiq mizāj har yaki az marīẓ az ṣadaqāt haẓrat Jahan Panāh dar shafakhāna muhaiya mi bāshad wa ba-maṣraf mi rasad wa hamchunin az ihsān haẓrat saltanat anast ke dīwān khairāt mustaqīm kardanidah wa aṣhāb dīwān mardum mutadin wa kāfi naṣb farmudah wa amwāl sahmu tazwīj az suhamu awqāf imlāk khāṣ muhai'ya kardah . . .[28]

(For the treatment of every kind of diseases both single and compound medicines are made available in the hospital of Firuz Shah. Patients and infirms, nobles and plebeians, masters and slaves, of near and distant get treatment. And food and diet according to the need of each patient is made available and served in the hospital from the royal endowment. And so great is the largesse of his royal majesty that a Department of Charity has been established. And efficient and upright officials were posted there, and portions of wealth from the properties of the waqfs were allocated. . . .)

Sirat-i Firuz Shahi further writes:

Az āsār haẓrat Jahān Panāh khallada mulkahu istiqāmat dar-ush shafa wa marastānai bimaristān dar haẓar wa safar wa aṯibba māhir muai'yan farmud ta mulazim dar-ush-

shafa bashand wa adwiya az har ṣinf ke brai anwa' marẓ mufid bāshad muhaiya dārand. Chunanke barai munafa' chashm . . . barai dafa' ṣafra . . . brai pak kardan me'dah . . . barai dafa' dard-o suparz . . . barai dafa' zahmathāi' masana wa gurda . . . barai kushtan kirm-i shikam wa kaddu-dana . . . barai dafa' dard-i sar . . . barai muhafaẓat mui wa darāz kardan wa siyāh kardanidan . . . barai khārish . . . barai quwah bāh . . . barai dafa' surfa . . . barai nishadan suddaha. . . .[29]

(Of the relics of His Majesty, his kingdom may perpetuate, the establishment of the *dar-ush-shafa'* and hospital, i.e. Bimaristan, while station or in journey, the efficient physicians were appointed so that they became the employees of the *dar-ush-shafa'*. And the medicines of every kind which could be useful for the treatment of various diseases were made available; for instance, for the benefits [treatment] of eyes . . . for the curing of the bile . . . for purging the bowels . . . for healing the pain of liver and spleen . . . for treatment of the diseases of bladder and kidney . . . for exterminating the intestinal worms and ulcers . . . for expelling headache . . . for nourishing hair and make it longer and black . . . for itching . . . for strength and potency . . . for curing cough . . . for clearing obstruction [severe constipation]. . . .)

Sirat-i Firuz Shahi has given a detailed description of human anatomy, known as *tashri-ul abdān*. Regarding Firuz Shah's expertise in setting fractured bones of hands and legs, it informs:

. . . Wa ba'aẓi ke dar siyāq wa ṣayd az markab uftadah wa uẓẓām wa a'ẓa' dast wa pa shikastah har say'i ke mahirān īn kār wa isatizah kabār natawanand badast-i mubarak khud ān-ra bastah wa ba-bastan ān irshād namudah dar muddat qarīb az ibtila' inkisār rastah wa bil-jabbār badal gashtah. . . .[30]

(. . . and some who have fallen from the horse while riding or hunting and broken limbs or bones of hands or legs, after all efforts of the experts and specialists in this work could not be successful [his royal majesty], with his own august hands set them [the fractured bones] and after setting [accomplishing the setting work] pleased to say that very soon [the patient] would become free from infliction and the bone was [thus] set).

Sirat-i Firuz Shahi also says that on personal instruction and training of Firuz Shah a collyrium was prepared that was used for cataract or *ab-i marwarīd*. It says:

. . . wa Kuhl Firuz Shahi ke mansub ba-farmayish khās murakkab pi charm-i mār-i siyāh wa adwiya digar wa dar dar-ush shafa barai 'ilāj 'amma mua'iyan dārand. . . .[31]

(. . . and Kuhl Firuz Shahi that relates to his royal majesty's special instruction, a compound [medicine prepared] with slough of black cobra and other herbs and kept available for the treatment of the common people in the hospital. . . .)

The next very significant work which remained as a reference book in Unani-tibb up to the nineteenth century in India, was *Ma'adan-ush Shifa* or *Tibb-i Sikandari*, an encyclopaedic work on Indian Materia Medica: composed in AH 918/AD 1512 by Mian Bhowa. He devoted a portion of his work to surgery in section I—that is *ilm-i tibb* or science of medicine. He has extensively drawn from *Suśruta Saṁhitā* and has given the details regarding the surgical instruments and various stages of surgical operations. He has also discussed human anatomy, various limbs and organs as well as veins and their origins.[32]

Surgery enjoyed promotion during the Mughal period as well. Syed Tabib Khurasani and Ataka Bakhshi were very prominent surgeons during Babur's time. The former had treated the Emperor's mother, Qutlugh Nigar Khanum who once became seriously ill and had a fatal disease. Atka Bakshi could perform any kind of surgery including that of the brain. He accompanied Babur in battles and served as military surgeon. He was a skilled bone-setter also.[33] Hakim Bina was an experienced surgeon during the time of Akbar. He operated on and cured several persons who had serious wounds. He also composed a work that he named *Khulasa-i Bina*. Emperor Jahangir took a keen personal interest in the growth of medicine and surgery. He even conducted several experiments in this regard: once when the Emperor shot a lion during hunting, he ordered for the lion's body to be dissected in order to ascertain whether its gall bladder was indeed inside its liver like that of other animals. He found that the lion's gall bladder was inside its liver and concluded that this might be the reason for the bravery of the animal.[34]

Muqarrab Khan was a renowned surgeon during the time of Jahangir and Shah Jahan. Recognizing his skill of treatment Jahangir wrote, '. . . *wa dar 'ilm-i jarrahi be-badl zaman khud ast wa peshawān guft ke dar in 'ilm u sāhib-i ṯarz ast* . . .'[35] (in the science of surgery he was unparalleled in his time, and his followers said that in this science, he had his own technique). When Jahangir suffered from *khun-para* or blood congestion (known as arteriosclerosis in modern medicine), he was bled from the left arm and had to lose about a *ser* of his blood on the advice of Muqarrab Khan.[36]

It is noteworthy that Babur died of an illness which could not be cured by any physician. Humayun fell from the stairs of his library in Delhi and broke his limbs and skull and passed away. Akbar died of blood dysentery. His court physician Ali Gilani did not prescribe any medicine for eight days; after eight days he gave him wrong medicines as a result of which the Emperor succumbed to his disease.[37] Jahangir and Shah Jahan suffered from urine retention problem—Hakim Momena had treated Jahangir while Taqarrub Khan gave *shir-i khisht* to Shah Jahan to cure him.[38] Jahangir's son Khusrau died of *qulanj* or the colic pain.[39] Mumtaz Mahal, the wife of Shah Jahan, died of excessive bleeding and labour pain while giving birth to her fourteenth child at the age of forty. Nadira Begum, the wife of Dara Shikoh, died at a young age suffering from dysentery and vexation. Mir Jumla also died of dysentery in Bengal.[40] In 1644, when Jahanara, Shah Jahan's daughter, caught fire by an accident, Hakim Sadr along with some other physicians were called in for treatment. But when she could not be cured by them, an English surgeon Dr Gabriel Boughton was invited from Surat who treated and cured her. Shah Jahan was so happy that he asked the doctor to make any wish and the doctor requested for duty free trade in Bengal for the East India Company which was granted in 1651. Similarly, the English surgeon William Hamilton treated the swellings in the groin of Farrukh Siyar and became successful in obtaining from the Emperor in 1717, the famous *farman* or royal order that is treated as magna carta for the English right to trade and settlement in India.

Every ruler had surgeons in their army both during the Sultanate and Mughal periods. These surgeons were efficient in extracting arrows, spears, swords, lances and other such weapons which got embedded in flesh, bone or ligament of the body of a wounded soldier. Yet, although they knew well how to extract these foreign elements from the body, all their knowledge was based on the ancient classical works like *Suśruta Saṁhitā*, *Ashtangahridaya* as well as *Kitab Al-Tasrif* of Abul Qasim Al-Zahrawi.[41] Tables 3.1, 3.2 and 3.3 give the names of prominent physicians and surgeons during the Sultanate and Mughal periods including the Provincial Sultanates. But what these Tables and available evidences establish is that surgeons were few, most of them being physicians. The books on medicine composed during the entire medieval period were mostly on pharmacology while the portion on surgery discussed in some of the works was confined to the description on human anatomy.[42] The surgical instruments which have been discussed in *Suśruta Saṁhitā* and *Kitab Al-Tasrif* were the first and the last original works in Ayurveda and Unani-tibb respectively. One does not come across any new work describing any new medical tool or the improvement of the old ones that had already been discussed in these two classical works on surgery. It was perhaps this state of surgery that provoked Manucci to comment that Persian physicians were guided by ancient books and had no idea of the new trends and developments; that they followed the centuries old process of treatment.[43] But it may be noted here that Manucci is also called a quack as he had not obtained a degree in medical science. However, the comments of the French physician François Bernier, who had obtained medical degree from the University of Montpellier, France in 1652, reflect that there was a tendency among the Western physician-surgeons (who came to Mughal India and were invited for treatment to the Mughal royal house and the houses of some nobles) that depicted 'a developing gap between European medical practice and that prevalent in India'.[44]

There was no provision for formal education, awarding of degrees or issuance of licences in the indigenous medical systems of pre-modern times, and the art of healing, particularly surgery, was the family cartel of practicing vaidyas and hakims—as is noted by John Fryer and John Ovington.[45] Taboo against contact with dead bodies in both Hindu and Muslim society has also been raised as a factor for the slow progress of study of human anatomy in India. In spite of this, details of human anatomy with illustrations are found in several classical works of Unani-tibb in Arabic, Persian and Sanskrit. Michael Pearson has pointed out that:

> . . . dissection had been considered to be antithetical not just to the Muslim tradition but also to the Jewish and Christian, though in fact some dissections had been undertaken

in Christian Europe long before Vesalius. The common dislike of vivisection meant that in both Christian and Muslim areas, surgeons, in terms of status, were far inferior to physicians. Great physicians like Ibn Sina disliked the very notion of surgery, and left it to surgeons and bone-setters.[46]

It is also said that Indian physicians remained dependent on physicians like Galen and Avicenna whose works were reproduced by translating and writing commentaries, and bloodletting was still treated as a cure for several diseases. But it is notable that:

> Galen remained a prescribed text at the Cambridge medical school until the middle of the nineteenth century, and the notion of the four humours remained influential into the nineteenth century. Bloodletting also continued. The great surgeon Paré was a ferocious bleeder. As late as the 1830s there was a bleeding craze in France, and some 20 million leeches a year were required to keep up with the demand.[47]

In Europe, smallpox affected all levels of society. 400,000 people annually died of smallpox in Europe in the eighteenth century and one-third of the survivors went blind.[48] In view of this, the claim that European medicine and surgery was greatly advanced in pre-modern period is challenged here. Michael Pearson has rightly remarked that it was François Bernier who was attached to the Mughal court, widely travelling in India between 1659 and 1667 and it was Bernier who made comments on India's indigenous medical systems, propounding the theory of Europe's advancement in medical science over Asians. It is notable that Bernier remained the focus of research and debate for decades in Indian history for his theory of sluggishness and depredation of Indian economy calling it 'Asiatic despotism'. In fact, most of the European travellers in India nurtured an assumed superiority over Asians in every field including science and technology and had the idea that 'borrowers could not invent or discover'.[49] Bernier charged that Indian surgeons did nothing about anatomy and surgery. Narrating Danishmund Khan, the surgeon of the time of Aurangzeb, about the circulation of blood he commented:

> It is not surprising that the *Gentiles* understand nothing of anatomy. They never open the body either of man or beast, and those in our household always ran away, with amazement and horror, whenever I opened a living goat or sheep for the purpose of explaining to my *Agah* [patron] the circulation of the blood, and showing him the vessels, discovered by *Pecquet*, through which the chyle is conveyed to the right ventricle of the heart. Yet notwithstanding their profound ignorance of the subject, they affirm that the number of veins in the human body is five thousand, neither more nor less, just as if they had carefully reckoned them.[50]

It was noted that plastic surgery was already done in ancient India as is known from *Suśruta Saṁhitā*. It was also performed during the medieval period, as is known from the accounts of the foreign travellers. Manucci who has criticized the Indian physicians for their medical practice based on old and traditional knowledge, has elsewhere praised the Indian surgeons for their efficiency in plastic surgery. He informed how the surgeons of Bijapur would cut the skin of a person near the eyebrows and provide for an artificial nose when the nose was cut off as a punishment by the local ruler.[51] Inoculation or sacrifications by a sharp needle for the treatment of smallpox was introduced during the Mughal period. Muhammad Akbar Arzani, a surgeon in the early eighteenth century further developed the treatment of smallpox when he used a gold needle to prick for draining out the vesicles.[52]

In Europe and London, barbers and surgeons were clubbed together up to the seventeenth century. In India, the *hajjam* or barber performed leeching, circumcising and bone-setting, while the *jarrah* or surgeon, apart from doing the work of bone-setting, would also perform operations and take care of the healing of wounds, extraction of foreign objects or part of a weapon embedded in the body—as also the work of skin-grafting for deformities of the face, low-lithotomy and couching the eye for cataract. Surgeons in England and France were separated from barber's guilds only in the 1740s.[53] In fact, medicine and surgery in Europe had the same position and status as it did in India and other Asiatic countries. It was only after the invention of modern form of vaccination in 1796 by Edward Jenner, a British physician, that Western medicine and surgery entered into a new phase of revolution; such inventions were unheard of in indigenous medicine in India. In fact, maintaining the balance of humours (or *tridosha* and *akhlat*) has been the chief thrust in India's indigenous medical stystems, both in Ayurveda and Unani-tibb. This could have been the reason for emphasis on care and preservation of health in both the systems rather than on treatment and cure. This could also have been a reason that surgery became inert in the indigenous medical systems of India.

Notes

1. R.L. Verma, 'The Growth of Greco-Arabian Medicine in Medieval India', *Indian Journal of History of Science*, vol. 5, no. 2, November 1973, p. 348.
2. Catalogue of Arabic Mss at the British Library, London, MSS no. Arundel Or. 41, pp. 217–21.
3. Hakim Md. Ajmal Khan, *Fihrist Kutub Arabi Kitabkhana-i Riyasat Rampur*, MSS no. 171, Rampur, 1902, p. 489.
4. Uri's Catalogue of Arabic MSS at the Bodleian Library, Oxford, vol. 1, MSS no. Marshman 413, p. 578.
5. Abul Hasan Ali bin Sahl Rabban Al-Tabari, 'Firdausal-Hikmat or Paradise of Wisdom', ed. M.Z. Siddiqui, Berlin: Sonne Press, 1928, pp. 557–624; M.S. Khan, 'Ali Ibn Rabban Al-Tabari: A Ninth Century Arab Physician, on The Ayurveda', *Indian Journal of History of Science*, vol. 25, nos. 1–4, 1990, pp. 20–33.
6. Ibn al-Nadeem, *Kitab Al-Fihist*, ed. Gustav Flugel, Leipzig, 1872; Beirut repr., n.d.; M.Z. Siddiqui, *Studies in Arabic and Persian Medical Literatue*, Calcutta, 1958, pp. 30–45.

7. G.N. Chaturvedi and K.P. Singh, 'Impact of Ibn Sina on Pulse Examination and Materia Medica of Medieval Period of Ayurveda', *Indian Journal of History of Science*, vol. 21, no. 4, 1986, pp. 358–62.
8. P.B. Adamson, 'Surgery in Ancient Mesopotamia', *Medieval History*, vol. 35, no. 4, 1991, pp. 428–35.
9. Archaeologists unearthed the tomb of ancient Egyptian doctor (2001). Available www.arabicnews.com, accessed on 25 August 2013.
10. Original manuscript of *Suśruta Saṁhitā* has not survived, and only 'copies of copies and revisions of revisions' exist. However, the Bower manuscript that is written on birch-bark and dated fourth century AD, was discovered by Hamilton Bower in 1890 from Kuchar, in eastern Turkestan. Now it is preserved in the Bodleian Library, Oxford. It was translated into English, in parts only, by U.C. Dutta (1883), A. Chattopadhyaya (1891), and A.F.R. Hoernle (1897). K.K.L. Bhisagaratna translated it in full between the years 1908 and 1917 and it is this translation which is now available.
11. K.K.L. Bhishagratna, *The Suśruta Saṁhitā* (English translation based on the original Sanskrit text), vol. I, repr., Varanasi: Chowkhamba Sanskrit Series Office, 1963, K. Natrajan, 'Surgical Instruments and Endoscopes of Susruta: The Sage Surgeon of Ancient India', *Indian Journal of Surgery*, vol. 70, October 2008, pp. 219–23; M. Tewari and H.S. Shukla, 'Sushruta: The Father of Indian Surgery', *Indian Journal of Surgery*, vol. 67, issue 4, August 2005, pp. 229–30.
12. David W. Tschanz, 'Arab Roots of European Medicine', *History of Medicine*, vol. 4, issue 2, 2003, p. 9, also may be checked at http://www.heartviews.org/text.asp?2003/4/2/9/64472.
13. Mostafa Shehata, 'Medical Instruments in Islamic Medicine', *Journal of the International Society for the History of Islamic Medicine* (*JISHIM*), vols. 6–7, nos. 11–14, 2007–8, pp. 60–6.
14. The earliest version of the manuscript dated 444 AH/AD 1052 is preserved in the Aga Khan Museum, Geneva bearing accession no. AKM00510. It carries 32 images.
15. Tschanz, op. cit.
16. Shehata, op. cit.
17. Ibid.
18. Henry Azar, *The Sage of Seville: Ibn Zuhr, His Time, and His Medical Legacy*, Cairo: American University in Cairo Press, 2008.
19. Peter E. Pormann and Emilie Savage Smith, *Medieval Islamic Medicine*, Edinburgh: Edinburgh University Press, 2007, p. 61.
20. Tschanz, op. cit.
21. Rabie E. Abdel Halim, 'Experimental Medicine 1000 Years Ago', *Urology Annals*, vol. 3, issue 2, May–August 2011, pp. 55–61.
22. Rachel Hajar, 'Animal Testing and Medicine', *Heart Views*, vol. 12, issue 1, January–March 2011, p. 42.
23. Missouri Brunetto, Giacoma M. and Maurizio Domenicucci, 'Origin of the Cannula for Tracheotomy during the Middle Ages and Renaissance', *World Journal of Surgery*, vol. 36, issue 4, 7 February 2012, pp. 928–34.
24. M. Al-Khoori, ed. and tr., *Kitab Al-Taisir Fi Al-Mudawat Wa Al-Tadbeer* of Ibn Zuhr (Avenzoar), Damascus: Darul Fikr Press for the Arab Educational Scientific and Cultural Organization, 1983, p. 149; Rabie E. Abdel Halim, op. cit.
25. M. Al-Khoori, op. cit., p. 129; Rabie E. Abdel Halim, op. cit.
26. Iqtidar Husain Siddiqui, 'Science of the Medicine and Hospitals in India during the Delhi Sultanate Period', *Indian Historical Review*, vol. 39, no. 1, 2012, pp. 11–18.
27. S. Ali Nadim Rezavi, 'Physicians as Professional in Medieval India', in *Disease and Medicine in India: A Historical Overview*, ed. Deepak Kumar, New Delhi: Tulika Books, 2001, pp. 40–65.

28. امراض بر نوع دوای مفرد و مرکب در شفاخانہ فیروزشاہی مہیا
می دارند۔ مریض و سقیم و وضیع و شریف و احرار و عبید و قریب و
بعید اشفاع حاصل می کردد و اطعمہ و اغذیہ موافق مزاج ہر یکی از
مریض از صدقات حضرت جہانپناہ در شفاخانہ مہیا می باشد و بمصرف
می رسد و ہمچنین از احسان حضرت سلطنت آنست کہ دیوان خیرات
مستقیم کردانیدہ و اصحاب دیوان مردم متدین و کافی نصب فرمودہ و
اموال سہم تزویج از سہام اوقاف املاک خاص معین کردہ ـــ

Sirat-i Firuz Shahi, MSS no. H.L. 99, Khuda Bakhsh Library, Patna, ff. 241–2.

29. از آثار حضرت جہانپناہ خلد ملکہ استقامت داراشفاً و مارستان ای
بیمارستان در حضر و سفر و اطباً ماہر را معین فرمود تا ملازم دارالشفاء
باشند و ادویہ از ہر صنف کہ برای انواع مرض مفید باشد مہیا دارند۔
چنانکہ برای منافع چشم۔برای دفع صفرا۔برای پاک کردن معدہ۔برای
دفع دررد جگروسپرز۔برای دفع زحمتہای مثانہ و گردہ۔برای کشتن کرم
شکم و کدودانہ۔برای دفع درد سر۔برای محافظت موی و دراز کردن و
سیاہ کردانیدن۔برای خارش۔برای قوہ باہ۔برای دفع سرفہ۔برای نشادن
سدّھا۔۔

Sirat-i Firuz Shahi, ff. 235–41.

30. ۔۔ و بعضی کہ در سیاق و صید از مرکب افتادہ و عظام و اعضاًء دست
و پا شکستہ ہر سعی کہ ماہران این کار و اساتذہ کبار نتوانند بدست مبارک
خود انرا بستہ و با بستن ان ارشاد نمودہ در مدت قریب از ابتلاء انکسار
رستہ و بالجبار بدل گشتہ۔۔۔

Sirat-i Firuz Shahi, f. 333.

31. ۔۔۔ و کحل فیروز شاہی کہ منسوب بفرمایش خاص مرکب پی چرم مار
سیاہ و ادویہ دیگر و در دارالشفاء برائے علاج عامہ معین دارند۔۔۔

Sirat-i Firuz Shahi, ff. 334, 338.

32. Syed Hasan Askari, 'Medicines and Hospitals in Muslim India', *PIHC*, 20th Session, Bombay, 1957 (Bombay, 1958), p. 173; Altaf Ahmad Azmi, 'Unani Medicine: Hakims and Their Treatises', in *History of Science, Philosophy and Culture in Indian Civilization*, ed. B.V. Subbarayappa, vol. IV, part II—*Medicine and Life Sciences in India*, New Delhi: Munshiram Manoharlal, 2001; repr. 2009, pp. 332–3.
33. Zahiruddin Muhammad Babur, *The Tuzuk-i Baburi* or *Memoirs of Babur*, ed. and tr. A.S. Beveridge, repr., Delhi, 2006, pp. 169–70, 246.
34. Nuruddin Muhammad Jahangir, *The Tuzuk-i Jahangiri* or *Memoirs of Jahangir*, tr. Alexander Rogers and ed. Henry Beveridge, vol. I, Delhi: Low Price Publications, 2006, repr., p. 351.

35. ۔۔ و در علم جرّاحی بی بدل زمان خود است و پیشوان گفت کہ درین علم
او صاحب طرز است۔۔۔

Jahangir Nama (Khuda Bakhsh Library, Patna, H.L. 43), ff. 45b–46a.

36. *Memoirs of Jahangir*, vol. I, pp. 225–6; Syed Ali Nadeem Rezavi, 'An Aristocratic Surgeon of Mughal India: Muqarrab Khan', in *Medieval India 1: Researches in the History of India 1200–1750*, ed. Irfan Habib, Delhi: Oxford India Paperbacks, 1999, p. 159.
37. *Jahangir Nama*, ff. 90a–92b.
38. Syed Zillur Rahman, 'Indian Hakims: Their Role in the Medical Care of India', in *History of Science, Philosophy and Culture in Indian Civilization*, ed. B.V. Subbarayappa, vol. IV, part II—*Medicine and Life Sciences in India*, p. 384.
39. *Memoirs of Jahangir*, vol. II, p. 228.
40. Francois Bernier, *Travels in the Mogul Empire*, AD *1656–1668*, Delhi: Low Price Publications, 2008, repr., pp. 103, n. 2, 173.
41. K.K. Thakral, 'Techniques for Extraction of Foreign Bodies from War Wounds in Medieval India', *Indian Journal of History of Science*, vol. 16, no. 1, May 1981, pp. 11–16.
42. The author has consulted the published catalogues of Khuda Bakhsh Library, Patna; Raza Library, Rampur; The Asiatic Society, Kolkata; Salarjung Mesuem, Hyderabad; India Office Library, London and various other libraries like National Libarary, Kolkata; Hazar Duary Library, Murshidabad; National Archives, New Delhi; Maulana Azad Library, Aligarh Muslim University, Aligarh; Central Library, Benares Hindu University, Varanasi; Central Library, Patna University, Patna and found that there are many manuscripts and published works in Arabic, Persian and Urdu on Unani medicine. The author was not able to consult some other libraries and museums including the Hamdard Library, New Delhi. Also may be consulted, Rahman A. et al., *Science and Technology in Medieval India: A Bibliography of Source Material in Sanskrit, Arabic and Persian*, New Delhi: Indian National Science Academy, 1982; Rezavi, op. cit.
43. Niccolio Manucci, 'Mogul India, or, Storia Do Mogor: 1653–1708', vol. III, ed. & tr. William Irvine, repr., Delhi, 2005, pp. 332–3.
44. Michael Pearson, 'The Thin End of the Wedge: Medical Relativities as a Paradigm of Early Modern Indian-European Relations', *Modern Asian Studies*, vol. XXIX, no. l, 1995, pp. 141–70; Michael Pearson, 'Early Modern Medical Regimes of Knowledge: Europe and India Compared', unpublished but available on Google search, accessed on 1 October 2013, pp. 1–30.
45. Dr John Fryer, *A New Account of East India and Persia*, 3 vols., no. I, ed. W. Crooke, London: Hakluyt Society, 1909–15, p. 286; John Ovington, *A Voyage to Surat, in the Year 1689*, ed. H.G. Rawlinson, London: Humphrey Milford, 1929, p. 205.
46. Michael Pearson, 'Early Modern Medical Regimes of Knowledge: Europe and India Compared', p. 21.
47. Ibid., p. 23.
48. Stefan Riedel, 'Edward Jenner and the History of Smallpox and Vaccination', *Proceedings*, vol. 18, no. 1, Dallas, Texas: Baylor University, Medical Center, January 2005, pp. 21–5.
49. Michael Adas, *Machines as the Measure of Men: Science, Technology, and Ideologies of Western Dominance*, New York: Cornell University Press, 1989, p. 385.
50. Bernier, op. cit., p. 339.
51. *Storia Do Mogor*, vol. II, p. 282.
52. Ishrat Alam, 'Smallpox and Its Treatment in Pre-Modern India', in *Disease and Medicine in India*, ed. Deepak Kumar, p. 91; Irfan Habib, 'Inside and Outside the Systems: Change and Innovation in Medical and Surgical Practice in Mughal India', Deepak Kumar, ed., *Disease and Medicine in India*, p. 75.
53. Michael Pearson, 'Early Modern Medical Regimes of Knowledge: Europe and India Compared', p. 6.

4

Medical System during the Time of Jahangir

A Study

DEBRAJ CHAKRABORTY

INDIA HAS A rich indigenous medical tradition from ancient period. This medical system is known as Ayurveda. The Ayurvedic medical therapies have modified in course of time and several new concepts and therapies have been incorporated within it. With the establishment and expansion of Turkish rule in India, a new stream of medical science came to the fore. This new medical tradition was Unani. Ayurveda and Unani continued to progress in two parallel lines but neither of them were contradictory to each other. Instead, they comprehended and complemented each other in the Indian eco-botanical climate. Unani rapidly grew in India by the thirteenth and fourteenth centuries. Under the Mughals, medical system appeared as an important branch of knowledge. Babur (r.1526–30), the founder ruler, had great zeal in medical science and even he took interest in India's conventional medical system. This tradition even continued during the time of Humayun (r.1530–40/1555–6) and Akbar (r.1556–1605). But considerable progress in this field could be seen during the reign of Jahangir (r.1605–27). He was not only interested in the development of medical science but he had his own observation regarding the causes of different diseases. His autobiography, known as *Jahangirnama*, gives an insight in this genre. This essay tries to examine the development in the field of medical science and growth in public health system at the time of Jahangir.

Pre-Mughal India can be best studied, to understand the measures which were taken by the Mughals particularly at the time of Jahangir, for the development in medical science and public health system. The Sultanate rulers of Delhi had extended support and patronage to the learned scholars and talented physicians. Introduction and growth of new medical tradition in India had a wide extent impact on society. A new professional class, called medical practitioners, gradually emerged and they were commonly known as hakims. At the early stage physicians got royal patronage and support and in most of the cases they were attached to the royal families.[1] However, in course of time it gradually became a popular medical system when rulers paid attention to the public health system. A good number of hospitals were established by the Sultanate rulers of Delhi and it was a noteworthy step to promote public health system in medieval India.[2] A hospital was usually called *Dar-ush shifa*, *Shifa-Khana*, *Sihat-Khana*, *Bimar-Khana* or *Bimaristan*. The dispensaries attached to the hospitals were known as *Dawa-Khana* or *Daru-Khana*. It is mentioned by Barani that there were at least 70 *Dar-ush shifa* or hospitals in Delhi where about 1,200 skilled physicians worked.[3] However, famous chronicler Muhammad Qasim Farishta has said that Firuz Shah established 115 hospitals.[4] This figure of hospitals given by Farishta appears to be a sheer exaggeration. Afif has enlightened us that these hospitals were open not only for the elites but also for the common and poor.[5] Both simple and compound types of medicine were kept in the hospital for the treatment. Not only medicines but sometimes foods too were provided to the poor and afflicted.[6]

Not only the central authorities, but also some provincial rulers took interests during that period for the development of medical science and public health system. Farishta has mentioned that the Bahmanid Sultan Alauddin II (r.1436–58) had established a hospital at Bidar. Both Hindu and Muslim physicians were appointed in this hospital to ensure medical facilities to his subjects. It is important to note that along with the medicines, food and drink were also provided to the patients free of cost. The famous *Dar-ush shifa* which is still running near Char Minar at Hyderabad was established in 1595 by Sultan Muhammad Quli Qutb Shah (r.1580–1611). It was not only a hospital but also a learning centre for medical science. It had the capacity of 400 patients and, medicines and diet were provided by the hospital. Experienced and skilled physicians were appointed in this hospital.[7]

During the Sultanate period, rulers have taken some zeal in medical science. Not only eminent physicians were invited from Central Asia but also in many cases rulers had taken interests in medical science. It was Sultan Firuz Shah who had great passion for medical science. *Sirat-i-Firuz Shahi* informs that he was an expert in joining fractured bones.[8] He not only had the knowledge of Unani but sometimes he examined patients also. This study shows that the Sultans of Delhi took serious measures for the development of medical science and public health system in pre-Mughal India.

II

Medical science and public health system got prime importance under the Mughals. Babur, the founder of the Mughal rule in India, was interested in medical science and he had a number of expert physicians in his court.[9] In his memoirs, Babur has recorded information about some medicinal herbs and fruits produced in India.[10] Some eminent physicians came to join the service of Babur from Central Asia and Persia. They were the best ones of the time and experts in different branches of Unani. The period of Humayun was equally important for the development of medical science. He took personal interests and effort for its development. During the regime of Akbar, the art of healing got royal support and patronage which paved the way for the development of different branches of medicine. Medical science and public health system received prime importance during the time of Jahangir. Among the Mughal rulers, Jahangir is known for his interests in nature and environment. Even he had great passion for medical science. He was the first ruler in Mughal line who attempted to make a connection between environment and health. He noticed that the environment of Agra was responsible for some diseases in the city. In his Memoirs, he wrote: 'The air of Agra is warm and dry; physicians say that it depresses the spirits and induces weakness. It is unsuitable to most temperaments, except to the phlegmatic and melancholy, which are safe from its bad effects.'[11] It is well known that the Emperor Jahangir was wine and opium addicted. A hakim advised him to disband these practices for the betterment of his health. So in 1617, Jahangir passed a royal order that 'no one should smoke because of harmful effects of tobacco'. It is interesting to note that the Persian ruler Shah Abbas had already issued orders against the use of tobacco in Persia.[12]

In 1609, Jahangir was in Gujarat where he had fever due to excessive heat, pollution, dust and stagnant water. He wrote in his Memoirs that as a result of the great heat (*Shiddat-i garma*) and the corruption of the air (*Ufunat-i hawa*), sickness had broken among the people of the city and even in the camp. They were attacked by inflammatory fever (*tap-i muharraq*) or sometimes they suffered from pains in the limbs (*dard-i a'aza*) and they became ill and sick for the next three-four days. The emperor was very disappointed with that type of environment as he addressed the city as *Bimaristan* and *Jahannumabad.*[13] He writes:

I have suffered from fever for a day and night only but have become so weak as if I have been bed-ridden for a long time. I have lost appetite completely and have no desire for food. I wonder what beauty and goodness did the founder of this city find that he built a city in this wretched place and after him others have passed their life in this dustbin. Its climate is poisoned (polluted); its land is sandy having little water and much dust and sand as described before; water is very bad and unpleasant; the river near the city is always dry except in rainy season; the water of its wells is mostly saltish and bitter; and the water of ponds of the city has become muddy due to the soap used by washer men. The rich people have built storage-tank in their houses, which are filled with rain-water and used for drinking until the next rainy season. The harmful effect of water, which has no access to air and no way for removal of vapours, is quite clear. There is a jungle of thorny bushes, instead of grass and flowers, outside the city and the bad effect of the air, which blows over the prickly bushes, is also evident. O thee! What name should I give you which is full of these qualities. I have called Ahmedabad before as *Gardabad* (place of dust), now I do not know whether to call it a place of poison or *Bimaristan* (place of patients) or field of prickly (thorny) bushes or *Jahannumabad* (hellish place), which possess all these qualities. Had rainy season not started, I would not have stayed in this place of hardships even for a day and would have hastened out the city on the carpet of air like Solomon.'[14]

Jahangir was perhaps aware of the theory of Baghdad's renowned physician, Zakariya Razi (d.926) who first wrote about the climatic effects on human body and health.

When a plague broke out in some parts of the country during his time the emperor questioned the learned physicians about the cause of this disease. He narrated:

> In this year, or rather in the 10th year after my accession, a great pestilence appeared in some places in Hindustan. The commencement of this calamity was in the parganahs of the Punjab, and by degrees the contagion spread to the city of Lahore. Many of the people, Musalmans and Hindus, died because of this. After this, it spread to Sirhind and the Duab, until it reached Delhi and the surrounding pargahanas and villages, and desolated them. At this day it had greatly diminished. It became known from men of great age and from old histories that this disease had never shown itself in this country. Physicians and learned men were questioned as to its cause. Some said that it came because there had been drought for two years in succession and little rain fell; others said it was on account of the corruption of the air which occurred through the drought and scarcity. Some attributed it to other causes.[15]

When the plague (*waba*) hit the city of Agra in his thirteenth regnal year (7 January 1619) and many people began to die, Jahangir noted, 'At this time, again, it appeared from the reports of the loyal that the disease of the plague was prevalent in Agra, so that daily about 100 people, more or less, were dying of it. Under the armpits, or in the groin, or below the throat, buboes formed, and they died.'[16]

III

Several skilled physicians were appointed at the royal service during the time of Jahangir. Among them Hakim Rukna Kashi, Hakim Sadr, Hakim Momena, Hakim Hamiduddin, Hakim Ruhullah, Abdus-sh Shakur, Muqarrab Khan and Hakim Amanullah Khan were leading Unani practitioners.

Hakim Rukna Kashi (d.1656) who came from Shiraz had earlier served as physician at the court of Shah Abbas of Persia. Later, he migrated to India and was appointed as the physician at the court of Akbar.[17] When Jahangir fell ill in Kashmir in 1623, Hakim Kashi was called for his treatment from Agra. He went to Kashmir and started treatment.[18] Unfortunately, Jahangir was not satisfied with the process of his treatment so he dismissed him from the post. But during the reign of Shahjahan, he again entered the royal service. Contemporary sources have mentioned that he was a skilled physician who had good knowledge of medical science as well as the art of healing. The *Amal-i Saleh* has described about his professional skills. It says that, 'He was perfect in the art of medicine especially in the treatment and had a cure for every difficult ailment. . . .'[19]

Maathir ul-Umra has referred to him as the most celebrated physician of the time.[20] The *Tabaqat-i Shahjahani* admired the knowledge and experience of this hakim in medical science.

Hakim Sadr was the son of Hakim Fakhruddin Shirazi.[21] He belonged to an affluent family popular in Central Asia for their excellent knowledge of medical science. He came to India in 1603. Here, he served under the famous Hakim, Ali Gilani. He joined as the Mughal court physician under Jahangir. Jahangir was satisfied with his skill and knowledge of medical science and gave him the title of *Masihu-z-Zaman* or 'Physician of his Age' and a *mansab* of 5,000 with 30 horses.[22] In his Memoirs he mentioned,

> It has been recorded with regard to the case of *Masihu-z-Zaman* that, notwithstanding what was due from him for his brining-up and my kindness to him, he had not the grace to attend upon me in such an illness; and more strange still is it that he suddenly threw off the veil of modesty and asked for leave to undertake a journey to the Hijiz. . . .

Jahangir still sanctioned Rs. 20,000 for his journey.[23] He continued to be a royal physician of Shahjahan (r.1627–58) also. When Jahanara, Shah Jahan's daughter, accidentally caught fire and was burnt badly, Hakim Sadr along with some other physicians was called for treatment. Hakim Sadr compiled two books, *Hidayat al-Hikmat* and *Hifz al-Sihhat*. The second work was dedicated to Prince Aurangzeb.[24]

Hakim Momin Shirazi was a famous physician of the time of Jahangir, Shah Jahan and Aurangzeb (r.1658–1707).[25] He enjoyed royal prestige and honour for his contribution in medical science. He had been credited for the treatment of Aurangzeb when he was ill in the last days of his life.[26] When Jahangir suffered from the retention of urine which was distressing, Hakim Momena tried his best to cure the sick emperor and some relief was noticed after his treatment but some other problems soon appeared.[27]*Amal-i Saleh* has mentioned him as a good and experienced physician. Hakim Hamiduddin and Hakim Ruhullah were prominent Unani practitioners of Gujarat. Both were inducted into the royal service by Jahangir. The former was granted a village for his maintenance. In his Memoirs Jahangir said, 'I gave him and his sons 1,000 rupees and some shawls, and set aside a whole village for his maintenance. . . .'[28] Hakim Ruhullah was very respected and renowned physician of his time. He treated Empress Nurjahan when she fell sick.

Hakim Abdus-sh Shakur was a skilful physician and had commendable knowledge of medical science. He was one of the trustworthy physicians of Jahangir. He cured the emperor when he was seriously ill and got weakness.[29] Sheikh Hasan was a very personal physician of Jahangir who conferred upon him the title of Muqarrab Khan. He was very efficient surgeon and Jahangir was satisfied with his skill and methods of treatment.[30] Muqarrab Khan was appointed to different responsible administrative posts and always remained close to the imperial power. Jahangir has acknowledged him as one of the top surgeons during his time. In 1612, when Muqarrab Khan was posted in

Delhi, he treated the emperor who was suffering from *khun-para* or congestion of blood. On his suggestion, Jahangir was bled and about a *ser* of blood was taken out from his left arm. The operation was successfully carried out by Muqurrab Khan.[31] Muqarrab Khan wrote a book entitled *Anis al-Kahhal* on eye diseases. He was also in contact with the European physicians who visited India and learnt many things from them.

Hakim Amanullah Khan was a famous physician and a great scholar. His work *Ganj-i Badaward* included a large list of different types of drugs as well an exhaustive bibliography on medical works he had consulted. He went through approximately 105 Arabic and Persian texts and some Sanskrit works as well. The manuscript is preserved in Aligarh Muslim University Library. Hakim Amanullah translated *Madan Vinod*, a Sanskrit book, into Persian named it *Dastur al-Hunud* wherein he discussed the principles and theories of Ayurveda and explained the Ayurvedic terms. *Umm al-Ilaj* was his another contribution in which different aspects linked to the medical treatment like age of the patients, dose of medicine, nature of disease and most importantly seasonal effects on human life have been discussed in detail.[32]

IV

Public health system was of prime concern for the Mughal rulers. Evidences are available in the contemporary documents relating to the establishment of charitable hospitals for the people who were unable to bear the cost of the treatment. As a result of which Akbar built public hospitals at different places. A hospital was built in his capital—*Akbarabad* in Agra, which was known as *Shifa Khana-i Akbarabad*.[33] Two other hospitals, one at Agra and the other at Fatehpur Sikri were built. Medicine and food were given free of cost to the patients in both the hospitals.[34] Akbar had built a big hospital in Ahmedabad also.[35] This tradition received new force when at the early age of his accession Jahangir issued his famous twelve ordinance, one of which clearly mentions 'Hospitals were to be built in large cities and physicians were to be appointed to attend the sick. The expenses were to be paid from the royal treasury.'[36] In these hospitals, a number of skilled physicians and surgeons were recruited by the state and usually they were under the charge of a chief physician, called *darogha-i dar-ush shifa* or the superintendent of the hospital. A number of *mutasaddis* or clerks and other staffs were appointed in these hospitals to assist the superintendent.[37] Physicians along with the other staffs of these hospitals were paid from the treasury on daily basis. The physicians serving the government hospital had to submit an attendance certificate before their salary was released. Some nobles and provincial governors took personal interests in establishing charitable hospitals.

Noticeable changes took place in the field of Unani medical tradition and one could mark that Unani, during the Mughal period particularly, shifted from the domain of aristocracy to the sphere of the common man. An interesting miniature painting displays that physicians used to sit on roadside also providing medical facility to the common people. In one such painting of Abul Hasan during the time of Jahangir, a physician surrounded by some bottles, jars, cups, bags and some other medicinal substances like *sufuf* (powder), *sharbat* (syrup) and *arq* (liquid medicine) is found sitting near a house on a roadside platform under a *shamiana* or canopy and advising an old patient. There are two books on his right side and perhaps these are medical books or some notebook for the physician to make notes regarding his personal experience when he examined a patient. There is a small mortar and pestle to mix the medicine (arrow marked). It is also interesting to note that every bag and bottle is labelled. Behind the physician there is a boy who probably is his assistant or disciple (Fig. 4.1).[38] This miniature provides some information about the bazaar medical tradition of the Mughal India and also highlights medical facility for the commoners.

The public health system in pre-colonial India is a debatable issue. A group of European scholars think that in Britain the concept of public health developed in an organized way by the mid-seventeenth century. They found that the scenario was different in India. The concept of public health system did not develop in India during that period. However, public health has received prime importance in India from ancient period. During the time of Jahangir, building and maintenance of charitable hospitals was the concern of the state. Being a vast country, India has maintained a very huge population. Provision of medical facility in such a vast nation in pre-modern period was indeed a difficult task. Despite all limitations at the time of Jahangir, public health has incorporated with the state policies. Not only government supported hospitals but some charitable hospitals were also constructed by the nobles and aristocrats of the society. It is also evident that physicians were developed as a professional group in entire Mughal India. The extent of the physicians was not only limited to the court or royal houses but another group of physician was developed

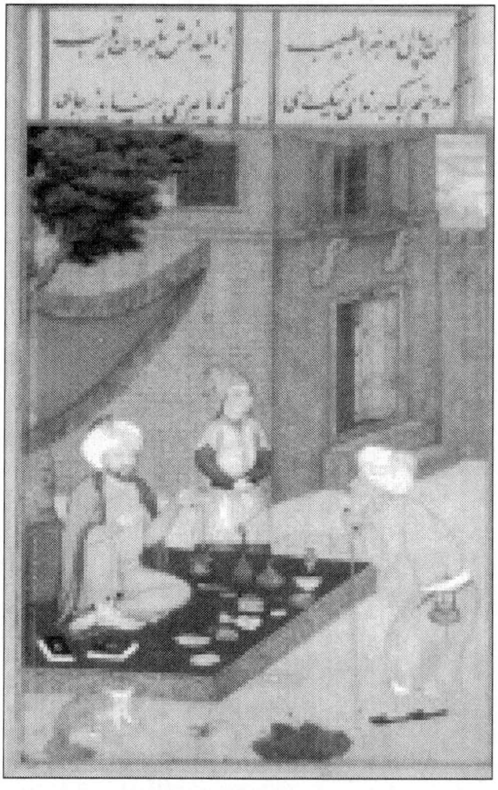

Fig. 4.1: Medical facility for the commoners
Courtesy: Aboulala Soudavar Collection, New York

for the purpose of treatment of common man and they were called bazaar physicians. Therefore, two things clearly emerge that under Jahangir a sophisticated and improved medical system was introduced and that he himself took interest for its development and that public health system has been projected as a part of welfare state policy.

Notes

1. A. Rahman et al., *Science and Technology in Medieval India—A Bibliography of Source Materials in Sanskrit, Arabic and Persian*, New Delhi, 1982; Iqtidar Alam Khan, 'The Middle Class in the Mughal Empire', *Social Scientist*, vol. 5, no. 1, August 1976, pp. 28–49; S. Ali Nadeem Rezavi, 'Physicians as Professionals in Medieval India', in *Disease and Medicine in India: A Historical Overview*, ed. Deepak Kumar, New Delhi, 2001, pp. 40–65.
2. S.H. Askari, 'Medicines and Hospitals in Muslim India', *Journal of Bihar Research Society*, vol. XLIII, nos. 1–2, 1957, pp. 7–21.
3. Ziya Uddin Barani, *Tarikh-i Firuz Shahi*, ed. Sir Syed Ahmad, Calcutta: B.I. Series, 1862, pp. 352–66.
4. Farishta, *Tarikh-i Farishta*, vol. I, Lucknow, 1864, p. 151; A.A. Azmi, *History of Unani Medicine in India*, New Delhi, 2004, p. 13.
5. Shams Siraj Afif, *Tarikh-i Firuz Shahi*, ed. Wilayat Hussain, Calcutta: B.I. Series, 1891, pp. 359–60.
6. *Sirat-i Firuz Shahi* (Persian MS. 547), Khuda Bakhsh Oriental Public Library, Patna, ff. 161–70; Azmi, op. cit., p. 14.
7. H.K. Sherwani, *History of Qutb Shahi Dynasty*, New Delhi, 1974, p. 314.
8. *Sirat-i Firuz Shahi*, Chapter IV, f. 165a; S.H. Askari, 'Medicines and Hospitals in Muslim India', p. 12; R.L. Verma, 'The Growth of Greco-Arabian Medicine in Medieval India', *Journal of History of Science*, vol. 5, no. 2, p. 350.
9. Zahiruddin Muhammad Babur, *Babur-Nama or Memoirs of Babur*, ed. and tr. into English by A.S. Beveridge, repr., Delhi, 2006, pp. 169–70.
10. Ibid., p. 82 (medicinal qualities of the plum of Bukhra), 246, 399, 511, 607–8, 660.
11. Jahangir, *Tuzuk-i Jahangiri* (Memoirs of Jahangir), vol. I, ed. H. Beveridge, tr. A. Rogers, repr., Delhi, 1999, p. 4.
12. S.P. Sangar, 'Intoxication in Mughal India', *Indian Journal of History of Science*, vol. 16, no. 2, November 1981, p. 210.
13. Jahangir, *Tuzuk-i Jahangiri*, ed. Sir Syed Ahmad, Aligarh, 1864, pp. 229–31.
14. Ibid., p. 231.
15. Jahangir, *Tuzuk-i Jahangiri*, vol. I, p. 330.
16. Ibid., vol. II, pp. 6, 65.
17. Nawab Samsuddaula Shahnawaz Khan, *Maathir ul Umara*, vol. II, ed. and tr. H. Beveridge and Baini Prasad, repr., Calcutta: B.I. Series, 1952, p. 283; Abdul Hamid Lahori, *Padshshanama*, 2 vols., Calcutta: B.I. Series, 1866–72, vol. I is divided into two parts (i) and (ii), vol. 2, 1867, p. 349.
18. Jahangir, *Tuzuk-i Jahangiri*, vol. II, p. 211.
19. Muhammad Saleh Kunbuh, *Amal-i Saleh*, vol. III, Calcutta, 1812, p. 387; Azmi, op. cit., p. 152.
20. Shahnawaz Khan, op. cit., p. 283.
21. Khafi Kahn, *Muntakhab-ul lubab*, vol. I, ed. and tr. Kabiruddin Ahmad and W. Haig, Calcutta: B.I. Series, 1865–73, p. 508.
22. Jahangir, *Tuzuk-i Jahangiri*, vol. I, pp. 154–5.

23. Ibid., vol. II, p. 217.
24. C.A. Storey, *Persian Literature: A Bio-Bibliographical Survey*, vol. II, London, 1971, p. 267.
25. Azmi, op. cit., p. 158.
26. Munshi Muhammad Kazim, *Alamgir Nama*, Calcutta, 1868, p. 926, cited in Azmi, op. cit., p. 159.
27. Jahangir, *Tuzuk-i Jahangiri*, Ghazipur edn., p. 380; Azmi, ibid., p. 159.
28. Jahangir, *Tuzuk-i Jahangiri*, vol. I, p. 189.
29. Ibid., p. 267.
30. Ibid., pp. 27–8.
31. Ibid., p. 226; Syed Ali Nadeem Rezavi, 'An Aristocratic Surgeon of Mughal India: Muqarrab Khan', in *Medieval India: Researches in the History of India 1200–1750*, ed. Irfan Habib, repr., New Delhi, 2000, pp. 154–65.
32. *Ummu'l-i-Ilaz* (Persian MS no. 1554), Kolkata: The Asiatic Society, f. 3v; William Ivanow (Compiled), *Concise Descriptive Catalogue of the Persian Manuscripts in the collection of the Asiatic Society of Bengal*, repr., Calcutta: B.I. Series, 1984, pp. 724–5; Azmi, op. cit., pp. 167–79.
33. Ibid., p. 62.
34. Ibid.
35. Ibid.
36. Jahangir, *Tuzuk-i Jahangiri*, vol. I, p. 4; Verma, op. cit., p. 357; Rezavi, op. cit., p. 47.
37. Reference relating to mutasuddis and kotwal in government hospitals is available in Gopal Rai Surdaj, *Dur-rul Ulum*, MS. Bodleian Library, oxford, f. 45b cited in Rezavi, op. cit., n. 59.
38. 'An Old Man Consults a Doctor', *Bustan-i Sa'adi*, Aboulala Soudavar Collection, New York, f.176r; S.C. Welch and Annemarir Schimmel, *The Emperor's Album: Images of Mughal India*, New York, 1987, fig. 25; Rezavi, op. cit., Plate 2, fn. 95. Syed Ali Nadeem Rezavi, 'Representation of the Middle Class Professionals in Mughal Visual Art', in *The Varied Facets of History: Essays in Honour of Aniruddha Ray*, ed. Ishrat Alam and Syed Ejaz Hussain, Delhi: Primus Books, 2011, pp. 159–94, see p. 188, plate VII.

5

Situating Traditional Medicine in Modern Times

Ayurveda in Colonial Bengal

Achintya Kumar Dutta

Indian traditional medicine does not mean any single system of cure. It consists of different types of cure—Ayurveda, Unani, Siddha, Yoga, folk medicine, etc. This essay is a modest attempt to focus on the efficacy or inefficacy of Ayurveda in modern times, specially in the nineteenth and twentieth centuries, and how reputed Ayurvedic physicians did see through the nature of Ayurveda during the colonial period, when medical encounter took place between the East and the West. It is often argued that Ayurveda could tackle successfully only some elemental diseases like amoebiasis, rheumatism, etc., and was unable to cope with epidemics and unknown diseases caused by protozoa and bacteria, and the Ayurvedic physicians could not save the epidemic victims. Thus, the efficacy of Ayurveda in tackling the fatal diseases has repeatedly been questioned in official and non-official publications. The decay of Ayurveda has been reflected in the medical literature in the nineteenth and twentieth centuries. The situation does raise certain questions as to why did it decay? Who was responsible for it? Was Ayurveda an archaic or unscientific irrational system that caused its decline? These are some of the questions that have been addressed in this essay.

Ayurvedic medicine was taught and practised in the traditional way in Bengal at the beginning of the nineteenth century. The physician was called a kaviraj, prince of verse, referring to his mastery of Sanskrit texts. In Ayurveda, disease was conceptualized as the result of a derangement or imbalance among the three humours (*tridosha*)—wind, bile and phlegm, which jointly governed the physiological processes of the body. In a healthy individual, all three humours existed in harmony; sickness arose from an excess or disorder of one humour.

Ayurveda in general provided a broad cultural framework of healthy living and treatment for curing chronic and elemental diseases including remittent and intermittent fever, leprosy, epilepsy and even insanity. Inoculation and hydropathy were applied in various forms. The Ayurvedic physicians also used their traditional drugs for the treatment of cholera, malaria, smallpox, kala-azar, and beriberi. Kabiranjan Satyacharan Sengupta, a well-known vaidya in twentieth century in Ranaghat, acknowledged that though the name malaria seemed to be new, it could be brought within the domain of a disease named *bisamjwara* in Ayurveda. Ayurvedic physicians could completely cure it and used *nata* and *harital* for such cases.[1] A gentleman named Satischandra Bandopadhyay, who himself was cured of influenza by Ayurvedic drugs, has also asserted the efficacy of Ayurveda in curing influenza. Drugs like *visweshwar rasa* was used in cases of influenza.[2] It has been mentioned in a medical journal, *Ayurvijnan*, that during the influenza epidemic of 1918–19, about 95 per cent patients received this treatment and were cured of this ailment.[3] Kaviraj Satya Charan Sengupta reported in Ayurveda, a journal in 1916 that Ayurveda could successfully treat cholera cases by drugs like *chitrakadiguri* and *bajrakshara*, though most of the people believed in allopathy and homoeopathy for its treatment and hardly relied on Ayurveda.[4] During the early cholera epidemics, vaidyas and hakims supplied those who sought their assistance with treatment and medicines in accordance with their humoural pathologies.[5] The physicians administered purgatives, like calomel, to rid the body of its poison, followed by cooling drinks of rosewater and lime juice, or advised embrocations of turpentine and other fluids to relieve the cramps. The vaidyas prescribed medicines composed of black pepper, bora, asafetida, aniseed, ginger and cloves; some incorporated opium or Indian hemp to dull the pain and relax the body. Even the Bengal Medical Board informed its practitioners during the epidemic in the early nineteenth century that, where Western drugs were not available or seemed inappropriate, local ones could be used. The Board sometimes even chose indigenous physicians in Calcutta to administer their medicines for cholera.[6] Even the British doctors, despite their cultural reservations, borrowed from the vaidyas and hakims and employed almost identical drugs and treatments. [7]

Like other diseases in the Ayurvedic corpus, smallpox or pastule (*masurika*) was understood in terms of a humoural construction of the body. The experienced vaidya after identifying the specific form of the disease, principally through the character of the pastules, could administer purgatives to flush the body of its poisons, and prohibit foods likely to produce or prolong the derangement of the humours. But the general impression in the nineteenth century was that the disease was considered, even by the physicians themselves, to be beyond their powers to prevent or to relieve.[8] The only appropriate course was to seek the mercy of Goddess Sitala, a deity who had crept into Ayurvedic texts later. Interestingly, when the nature of the disease was known, kaviraj retired and *malakar* (attendant of Sitala) was summoned and the smallpox patient was thus left at the mercy of the Goddess. However, one way of protecting the people from its ravages was through inoculation or tika. This was among the commonest and most effective forms of indigenous medical practice in India until it was displaced by Jennerian vaccine in the second half of the nineteenth century, though the indigenous method of variolation is seen, in many contemporary accounts, as a religious ceremony and a ritual invocation of Sitala than as a medical procedure as such.[9] In 1923, a contemporary Kaviraj Sachindranath Vidyabhusan claimed that Ayurveda could also cure kala-azar which was included within the category of *bisamjwara*, which was claimed to be curable by Ayurveda. During this time, Kaviraj Surendranath Dasgupta Kavyatirtha treated many kala-azar cases successfully at some places in Calcutta where allopathic doctors were giving antimony injection to the kala-azar patients.[10] Ayurvedic physicians also claimed that they could cure disease like beriberi and provided its remedy at a time when modern doctors failed to tackle it. They used *pipulchurna*, *makaradhwaja*, *arjuna*, etc., for its treatment and advised to take specific foods full of protein and vitamins, such as *dhenki*-husked rice, masur dal, lemon, sugar, etc., for quick recovery from this disease.[11] They also used *chalmugra* for the treatment of leprosy cases.

It is, thus, evident that Ayurveda was not only concerned with elemental diseases but could also treat fatal diseases like cholera, smallpox, kala-azar, beriberi, etc. It travelled far and wide, providing prescription for maintaining good health to curing severe diseases. However, it failed to demonstrate its efficacy when epidemics broke out during the colonial rule. Western medicine in India in the seventeenth and eighteenth centuries was rudimentary and Ayurvedic physicians were respected for their knowledge. Many of them also received the patronage of local rulers, but they kept losing ground steadily in the nineteenth century when allopathy (mainly) and homoeopathy, the two alien medical systems, penetrated the Indian soil. Finding it badly mauled and let down, the Ayurveda system went into a sulky withdrawal, instead of confronting the new challenge. That the vaidyas were losing their influence is evident from the fact that more and more patients were flocking to the government hospitals and dispensaries. The people were attracted to a newer mode of treatment because of its superior methodology in curing a disease in a novel manner.[12] The vaidyas and kavirajs held the British rule responsible for the decline of Ayurveda. However, their weaknesses cannot be ignored.

Ayurveda had a popular strength in rural Bengal. It was cheaper than allopathy and also easily available. Very few people, hardly 10 per cent could receive allopathic treatment in Bengal. Most of the villagers did not have the capacity to receive it, as it was too costly. The government did not have adequate infrastructure to bring all the villagers within the purview of modern health care service. The number of doctors was very small and majority of the people hardly received any medical care from them. The village people usually thought that the government doctors were avaricious, and that the people in charge at primary health centres were neglectful, dishonest, and insulting. Even though government workers might occasionally treat them with respect and provide inexpensive care, villagers often considered them to be a last resort.[13] Consequently, the rural people had to depend on Ayurvedic physicians. The common religious background brought the kaviraj close to the patient. The kavirajs were orthodox Hindus whose way of life followed strict religious rules. Thus, orthodox patients preferred a kaviraj to an allopathic doctor, and devout Brahmins and widows could not accept allopathic medicines.[14] But compared to efficacy and methodology of treatment, Ayurveda was less systematic, methodical, pervasive and penetrative than the colonial medicine. Consequently, it gradually appeared to be an ineffective system of medicine and people also lost faith in it.

G.C. Roy, in his report on Burdwan fever, pointed out that the kavirajs used *atees* and *neem* for such fever, but their effect was too slow and uncertain. Arsenic was in vogue amongst the kavirajs in acute as well as chronic fevers. But its action was slow; several days' administration was necessary to produce a perceptible effect.[15] It was contraindicated in remittent congestive cases or those in which the liver and spleen or any other internal organs are congested. Neither the zamindar nor the common people relied on the kavirajs, because they could not prepare proper drugs for fever or cholera. Acharya Jogesh Chandra Roy Vidyanidhi in his autobiography, *Atmacharita*, has described the horrible effects of Burdwan fever in Bankura and asserted that *dasmul pachan* and *bhaskar laban* of the village vaidyas could not control the fever.[16]

Ayurveda was, thus, gradually losing its hold over the rural society. In fact, it had certain inherent defects which had reduced its efficacy and caused its decline. It remained crude and unimprovised. The Materia Medica was not standardized. Each individual was considered unique and the treatment was person specific. Ayurveda was unable to cope with epidemics and combat unknown diseases. It had no answer to the newly discovered parasites, new diagnostics and novel vaccines. The kaviraj or vaidya could not transcend the traditional way of practice. Patients consulted them at home, and they took personal interest in the patients. They observed the outward appearance and behaviour of patients and then after clinical examination diagnosed. They prepared their own medicine, considering it the secret of their material success and thus exploiting its commercial value.[17] Instead of confronting the new challenge, they had accepted their system's backwardness and stagnation in the sphere of medical research. There was no professional scientific knowledge through research. Ayurveda practitioners were physicians and their science emerged out of their medical practice. There was lack of spirit of enquiry among them. They stuck to their defence of *nidana* (treatment), putting emphasis on the power of resistance of human body.

The kavirajs made no attempt to change their traditional mode of medical education throughout the nineteenth century. Conventional Ayurvedic education continued in the private homes of the kavirajs. The tol system was used to educate physicians.[18] However, even the modest tols could not be compared to the splendid, well-equipped college that offered many training possibilities. Naturally, young boys who wanted to become physicians did not want to enter the tols, but were attracted to allopathic medicine.[19] British policy encouraged this trend by granting scholarships and by distributing free medical books, charts and models. Moreover, the students who studied allopathy had much better chances of achieving a good position in life than those trained in the old tols. The only medical topic taught in the traditional tols was internal medicine (*Kayacikitsa*), not the *astanga ayurveda* or eight branches of knowledge. The seven other branches were: *Shalya tantra* (surgery), *Shalakya tantra* (opthalmology, ear, nose, dentistry, etc.), *Agada tantra* (toxology or poison related therapy), *Bhoota vidya* (psychiatry), *Kumarbhritya tantra* (paediatrics and midwifery), *Rasa tantra* or *Rasāyana* (pharmacology and alchemy), *Bajikarana tantra* (science of aphrodisiac or reproduction).[20] Their lack of enthusiasm for the institutional promotion of their knowledge appears more glaring when homeopathy, despite numerous constraints and allopathic rivalries, could boast of a handful of medical schools and colleges by the 1880s.[21]

Interestingly, some of the well-known kavirajs of Bengal held the vaidyas or kavirajs responsible for the decline and the degenerated state of Ayurveda and that view has been reflected in a number of medical journals, such as *Ayurveda, Ayurvijnan, Ayurvijnan Sammilani* and so on. They have pointed out that kavirajs gradually lost their expertise and consequently efficacy of their treatment got reduced. Kaviraj Shakticharan Visharad had attributed the failure of Ayurveda to the wrong treatment of most of the cases by kavirajs.[22] Ayurvedic physicians did not learn anatomy and surgery; good students did not get themselves inclined to study it; and they were rather in search of government jobs.[23]

To the reputed Ayurvedic physicians, Ayurveda meant astanga Ayurveda which includes anatomy, physiology and surgery. In other words, it consists of theoretical as well as practical knowledge of human body. But most of the vaidyas or kavirajs practised Ayurveda only on the basis of their traditional theoretical knowledge, which was also not very sound. They did not learn Ayurveda in the way Gangadhar Ray and other celebrated kavirajs did. Ancient practice of dissection or anatomy and surgery had been abandoned and forgotten by most of them. Consequently, vaidyas remained profoundly ignorant of human anatomy and body's internal functions and disorders. They felt pride of their incomplete inherited knowledge, disregarding its further advancement by research and experiments.[24] They were not the vaidyas in the real sense of the term. Most of the vaidyas treated the patient symptomatically on the basis of their knowledge of internal medicine (*Kayacikitsa*). In the nineteenth century, Revd Lal Behari Day wrote:

> For modern medicine, he (the village kaviraj) had a perfect contempt and it was one of his constant sayings that European doctors did not at all understand the treatment of Indian fever. He admitted the superiority of English to native doctors in surgery, but then it was his opinion that surgery formed no part of the functions of a medical man, as surgical operations belonged, properly speaking, to the province of the barber.[25]

Surprisingly, they disdained allopathic doctors as dead-body dissecting doctors.[26] Thus, they virtually turned to be quacks in rural Bengal and professed Ayurveda just as a means of livelihood only, not guided by any idea of social service. Satish Chandra Bandopadhyay, who himself was attacked by influenza during the epidemic phase between 1917 and 1918 and was cured by a qualified Ayurvedic physician of a town, Barishal, lamented that there were a number of quack vaidyas in his village, but not a single good and qualified physician.[27] In fact, the efficient and well trained vaidyas were few in number and they usually lived in the towns or metropolis of Calcutta, where they could easily make their fortune and live comfortably. Consequently, the vaidyas could hardly come to the aid of epidemic victims in rural Bengal.

In 1918, the Ayurveda Sahba observed that when malaria broke out in severe epidemic form, taking a heavy toll of human lives, the kavirajs remained as passive onlookers and demonstrated their inability to tackle this disease.[28] At this juncture, the allopathic doctors came forward with quinine to provide relief to the sufferers. More importantly, the vaidyas and kavirajs became sceptic of the use of quinine by the doctors, and started selling quinine under a new label for earning money. Thus, the so-called ignorant and selfish kavirajs had actually caused the decline of status of Ayurveda in Bengal.

Ayurveda practice became the monopoly of the Baidya caste, the physician caste of Bengal. There were several families of this caste in rural Bengal and mostly the male members of the caste had in succession been practicing Ayurvedic medicine, as if it was their hereditary right. Very few people from other castes would come to study Ayurveda. But like the people of other Bengali castes, many of the vaidyas gradually switched over to other respectable professions in the colonial milieu, leaving their traditional ancestral occupation of Ayurveda practising. During 1933–4, when Tara Krishna Basu first revisited Kanchanpur (the village of Revd Lal Behari Day), he noted that 'the kavirajs of the village have fallen on evil days. One part of the village is known as kaviraj para, or the ward of the kaviraj. But most of the families have now (1950s) given up their hereditary occupations. . . .'[29] By the 1950s, the descendants of the kavirajs had taken to other occupations and there was none in the village to practise Ayurveda. More importantly, many of the vaidyas looked forward to becoming modern doctors and therefore studied allopathy, since as allopath doctors they could easily make their fortune and earned prestige. Surprisingly, only the dull, unintelligent and less equipped male members from Baidya family pursued Ayurveda.[30] This undoubtedly reduced the status of Ayurveda.

The value of Ayurveda system was reiterated not only by the vaidyas and kavirajs, but also by the Western medical practitioners. While teaching physiology in Calcutta Medical College, Sir Charles Havelock mentioned that what he taught was completely imbibed and described by the ancient Hindu sages.[31] Sir Pardy Lukis, Director General of the IMS (1910–17) echoed almost the same voice, acknowledging the contribution of the ancient saints to Ayurveda. He also remarked that 'if I were ill . . . I would prefer to be treated by a good *vaid* or *hakim* than a bad doctor'.[32] That Ayurveda was a system of medicine with great potentialities can hardly be denied. On many occasions in rural Bengal, it was found to be successful in curing a number of chronic diseases of the people who were disgusted with allopathic treatment. But it remained undeveloped and turned to be backward and crude in the hands of the quack-vaidyas in nineteenth-century Bengal.

However, it would be unhistorical to deny that the process of decline of Ayurveda started long before the nineteenth century. It is argued that Ayurveda was neglected, if not ignored, to a great extent during the pre-colonial times, when Unani received more support of the state, and the process of decline started thereafter. During the period of Delhi Sultanate, the Unani system of medicine was patronized by a number of rulers—Md. Bin Tughluq and Firoz Shah. The period also witnessed the composition of Unani medical treatise like the *Rahat-al-insan* and *Shifa al-Khani*.[33] Though the Mughal rulers were not inimical to Ayurveda, the state did not sponsor its promotion. The people belonging to Baidya caste might have apprehended the loss of popularity of Ayurveda and contemplated to switch over to other lucrative professions. This process gathered momentum during the East India Company's rule when some new job opportunities were created in Bengal. Under the circumstances, these new jobs were found to be more attractive than the profession of a vaidya. Consequently, the Baidya caste students with higher calibre were inclined to the newly created jobs.

It is also revealed by scholars that compared to European medical science, medical science in India did not advance much during the middle ages, particularly in the seventeenth and eighteenth centuries. Rather, some of the delicate skills—surgical operations, for instance, the old expertise degenerated mainly because there were no proper provision for medical education.[34] Anatomy had also gradually degenerated during medieval times. No new works were being produced and even the old copies of medical treatises were becoming somewhat scarce. Ayurveda was almost getting lost in the eighteenth century, as William Jones regretted, who, despite his best effort, had hardly found a single original treatise in medicine.[35] This noble profession gradually passed from erudite practitioners and scientists into the hands of semi-ignorant people depending only on heresy knowledge or knowledge gathered from an imperfect comprehension of incomplete or incorrect texts. Indian medical men remained unconcerned about the scientific method of experiment and observation which became the basis of modern medical science. Actually science including medicine was more individualistic than institutionalized.[36] The only impulse required for its progress was demand and encouragement. But the pre-colonial socio-economic structure and intellectual atmosphere failed to supply it.

However, this does not imply that Ayurveda was an unscientific and ineffective system of medicine. One cannot blame the efficacy of Ayurveda for the deficiency of the kavirajs. Actually Ayurveda had required further development, but the vaidyas and kavirajs were satisfied with knowledge acquired at a very early period. With Ayurveda in decline, the people fell back on superstition and quackery. It is because of the mishandling of the cases by the village quacks (kavirajs) that there was no effective treatment and consequently people lost faith in this system.[37] It is known from an account of a High Court judge, Sir John Woodroff that one of his servants asked for allopathic medicine instead of ayurvedic when he fell ill.[38] In fact, lack of this confidence in Ayurveda affected this system of medicine to a large extent. The quack kavirajs and the ignorant vaidyas even lacked proper knowledge of herbal medicines and method of treatment. Most of the traditional vaidyas and kavirajs avoided practical training and surgery. This was the root cause of its decline. The absence of anatomy, physiology and surgery in Ayurveda had lowered its prestige and it appeared to be inferior to the Western medicine.[39] There was, in fact, no development of knowledge in Ayurveda which was rather found to be inert and tradition-bound. Though about 50,000 kavirajs were practicing in Bengal in the early twentieth century, they did have a few organization or journal to discuss or publish important issues on public health.[40] For centuries, the Portuguese, the Dutch and other Europeans had noted the value of certain drugs employed in India but unfamiliar to Europe. They collected knowledge from Indian system of medicine and utilized it for the advancement of their own systems. But there was no quest for modern medical knowledge amongst the vaidya*s*, no spirit of enquiry to explore the unknown.

At the same time, the British were unfair in rejecting Ayurveda as a viable alternative to Western medicine. They never considered it to be a part of scientific discipline. Claims of its therapeutic efficacy and contribution to modern medicine were always scoffed at.[41] Though the British-India government employed indigenous medical practitioners in the health service particularly during the situations of distress created by frequent outbreak of epidemics, it was unwilling to sponsor and promote traditional medicine through institutionalization. Nor did the government take any effective step for producing the number of qualified Ayurvedic physicians in the country who could have served the people during the inroads of severe diseases either in epidemic or endemic forms. When Kaviraj Raj Mohan Ray addressed a note to Sir Charles Elliot, Lt Governor of Bengal, urging the claims of Ayurveda to official encouragement and support and for founding a college for teaching Ayurveda with a hospital attached to it, the request was not complied with.[42] In fact, Indian medical traditions were completely ignored and the study of indigenous drugs found no place in medical curriculum of Indian universities.[43] W.B. O'Shaughnessy had drawn the government's attention to this neglect, but in vain. In 1894, while presiding over the section of Pharmacology at the first Indian Medical Congress, Kannai Lal Dey, a professor of chemistry at Calcutta Medical College, emphasized the study of indigenous drugs, their systematic cultivation and their increased use in medical depots.[44] However, the government did not pay any heed to it. In a medical conference in 1917, Dr Nilratan Sircar also advocated further investigation into Ayurvedic system, but was of no use. In 1917, Annie Beasant at the Calcutta session of the Indian National Congress advocated for the spread of Ayurveda, focusing on its intrinsic qualities and approaching the government for financial assistance for its rejuvenation.[45] However, even this invention was in vain.

Ayurveda had the intrinsic qualities as an alternative system of medicine, but it was suppressed by the politico-medical hegemonism of the West. The peaceful coexistence of Ayurveda and Western medicine ended from 1835. It has been observed by many scholars that before 1835, the British rulers did not interfere with the indigenous medical system. Western doctors learnt from Indian physicians and supported their modes of diagnosis and treatment; parallel instruction in Ayurveda and Unani medicine was started in Sanskrit College and Calcutta Madrasa along with the teaching of allopathy through translated Western texts; and more teachers were appointed to teach Ayurveda in these institutions. However, this policy of accommodation was given up in 1835, after the consolidation of British rule in Bengal which had given the British authorities the confidence to override the indigenous system and introduce allopathy firmly through the establishment of Calcutta Medical College (1835). Thus, a tendency to dismiss indigenous medicine grew. The introduction of Western education, particularly English education had further encouraged the authorities to stop teaching indigenous medicine in vernacular. The departments of indigenous medicine of Sanskrit College and Madrasa were abolished by the government order in 1835.[46]

Actually the official attitude was never enthusiastic. The official policy seems all along to have been directed towards the ultimate domination of Western medicine. The intention was not to promote indigenous medicine as an alternative to Western medicine, but to draw upon what was useful from indigenous therapeutics. The intention was to prove superiority of Western medicine and thereby its domination. There was an attempt of appropriation of indigenous medicine in British pharmacopoeia for the sake of medical superiority and that is why indigenous Materia Medica was tapped.[47] There was a process of subordination and marginalization by which Western medicine marked its conquest over indigenous systems of medicine. Western medicine assumed a position of clear authority over Indian medicine. Its attitude was monopolistic and not pluralistic.

Ayurveda faced a severe crisis when it was officially marginalized from 1835. However, attempts were made by a group of intelligentsia for the revival of Ayurveda from the late nineteenth century. Two very popular vaidya*s* of Calcutta, Gangaprasad Sen and Neelamber Sen started the process of Ayurvedic rejuvenation by publishing the sacred texts in Bengali. Later Gangaprasad Sen started the first Ayurvedic journal in Bengali called *Ayurvedic Sanjivani* with the purpose of upholding the prestige of the Indian system.[48] He also started manufacturing commercialized Ayurvedic medicines. Chandrakishore Sen published inexpensive books to propagate the scientific essentials of

Ayurveda. Manufacturing units of Ayurvedic medicines like N.N. Sen & Co. Private Limited, Calcutta; Sakti Ausadhalaya of Dacca; Sadhana Ausadhalaya and Kalpataru Ayurvedic Works flourished in Bengal by the first decade of the twentieth century. Attempts were also made to organize the kavirajs of Calcutta by setting up associations like Ayurvedic Sabha (1901) and to popularize Ayurveda with the establishment of institutions like Astanga Ayurvedic School, Vaidyasastrapith, Govindasundari Vidyalaya.[49] Kaviraj Jaminibhusan Roy also championed the cause of Ayurveda in Bengal through the development of Astanga Ayurvedic School by publishing journal and books, by setting up chemical laboratory, and by providing treatment to the people in the indoor hospital attached to this school.[50] Subsquently, Astanga Ayurveda College and Hospitals (1916), Govindasundari Ayurvedic College (1922), and Viswanath Ayurveda Mahavidyalaya (1932) were set up for further advancement of Ayurvedic education. In this way, a group of indigenous physicians tried to attract more students to Ayurveda and rejuvenate it in the midst of constraints. But unfortunately the attempts for revival were not found to be successful. The apathy of the government, health officials, and allopathic physicians caused a stagnation of Ayurveda, putting a stop to its regeneration. The only strategy that succeeded was the manufacture of Ayurvedic drugs on commercial scale by a few entrepreneurial ayurvedists and chemists. Thus, Ayurveda survived despite official patronage of Western medicine, but the dominance of Western medicine was virtually complete.

It is true that indigenous medical systems received very little official attention and government patronage during the British rule. But has there been any remarkable shift in independent India? Is it not the British legacy still being followed by the Government of India? From time to time, since India became independent in 1947, all government committees to review the state of Ayurvedic education were dominated by allopathic practitioners who were generally cold towards it in recommending official support of any kind. There was much fanfare in the country including in West Bengal Assembly leading to the passage of Ayurveda Bill, but with few practical consequences. There were always cuts in Central Government's subsidies to the states and this caused fiscal reduction in the states in medicine and health. The fund allocated for the development of indigenous medical systems is scanty. Infrastructure of Ayurvedic dispensaries or salaries of qualified Ayurvedic physicians seems to have not been remarkably altered. The majority of students coming out of the Ayurvedic institutions can neither get jobs within the state nor win the prestige required for successful private practice.[51] Even the number of Ayurvedic educational institution and dispensary of hospital are far from being satisfactory. In fact, the condition of indigenous medical systems is still deplorable. The plans which were not taken up during the colonial rule have not been adopted for implementation after India became independent. While a series of new plans and 'models' were often announced, specially in relation to the indigenous medical systems, these were rarely funded comprehensively or consistently supported by the government or even non-government organizations.

At present, there are more questions than answers about the traditional Indian medicine in general, and about Ayurveda in particular, and if one looks into it, more questions will arise as has been expressed by Johannes Laping.[52]

Notes

1. Satyacharan Sengupta, 'Ayurvede Olautha' (Cholera in Ayurveda), *Ayurveda*, 3 year, no. 8, Baisakh 1326 BY, pp. 313–16 (hereafter 'Ayurvede Olautha').
2. Satischandra Bandyopadhyay, 'Ayurveder Swapakshe Ekti Satya' ('A Truth in Favour of Ayurveda'), *Ayurveda*, 3 year, no. 9, Jaistha 1326 BY, pp. 351–5.
3. Shakticharan Bisharad, 'Ayurveder Prachar' ('Campaign of Ayurveda'), *Ayurvijnan*, 1 year, no. 10, Bhadra 1334, pp. 446–9.
4. Sengupta, op. cit., pp. 313–16.
5. David Arnold, *Colonizing the Body: State Medicine and Epidemic Disease in Nineteenth-Century India*, Delhi: Oxford University Press, 1993, p. 179.
6. Ibid., pp. 179–80.
7. Ibid., p. 181.
8. Ibid., p. 125.
9. Ibid.
10. Sachindranath Vidyabhusan, 'Kalajwar' (Black Fever), *Ayurveda*, 8 year, no. 2, Kartik 1330 BY, pp. 39–40.
11. Sachindranath Vidyabhusan, 'Beriberi Ba Byapak Soth' (Beriberi or Large Swelling), *Ayurvijnan*, 1 year, no. 1, Agrahayan 1333 BY, pp. 14–17.
12. Anil Kumar, *Medinine and the Raj: British Medical Policy in India 1835–1911*, New Delhi, 1998, p. 68.
13. Charles Leslie, 'Interpretations of Illness: Syncretism in Modern Ayurveda', in *Paths to Asian Medical Knowledge*, ed. Charles Leslie and Allan Young, California, 1992, pp. 177–208.
14. Brahmananda Gupta, 'Indigenous Medicine in Nineteenth and Twentieth Century Bengal', in *Asian Medical Systems: A Comparative Study*, ed. Charles Leslie, Delhi, 1998, pp. 368–78.
15. G.C. Roy, *Causes, Symptoms and Treatment of Burdwan Fever or the Epidemic Fever in Lower Bengal*, London, 1876, pp. 109–10.
16. Acharya Jogesh Chandra Roy, *Atmacharita*, quoted by Ajay Kumar Ghosh, 'British Shasita Bankuray Jwarer Yantrana' (Agony of Fever in British Bankura), *Bankurar Kheyali* (in Bengali), Bankura, 2009, pp. 112–16.
17. Chittabrata Palit, 'Modernity of Tradition: Ayurveda in Colonial Bengal', *Journal of History*, special issue, vol. XVIII, 2000–1, Department of History, Jadavpur University, Kolkata, pp. 175–87.
18. Gupta, op. cit., p. 368.
19. Ibid., p. 370.
20. Ibid., p. 375.
21. Kumar, op. cit., pp. 68–9.
22. Bisharad, op. cit., pp. 446–9.
23. 'Ayurvede Nabayug' (New Era in Ayurveda), *Ayurvijnan*, 1 year, no. 1, Agrahayan 1333 BY, pp. 4–5.

24. Sital Chandra Sharma, 'Ayurveder Katha' (About Ayurveda), *Ayurvijnan*, 1 year, no. 11, Ashwin 1334 BY, pp. 459–62; Birendra Kumar Sengupta, 'Samarjwar Ba Naba Influenza' (War Fever or New Influenza), *Ayurveda*, 3 year, no. 5, Magh 1325 BY, pp. 165–71.
25. Tara Krishna Basu, *The Bengal Peasants from Time to Time*, Calcutta, 1962, p. 68.
26. Sengupta, 'Ayurvediya Chikitsar Bartaman Abastha O Ayurvediya Chikitsar Unnatir Upay' (Present Condition of Ayurveda Treatment and the Way of Its Development), *Ayurveda*, 3 year, no. 6, Phalgun 1325 BY, pp. 201–9 (hereafter 'Ayurvediya Chikitsar Bartaman Abastha').
27. Bandyopadhyay, op. cit., pp. 351–5.
28. *Ayurveda*, year, no. 5, Magh 1325 BY, p. 194.
29. Basu, op. cit., p. 67.
30. *Ayurvijnan*, 1 year, no. 3, Magh 1333 BY, p. 98.
31. *Ayurvijnan*, 1 year, no. 2, Pous 1333, pp. 50–1.
32. Margaret Jones, 'A Bounded Medical Pluralism: Ayurveda and Western Medicine in Colonial and Independent Sri Lanka', in *The Development of Modern Medicine in Non-Western Countries: Historical Perspectives*, ed. Hormoz Ebrahimnejad, London: Routledge, 2009, pp. 108–59.
33. Zahir Baber, *The Science of Empire: Scientific Knowledge, Civilization, and Colonial Rule in India*, Delhi, 1998, pp. 78–9.
34. Satpal Sangwan, *Science, Technology and Colonisation: An Indian Experience 1757–1857*, Delhi, 1991, p. 4.
35. Ibid., p. 4.
36. Ibid., p. 10.
37. Bandyopadhyay, op. cit., pp. 351–5.
38. 'Arya Chikitsa' ('Aryan Treatment'), *Ayurveda*, Ashwin 1328, 6 year, no. 1, pp. 3–9.
39. Sengupta, 'Ayurvediya Chikitsar Bartaman Abastha', pp. 201–9.
40. Bimalananda Tarkatirtha, 'Ayurvijnan Sammilanir Path' (The Way of Ayurvijnan Sammilani), *Ayurvijnan Sammilani*, 1 year, no. 2, Sravan 1338 BY, p. 34.
41. Kumar, op. cit., p. 72.
42. Ibid., p. 72.
43. Deepak Kumar, *Science and the Raj 1857–1905*, New Delhi, 1997, p. 166.
44. Ibid., p. 166.
45. 'Bibidha Prasanga' (Miscellaneous), *Ayurved*, no. 12, Bhadra 1326 BY, p. 476.
46. For details, see Gupta, op. cit., pp. 370–1; Chittabrata Palit, op. cit., pp. 177–8.
47. Arnold, op. cit., p. 52.
48. Gupta, op. cit., p. 373.
49. For details about revival of Ayurveda and the revivalists, see Gupta, op. cit., pp. 371–6; *Ayurvijnan*, 1 year, no. 9, Sraban 1334 BY, pp. 387–8; Charles Leslie, 'Ambiguities of medical revivalism in modern India', in *Asian Medical System*, ed. Charles Leslie, Delhi, 1998, pp. 356–67.
50. For details, see *Ayurvijnan*, 1 year, no. 8, Asar 1334 BY, p. 376 and 1 year, no. 2, Magh 1333 BY, pp. 136–40.
51 Gupta, op. cit., p. 377.
52. Johannes Laping, 'Dialogue in research on traditional Indian Medicine', in *Studies on Indian Medical History*, ed. G. Jan Meulenbeld and Dominik Wujastyk, Delhi, 2001, repr. edn., pp. 219–21.

6

Ayurvedic Medicine in Colonial Bengal

Challenge and Response

SUJATA MUKHERJEE

THE LATE NINETEENTH and early twentieth centuries witnessed significant developments within the Ayurvedic system in colonial India. This essay makes an attempt to reopen the question of the causes and nature of these developments in Bengal and hopes to add to the existing knowledge. The colonial rule undoubtedly marked a watershed in the history of the age-old indigenous medical systems in India. One broad aim of the reforms undertaken by the protagonists of indigenous medicine in response to the challenge thrown by Western medicine was to redefine the relationship between the practitioners and the public. This aspect, however, has not been analysed adequately. It also needs to be emphasized that as a result of the different creative methods adopted by the Ayurvedic practitioners, in order to face the attack posed by biomedicine and survive, significant transformation took place within the system. This essay, therefore, seeks to reanalyse the processes of encounter between the Western and Ayurvedic medicine and the response of Ayurvedic practitioners in Bengal to the challenges posed by biomedicine in colonial Bengal in order to understand more deeply the dynamic nature of an age-old therapeutic system.

Advent of Colonial Rule and Indigenous Medicine

From the period of earliest contact with India, the Europeans found out that India had an age-old, vibrant and pluralistic pattern of therapeutic practices which could not be ignored. A number of European physicians had visited India between the sixteenth and eighteenth centuries and wrote extensively on Indian medicine. The Portuguese, Dutch and other Western powers noted the value of certain Indian drugs, which were unfamiliar to European pharmacopoeia.[1] Even then, when European physicians first encountered

Indian medicine in the sixteenth century, they found the system that was—in its broad features—completely recognizable.[2] Like the European system, the Indian Ayurveda presented a theoretical underpinning of humouralism. It also had a similar attitude to the use of plant medicines, and many exact in diagnosis and therapy.[3] During the early phase of colonial rule, the official attitude towards Indian medicine was prompted by an urge to learn about the efficacious therapies offered by different indigenous systems because it was believed that the diseases of Indian climate could be treated effectively by indigenous methods. Moreover, the epistemic similarities also encouraged this lenient approach.

British Policy: Three Stages

The policy of the British colonial regime towards indigenous medicine evolved through different stages. Researchers have pointed out that there were three stages of this evolution.[4] It should, however, be noted that there were overlaps in these stages and moreover, as pointed out by David Arnold:

> The relationship between Western and Indian medicine needs to be perceived at pluralistic and dialectical terms, terms that allow for a continuing interaction between the two during the long history of colonial rule in India or that express the relationship as a protracted epistemological struggle which says more about the nature of political and economic power under colonial rule, than about the abstract merits of two, contrasting, competing, but not wholly incompatible medical systems.[5]

The first phase extends from the late eighteenth century until the middle of the nineteenth century (and coincides with when the regime itself was simultaneously consolidating and expanding its rule). As pointed out by scholars, the willingness of Europeans to learn from indigenous medicine reflected epistemological similarities between European and Indian medical systems. In fact, until the mid-nineteenth century, Western medicine, Ayurvedic or Hindu medicine, and Unani or Islamic medicine, had much in common regarding basic notions of disease causation, treatment, and prevention.[6]

Many works of early orientalist scholars emphatically pointed out that an ancient system of medicine did exist in India which was worthy of investigation and also that a search for ancient Sanskrit manuscripts should be undertaken to rediscover this knowledge. In the words of William Jones, 'What their old books contain on this subject, we ought certainly to discover.'[7] Yet, the attitudes of the orientalist scholars were marked by certain degree of ambivalence,[8] which was caused by an appreciation of the ancient, and scepticism about the contemporary state of things in India. Jones, for example, did not hesitate to express the doubt that there existed in any Asian language a single 'original treatise on medicine considered as a science' as opposed to a 'mere empirical history of diseases and remedies'.[9]

John Forbes Royle, who came to India as an assistant surgeon, did valuable original research on the antiquity of Indian medicine. T.A. Wise's book contains a list of Hindu writers and their works on medicine. Whitelaw Ainslie's *Materia Medica* also mentions a large number of ancient Indian treatises on medicine. Ainslie writes, 'given the state of empirical obscurity in which the science (of medicine) is still sunk in India, it will readily be believed that many substances are daily prescribed but with trifling virtues, if indeed, any to recommend them'. Yet, the overall conclusion reached by Ainslie and others was that Indian and Greco-Roman civilization had 'proceeded from the same point' and that European and Indian medical systems had the same epistemological foundations which definitely boosted the supporters of indigenous medicine.

Most of the authors writing after Jones including J. Johnson (1813), B. Heyne (1814), H. Wilson (1825), W. Ainslie (1826), W. Turning (1832), G. Playfair (1833), J.R. Martin (1837, 1856), J.F. Royle (1837), and T.W. Wise (1845), compared the past glories and achievements of Hindu science and medicine with its later degeneration.

It seems that the orientalist discourse formulated a theory of decline in the field of medical knowledge in India, which accompanied the supposed decline in other cultural domains. It assumed a golden age of 'Hindu' medicine in the remote past. Gradually decline seemed to set in due to the Buddhist doctrine of ahimsa or non-violence, which was said to have caused dissection to be abandoned, leading to deterioration of surgery and anatomical knowledge.[10]

Further decline was attributed to Muslim rule and the introduction of a rival system of medicine. Still, however, the early decades of the nineteenth century witnessed an eagerness to learn about India's rich materia medica from medical texts and also by interrogating native practitioners.

Medical Education before 1835

Colonial official policy at its early stage, no doubt, tried to promote indigenous medical knowledge to utilize its efficacious therapeutics. There was an eagerness to learn about India's rich materia medica not only from medical texts but also by interrogating native practitioners. This has been termed as the 'utilitarian' approach of early colonial state towards Indian medicine. However, the 'hegemonic' approach put emphasis on direct clinical examination of the body. The latter became important from the 1840s onwards and ultimately displaced the reading of texts or the eliciting of information from 'native informants'.[11]

The earliest official involvement with medical education in India was prompted by an utilitarian approach and a need to provide expert apothecaries, compounders, and dressers in different hospitals. These would serve two purposes. These subordinate assistants would help European doctors and surgeons who looked after the health of European civilians and military employees and also reduce company's financial burdens by limiting the appointment of European doctors. The English East India Company established the Indian Medical Service as early as 1764 to look after European health in

British India. IMS officers headed military and civilian hospitals in Bombay, Calcutta, and Madras and also accompanied Company's ships and the armies.[12]

In 1822, the Medical Board to the Governor General-in-Council, submitted a proposal for starting an institution for training native doctors for the army. In their memorandum dated 1 May 1822 the Medical Board wrote:

The paucity and insufficiency of that very useful body, the Native Doctors, has been long matter of complaint in the Medical Department of the army. In former times, little difficulty was experienced in procuring qualified persons of this class. The General Hospitals, which were then established in different parts of the Country, afforded an excellent school of instruction, whence well-taught and experienced individuals could be at all times procured. The army was likewise then not nearly so extensive as it has since become, and the number of persons of this description required for its various establishments was comparatively inconsiderable.

Of late years, the case has greatly altered. The General Hospitals have been abolished, and every part of the army has been largely augmented, so that the demand for Native Doctors has, by a peculiar fatality, increased as the means of supplying them have been cut off. After this discontinuance of the General Hospitals, there being no longer any regular place of instruction for persons of this description, it became necessary when they were wanted, to seek them wherever they could be found. . . . In this way, the Native Doctors entertained within the last few years, have been persons of a very inferior description to those attached to the service in former times. . . .

Perhaps, the case now under representation cannot be placed in a stronger light, than by stating the fact, that the only Native Doctors now procurable, are so inexperienced and ill qualified, as to make it a matter of doubt, whether it would not be better to leave the sick to nature alone, than trust their lives to men so little capable of rightly treating them.[13]

The memorandum also stated:

It has appeared to the Medical Board, that the only means holding out a fair promise of remedying the evil, and of providing a numerous class of well-trained and skilful persons to serve as Native Doctors, will be found in the Institution of a regular school for their education, and the nomination of a skilful medical officer to instruct them in the most necessary branches of medical knowledge. . . . It is proposed to establish at the Presidency a class of Native pupils whose number shall never fall short of twenty; and whose vacancies be filled up as they occur.

The Governor General's order no. 41 dated 21 June 1822 established the School for Native Doctors or Native Medical Institution. It was placed under a Superintendent. The official order pointed out:

The duties of the Superintendent will embrace the whole Establishment; he is to direct the Studies, practical, and general Conduct of the students—to prepare manuals of the most necessary and intelligible parts of Medical Science, for their use, in the Native Language; to give demonstrations, and deliver Courses of Lectures to them on these subjects; and generally to take every available means of imparting to them, a practical acquaintance with the diseases of most frequent occurrence in India; the remedies best suited to their cure; and the proper mode of applying those remedies.[14]

It was decided that twenty students would be admitted to the Institution. Their age would not be below 18 or above 26. Hindus and Muslims were to be equally eligible, provided they came from respectable background. The candidates must be capable of reading and writing Hindustani either in the Nagree or the Persian character. The order further stipulated, 'The students are to be regularly enlisted as Soldiers; from the time of their admission they are to be supported at the expense of Government; when duly qualified, to obtain Certificates from the Medical Board; and are to succeed as Native Doctors on the occurrence of vacancies in the Army, or Civil Department.'[15]

The medical training at the NMI lasted 2–3 years. Junior students studied pharmacology, materia medica, physiology, and anatomy. The two senior classes were taught medicine and surgery.[16] The students would be attached to the Presidency General Hospital, the King's Hospital, the Native General Hospital and General Dispensary and were to be under the control of the medical staff there. After the death of James Jameson, who worked for less than a year (1822–3), Peter Breton became the next Superintendent (1823–30). He made translations of useful English medical treatises for the benefit of the students.[17] In Breton's opinion, the native therapeutic system contained many useful remedies which should not be ignored.[18] In 1830, Dr Breton died and John Tytler was appointed as the Superintendent. He compiled numerous tracts for the students and made translations of medical texts.

The Native Medical Institution has been much lauded as a noteworthy institution, which promoted parallel instructions in both Western and indigenous medical systems.[19] Its foundation in 1826 was followed by starting of medical classes at the Calcutta Sanskrit College and Calcutta Madrasa. At the former institution, Ayurvedic texts including *Caraka Saṁhitā* and *Suśruta Saṁhitā* were taught along with medical treatises written in Urdu. Students of the Calcutta Madrasa studied Unani-tibb system of medicine based on works of Arab physicians among others.[20] Some historians have, however, observed that it would be wrong to assume that the British official policy ever tried to promote 'indigenous medicine as an equal or alternative to the Western system but (as with Indian Materia Medica) to draw upon what was "useful" from indigenous therapeutics while encouraging students (by teaching the Western and Indian systems side by side) to discover for themselves the superiority of European medicine'.[21] William Adam, who made a survey of traditional education in Bengal in the 1830s suggested several measures to combine 'European theory and Indian experience'.[22] He proposed that medical textbooks should be written in Bengali, Hindi, and Sanskrit languages and free copies of these books would be distributed to learned Ayurvedic and Unani physicians. Periodical examinations for students would be held and special awards given to meritorious students as well as their teachers.

Liberalism in India

With the coming of Lord William Bentinck as Governor General in 1828, the British embarked upon a thorough-going programme of reform. A distinctive ideology of imperial governance shaped by the ideals of liberalism gained ascendancy till the time of Lord Dalhousie (1845–56).[23] A product of the industrial revolution and of Britain's almost worldwide predominance after the Napoleonic wars, liberalism provided a vision as well as strategy for the remaking of Britain as well as her empire. The liberal view of Indian society was expressed fully by James Mill in his *History of British India* first published in 1818. He was influenced by the historicist ideals of Scottish Enlightenment, which laid out a series of stages by which the degree of civilization of any society could be measured. Mill opposed the view of William Jones and pointed out that the Hindus never possessed 'a high state of civilization' and that they were rather a 'rude' people. According to him, there existed in India 'a hideous state of society' inferior even to that of the European feudal age. The mission of liberalism (and utilitarianism) was to civilize Indian society and culture and since it was thought that the contemporary European and especially British culture alone represented civilization, it necessarily meant that the goal was to transform the Indian into an Englishman. It was this liberal project itself that Macaulay described in his 1835 minute on education.

The liberal transformation of India meant, among other things, education in Western knowledge. Towards the end of 1833, a Committee was appointed by the Government of William Bentinck in Bengal to report on the state of medical education in the NMI, the Sanskrit College and Calcutta Madrasa.

The Committee was also to consider the question whether medical instruction would be confined solely to English lectures and whether only English treatises would be adopted for the class and Sanskrit medical books were to be totally discarded.[24] The Committee consisted of Dr John Grant as President and J.C.C. Sutherland, C.E. Trevelyan, Thomas Spens, Ramcomul Sen and M.J. Bramley as members.

When Dr Tytler's opinion was sought, he advocated continuation of the system and stated, 'I respectfully trust the Committee will not seriously contemplate a measure, which would be likely to cause the loss of many invaluable monuments of ancient learning.'[25] According to Tytler, the supply of European medicine was limited to urban areas. Majority of the Indian population depended on native drugs, which were cheaper and easily available. Moreover, drugs prescribed by Ayurvedic and Unani practitioners seemed to be better suited to the native constitution and the Indian materia medica contained many useful remedies of which European practitioners were not aware. Thus, in his opinion, it would not be expedient to abolish the Sanskrit medical class.

Dr Grant's Committee, however, criticized the medical education imparted at the NMI for its inappropriate nature of training and the examination system as well as for the absence of courses on practical anatomy. It found it appropriate to vote for the advancement of the European system and the English language 'because that language combines within itself the circle of all sciences, and incalculable, wealth of printed words and illustrations; circumstances that give it obvious advantages over the oriental languages, in which are only to be found the crudest elements of science, or the most irrational substitutes for it.' It also recommended the foundation of a new institute 'in which the various branches of medical science (European) should be taught'.[26]

The Committee submitted its report on 20 October 1834, where the anglicists' point of view finally prevailed over that of the orientalists. The defeat of the orientalists over the anglicists sealed the fate of the NMI and the medical classes in the Sanskrit College and the Calcutta Madrassa were abolished by the Government order of 28 January 1835. This recommendation soon followed by Macaulay's minute and Bentinck's resolution, sealed the fate of the school for native doctors and medical classes at the two leading oriental institutions of Calcutta.

It was followed by the order of 20 February which established the Medical College of Bengal with Dr M.J. Bramley as the Superintendent and Dr H.H. Goodeve and W.B. O'Shaughnessy as Professors. This ushered in a new era in the history of medical education in India. The CMC was the pioneer institution of the East for a systematic education in Western medicine. Its stated purpose was to train native youths aged between 14 and 20 irrespective of caste and creed in the principles and practices of medical sciences in accordance with the mode adopted in Europe. This undoubtedly marked the end of official patronage of indigenous medical learning.

Thus, from about 1835 to 1890, there was a clear attempt by the colonial state to establish the superiority of biomedicine. From the late 1870s, tropical medicine—its ideology European, its instrument the microscope, its epistemology the germ theory of disease—became the dominant mode serving the interests of the dominant economic groups and obscured the relationship of disease to social structure.[27] Concomitantly, it meant that the biomedical perspective of complete disdain for the traditional systems was consolidated during this phase. The biomedical tradition never fully conceded the possibility of any traditional system being thoroughly competent and comprehensive in itself; Ayurveda, Unani, etc., were 'unscientific' and obsolete forms of medical knowledge that needed to be discarded.

Reaction of Ayurvedic Practitioners

From this stage, i.e. late 1870s, the survival of both Ayurveda and Unani depended upon innovative and creative responses made by the practitioners of indigenous medicine on account of the impact of the powerful machinery of state supported Western medicine. The evidence shows that they were no passive recipients of colonial power. They responded to the challenge posed by the encounter with more advantageous group of the practitioners of biomedicine by adopting various methods. Broadly speaking, there were three methods: first, use of print media to publish journals and books for spread of knowledge and awareness about Ayurvedic therapeutic practice; second, creation of Ayurvedic clinics and new consumer-friendly products to utilize the new market opportunities, and third, establishment of educational institutions, national conferences and the associations trying to bring kavirajs (the name for Ayurvedic practitioners in Bengal; literally, the King of poets, from their mastery over the texts, which were in verse) as also other practitioners of therapeutic sytems like Unani together. This demonstrates the ways in which the practitioners of Ayurveda were seeking to defend what they perceived as their interests. They attempted to create a space for themselves, learnt how to zealously guard as well as grow in it, i.e. to create a modern space for themselves, so as to remain in contention within the locus of power.

The dissemination of knowledge available in the classics and later texts was conceived of as an urgent task by the protagonists of indigenous medicine. It was often assumed that the existing knowledge was not adequate even among the practitioners partly due to non-availability of texts. So attempts were made to disseminate knowledge about indigenous medicine through systematic collection and publication of texts. With the help of the printing infrastructure developed during the colonial period, the protagonists of indigenous medicine tried to transform the hitherto relatively inaccessible knowledge into social knowledge, as well as a shared system of knowledge. Publication of texts, popular commentaries and journals were undertaken in fairly large numbers in different parts of the country. From the beginning of the nineteenth century, different kinds of books and dictionaries were being published, which were translations from Sanskrit into Bengali. 'These books not only attempted to present Ayurveda as a systematic and organized form, they were also part of an effort to recognize Ayurveda through the techniques of modern education.'[28] By the end of the nineteenth century, there were as many as fifty medical journals in Indian languages.[29]

Several kavirajs made notable contributions in this regard. Gangadhara Ray (1789–1885) a renowned Kaviraj, wrote Sanskrit commentaries on 34 books, and himself composed 41 books. He made significant contribution to Ayurvedic scholarship by writing a commentary on the classic text of Caraka, called Jalpakalpalaru, Gangaprasad Sen (1824–96), another eminent Kaviraj, published the first Ayurvedic magazine in the Bengali language, *Ayurveda Sanjivani*.[30]

Bijoyratna Sen, a student of Gangaprasad Sen, translated the *Astangahridaya* of Vagbhatta into Bengali. This is one of the three primary classics of Ayurveda, and Bijoyratna published both his Bengali translation and the original Sanskrit text with accompanying introductions and suggestions. Bijoyratna supported the idea of cooperation between allopathy and Ayurveda, and inspired his favourite student, Jaminibhusan Ray, to establish a college where they were studied side by side.

Birth of the Ayurvedic Pharmaceutical

An inevitable development which took place during this period was the birth of the Ayurvedic pharmaceutical. Many well-known practitioners themselves took the initiative to prepare medicines on a larger scale than they had done so far, fix price lists and publish advertisements for them. It was understood that the popularity and effectiveness of Western medicine was largely dependent on its ready availability in the market. So if Ayurveda wished to offer an effective alternative to biomedicine, it had to develop a similar infrastructure. The end of the nineteenth century witnessed growth of the middle class, comprising of successful small traders, large landowners and emerging industrialists. This induced changing market opportunities and the profession responded to them.

Among the well-known practitioners, Gangaprasad Sen was apparently the first person to export Ayurvedic medicines to Europe and America.[31] Chandra Kishore Sen in Bengal opened a dispensary in 1878 in Calcutta for selling medicines at a cheap rate. His firm, C.K. Sen & Co., started large-scale production in 1898. So did N.N. Sen & Co. in 1884, and Shakti Aushadalaya of Dacca in 1901. Around 1884, a company called Kalpataru Ayurvedic Works established by Gananath Sen aimed to produce Ayurvedic medicines on a large scale, for sale at moderate prices, preparing them with the aid of modern machinery in the form of pills, tablets and powders.

In the early years of the twentieth century, particularly in the days of patriotic fervour following the partition of Bengal in 1905 when boycott of foreign goods was in full swing, many entrepreneurs sought to substitute colonial products with swadeshi products. In this enterprise, small industrial units opened by professional Bengalis played a pioneering role.[32] One of the swadeshi responses was setting up new Ayurvedic medicine manufacturing concerns and this gave another boost to the emergence of Ayurvedic pharmaceuticals in the early years of the twentieth century.

Ayurvedic Institutions and Associations

In 1907, the All India Ayurvedic Congress was formed which became the leading organization of the Ayurvedic practitioners in India. The All India Vedic and Unani Tibbi Conference (AIVUTC) first convened in 1910 remained 'an influential organization for Unani and, to a lesser extent, Ayurvedic practitioners until the 1920s, when its influence began to wane'.[33] The Conference had three main aims: first, to further the institutionalization of Unani and Ayurveda; second, to challenge the order of knowledge of indigenous medicine by breaking down traditional lines of transmission through families and encouraging the 'horizontal' dissemination of expertise among practitioners; and third, to provide a forum to lobby the government for the support of indigenous medicine. The Conference wished to transform and project Unani and Ayurveda as modern bodies of knowledge and professions.

An urgent necessity was felt to distinguish learned practice from irregular forms, denigrated as quackery, which were deemed to threaten the authority of practitioners, both with the public and with the state.

The teaching institution represented a powerful mechanism in the modernization of the profession, providing new forms of knowledge transmission. Calcutta Ayurvedic Institution was established in 1915 by Kaviraja Surrendra Nath Goswami, who had a Licentiate in allopathic medicine. In 1916, the Astanga Ayurveda College and Hospital was founded by Kaviraj Jaminibhusan Ray. Kaviraj Jaminibhusan was a scholar in both Ayurvedic and allopathic medicine. Since the only medical topic taught in the traditional Tols was internal medicine (*Kayacikitsa*), Jaminibhusan tried to revive the other branches of Ayurvedic learning by supplementing them with instruction in Western anatomy, physiology, surgery, and midwifery, along with physics, chemistry, and botany. Kaviraj Jaminibhusan was a new thinker of the period who particularly wanted to train Ayurvedic physicians knowledgeable in surgery and midwifery.

The Gobinda Sundari Ayurvedic College was started in 1922 by Kaviraj Ramchandra Mallick with the patronage of Sir Manindra Chandra Nandy, Maharaja of Cossimbazar. The course of study offered integrated Ayurvedic and allopathic medicine.The Viswanatha Ayurveda Mahavidyalaya was founded in 1932 by Kaviraj Gananath Sen, with the idea of restoring Ayurveda to a fully scientific basis by educating physicians trained in all branches of medicine. And in this institution, too, Ayurveda was taught side by side with allopathy.

Confrontation within the System and Logic of Market

In 1921, a national university of Bengal, Gaudiya Sarvavidyayatana, was founded as part of the Non-Cooperation movement, and the Vaidya Sastra Pitha was established as the Ayurvedic medical wing of this university. Kaviraj Shyamadas Vacaspati was the Founder-Principal of this institution. The students in his private tol shifted to this institution, which was initiated by a donation of Rs. 6,000 from the Tilak Swaraj Fund. Kaviraj Shyamada contributed towards the monthly expenditure of the college. After Shyamadasa Vacaspati died in 1934, a building was constructed for the college with the help of his son, Bimalananda Tarkatirtha, and the institution was renamed the Syamadas Vaidya Sastra Pitha. This school was a protest against the foreign-oriented education of the day and represented the views of the purists or those who favoured the Siddha system of traditional education and opposed integrating Western medical science with Ayurveda.

Thus, there developed a confrontation between the purists and the integrationists regarding the question of reform and adaptation. Curiously enough, despite the epistemological confrontation both the purists as well as those who advocated an integration of Western and Ayurvedic systems, had to address and shape their behaviour not by ignoring but taking into account the mechanism of the market. The most interesting aspect of this is that it was assumed that in the parameters of the market 'shuddh' and 'integrated' products, i.e. those made according to traditional formulae and those that were adapted from the pharmacology to make new medicines respectively, could co-exist without debate. None of the advocates of the either school could ignore the fact that they had to grapple with new problems and pressures faced by the profession and had to aim at reconfiguring the authority and rework its relation with the public. The practitioners were most concerned to present the credibility of their profession, to demonstrate to the public their authority, their capacities and their trustworthiness.

The tensions within the Ayurvedic profession—exemplified to some extent by the division between the purist and reformist strands—in fact speak volumes about the process of reform in Ayurveda, and the ways the practitioners were attempting to reformulate the practitioner's role in society. Evidently in the nineteenth and early twentieth centuries, the collapse of courtly patronage, the commodification of medical products, the use of print, the power of Western medical technologies, the emergence of new professional cultures and the exigencies of epidemic emergencies—all these created new challenges before the practitioners of indigenous medicine. In the colonial situation, the authority of the learned elite, hereditary practitioners of indigenous medical system like Ayurveda was constantly challenged by the emergence of new forms of professional structures in the drive to modernization. Medical practices, technologies and knowledge imported from outside India or developed within the Indian colonial context were reworked and adopted or contested in the negotiation of modernity in various Ayurvedic circles during this period. They had to confront a wider public in order to compete and survive. They reconfigured their knowledge and practices through the prisms of nationalist politics, changing social and moral norms, and colonial inspired models of legitimacy. The practitioners and advocates belonging to various schools were forced to take stock of what they thought to be good, authentic and legitimate, in order to represent this knowledge to the public on a vastly new scale, both to gain and maintain their trust and their custom, and in order to represent the credibility of their practices in new, less personalized administrative, legislative and political domains.

The new modes of reforming indigenous medicine in colonial India has often been interpreted primarily as a move to challenge the power of and seek equivalence with Western medicine through the emulation of its professional models. The practitioners of Ayurveda who sought to recast their profession were, no doubt, in many cases inspired by colonial-derived models—organizational, educational, conceptual, technological. But it is important to recognize that their adoption of these models was not a straightforward process. The evolving profession was engaged in various forms of dialogue: with itself (evident in the articulation of the competing interests of its own practitioners) with a variety of other medical practices and traditions folk, Unani, private and state-sponsored Western. The inner dynamics of reform, and the tensions within the profession motivated the will to reform. Most importantly as the public were its patrons, the practitioners sought to reach out to them.

There were tensions within a professional elite, whose sphere of authority until the colonial time was rooted in localized, familial and personal contexts, but through the late nineteenth century and into the twentieth century, professional elite woke up to the need to compete on a more global scale—through print, the mass production of medicines and professional organization. In this quest for recasting their identity and authority, the role played by the marketplace and public perception was of profound importance for the practitioners of indigenous medicine.

It may be asked whether the colonial era marked a radical and immediate disjuncture in the orientation of Ayurveda through the supplanting of pre-existing forms of instruction and legitimation. Pre-colonial era was marked by the importance of person-to-person transmission of knowledge, the power of family-based remedies, etc. In the colonial period, although family or teacher-pupil relations remained important, the authoritative practice of Ayurveda gradually ceased to be merely a local, family affair. Thus, the system underwent many transformations. Some notable aspects of this transformation are: medicines were not solely being dispensed to individual patients but were becoming available off the shelf. Moreover, instead of being made by a vaidya (practitioner of Ayurveda) in a small pharmacy, medicines were being mass produced by manufacturing companies. Ayurveda was no longer a knowledge system accessible only to the elite but was becoming disseminated to many through print media, etc. All these developments undoubtedly transformed the character of the Ayurvedic profession to a large extent. The personal relation was less important and reaching out to public sphere became more important than before. This remarkable transformation has become more and more prominent as years have gone by and ultimately has reached a point today where the Ayurveda is not the same as that during the pre-British times, since 'it has experienced a dramatic transformation in the last hundred years or so'.[34]

Notes

1. David Arnold, ed., 'Warm Climates and Western Medicine', *Clio Medica*, vol. 35, Amsterdam, 1996.
2. M.N. Pearson, 'The Thin Edge of the Wedge: Medical Relativities as a Paradigm of Early Modern Indian-European Relations', *Modern Asian Studies*, vol. 29, no. 1, 1995, pp. 141–70.
3. Dominik Wujastyk, *Root of Ayurveda: Selections from Sanskrit Medical Writings*, New Delhi, 1998. Deepak Kumar agrees, but also points out that their practices differed greatly. See Deepak Kumar, ed., *Disease and Medicine in India: A Historical Overview*, New Delhi, 2001, p. xvi.
4. Poonam Bala, *Imperialism and Medicine in Bengal: A Socio-historical Perspective*, New Delhi, 1991.

5. David Arnold, *Colonizing the Body: State Medicine and Epidemic Disease in Nineteenth-Century India*, Delhi, 1993, p. 14.
6. Mark Harrison, *Public Health in British India: Anglo-Indian Preventive Medicine 1859–1914*, New Delhi, 1994.
7. Arnold, *Colonizing the Body*, p. 45.
8. For an analysis of these attitudes see Arnold, ibid., pp. 33–50; Harrison, op. cit., pp. 36–58; Deepak Kumar, 'Unequal Contenders Uneven Ground Medical Encounters in British India, 1820–1920', in *Western Medicine as Contested Knowledge*, ed. Andrew Cunningham and Bridie Andrews, 1997, pp. 172–90.
9. Arnold, *The New Cambridge History of India*, vol. III, no. 5, *Science, Technology and Medicine in Colonial India*, Cambridge, 2000, pp. 66–7.
10. Charles Leslie, 'Ambiguities of Revivalism in Modern India', in *Asian Medical Systems: A Comparative Study*, ed. C. Leslie, Berkeley, 1976, pp. 356–67; Sujata Mukherjee, 'Women Medicine and Empire: Female Practitioners and Patterns of Health Care in Colonial Bengal', in *Modern Historical Studies*, vol. 2, Journal of Department of History, Rabindra Bharati University, March 2001.
11. Arnold, *Colonizing the Body*, p. 54.
12. A general hospital was built in Calcutta for Europeans as early as 1707. The Presidency General Hospital started in 1768 also accommodated only Europeans. In 1787, the Government built another hospital at Dum Dum chiefly for vaccine inoculation among soldiers and their families. Dispensaries became local centres for vaccination against smallpox and for conveying Western ideas about sanitation and hygiene.
13. The memorandum was signed by Dr Gillman, Dr Meik, Dr Russell, and Dr James Jameson, Secretary to the Medical Board and forwarded by the Secretary to Lieut. Colonel Casement, Secretary to Government in the Military Department under letter dated 9 May 1822, *Proceedings of the Medical Board*, National Archives of India, New Delhi, cited in S.N. Sen, *Scientific and Technical Education in India 1781–1900*, New Delhi, 1991, p. 129.
14. Ibid., p. 131.
15. Ibid.
16. O.P. Jaggi, *Medical Education and Research*, Delhi, 1979, p. 28.
17. The list of treatises prepared by Breton was appended by John Tytler's letter dated 30 March 1831 to James Hutchinson, Secretary of the Medical Board, *Proceedings of the Medical Board*, National Archives of India, New Delhi.
18. Letter dated 14 October 1824 from P. Breton to George Proctor, *Proceedings of the Medical Board*, National Archives of India, New Delhi.
19. Bala,, op. cit., p. 45.
20. Ibid., p. 44.
21. Arnold, *Colonizing the Body*, p. 55.
22. Leslie, op. cit., pp. 361–2.
23. Thomas R. Metcalf, *The New Cambridge History of India, vol. III, no. 4, Ideologies of the Raj*, New Delhi, 1995.
24. *Hundred Years of the University of Calcutta*, Calcutta, 1957, p. 35.
25. Letter dated 3 April 1834 from John Tytler to Major Troyer, *Minute Book of the Sanskrit College*, quoted in S.N. Sen, *Scientific and Technical Education in India*, op. cit., p. 152.
26. J.J.Richie, *Selections from Educational Records, Pt. II, 1840–59*, Calcutta 1922, p. 318; Vijay Govind, 'The Advent of Modern Medicine in British India (AD 1600–1900)', in *Western Colonial Policy*, ed. N.R. Ray, vol. II, Calcutta, 1983, p. 138.
27. Roy Macleod and Milton Lewis, eds., *Disease, Medicine and Empire: Perspectives on Western Medicine and the Experience of European Expansion*, London and New York, 1988.

28. Pradip Kumar Bose, ed., *Health and Society in Bengal: A Selection from late 19th Century Bengali Periodicals*, New Delhi, 2006, p. 22; Benoybhusan Roy, *Unish Satake Deshiyo Bhasay Chikitsavigyan Charcha*, Calcutta, 1995.
29. K.N. Panikkar, *Colonialism, Culture, and Resistance*, New Delhi, 2007, p. 182.
30. Brahmananda Gupta, 'Indigenous Medicine in Nineteenth and Twentieth-Century Bengal', in *Asian Medical Systems: A Comparative Study*, ed. Charles Leslie, London, 1976, pp. 368–77.
31. Ibid., p. 372.
32. Rajat Kanta Ray, *Entrepreneurship and Industry in India, 1800–1947*, New Delhi, 1992, p. 259.
33. See Guy Attewell, *Refiguring Unani Tibb: Plural Healing in Late Colonial India*, New Delhi, 2005.
34. Madhulika Banerjee, *Power, Knowledge, Medicine: Ayurvedic Pharmaceuticals at Home and in the World*, Hyderabad, 2009, p. 1.

7

The Old and the New of Ayurvedic Materia Medica

A Historical Perspective

Nupur Dasgupta

It was between the second century BC and second century CE that a burgeoning body of related knowledge on the workings of matter and materials, medicine and chemistry was observed to emerge especially in textual sources. This was the indirect result of pursuits into different branches of knowledge, the broader paradigms of which were connected and which foundationally converged upon the ancient Indian theories of atomism. These results or the contributions of different segments of early Indian intellectuals and professionals appeared unconnected on the surface, but had deeper epistemological links with each other. Trends in atomism had evolved quite early in the Buddhist, Jaina and Nyāya-Vaiśeṣika systems of philosophy. By the fourth–fifth centuries CE the metaphysics on creations had transcended into some advanced notions of matter, which may be termed as Naturalism.[1] Eventually, these got crystallized into proper premises in the Patañjali *Yogasūtra,* and in the late seventh to late eighth-centuries commentary on it in *Vyāsa Bhāṣya*—representing an enlightened concept of the *bhūta.*[2] In the meantime, as Kenneth Zysk has already suggested, the emperico-rational system of medicine flourished under the aegis of Buddhism,[3] which culminated, in a way, into the compilation of medical information in the *Caraka Saṁhitā.* This text, most probably a collation of information from several practising and travelling physicians or *Caraka* physicians, possibly śramanas[4] already referred to a philosophical basis for medical treatment. It began with deliberations on a deep knowledge of inner chemistry of organic matter, understood in terms of the metabolism of the animal body and the essences of the plant world. The *rasa,* as the essence of botanical and zoological ingredients, had also led on to *rasāyana*—arising out of the notion that the essences of medical ingredients would work with those of the animal/human body, and leading on to the system of the promotive Ayurvedic treatment for health. The meeting of these concepts on a broader cognitive paradigm enabled the contemporary developments in the philosophy of medical treatments and thereby in the processes of drug making. By the fourth–fifth centuries CE, the knowledge of materials had both widened and deepened as the chapters on *dravya* in the *Suśruta Saṁhitā* reveal. From then on, this influx of ideas and practices were rendered into a body of medical knowledge, one of the most proven aspects of which is contained in the observations on medicinal materials: *dravya* and *dravya rasa*. In fact, as one shall observe in the course of this discussion here, the knowledge related to *dravya* was put into the shape of a new discipline by the eleventh century and continued to dominate Ayurvedic practices till the mid-nineteenth century. In the nineteenth century, this body of traditional knowledge was incorporated by some of the Western scientists into the newly furbished scope of Western Materia Medica, in a colonial environment.

The early historical or even early medieval contexts of Ayurvedic practices quite naturally did not include scientific provenance tests. The foundation of this knowledge system was essentially based on clinical observations and applications, and repeated experiments with patients. However, in the medieval times, when other cultures of the world were experimenting with a more scientific paradigm, the discipline of Ayurveda was undergoing strict secrecy among its practitioners, without reference to innovations or new applications. It became replete with repetitive traditions untested and unmodified, legitimized only by virtue of repeatedly advertised tradition and claims to antiquity. The only refreshing element in this repetitive scene of dogma was the entry of the Unani system, and the adaptations of some medicinal and clinical practices from it into Ayurveda. The picture remained almost unchanged in the early part of the colonial times when, however, a number of inspired texts were being composed which were mere compilations of the Ayurvedic knowledge collated from different classical and less classical, rather derivative earlier texts. On the other hand, a growing interest was noted among Western scientists, especially physicians and botanists, in salvaging aspects of the knowledge system and their more epistemic analyses. However, this trend was short-lived, with the major governmental initiative for introducing Western medicine replacing traditional treatments. And yet, there was a major effort at redesigning the knowledge of Ayurveda according to the Western science norms by both European and Indian scientists and scholars in the late nineteenth century. So far as hard research-based practice is concerned, however, it is only from the fag end of the last century that real and hard experimental researches on some major Ayurvedic recipes for treatment have come up for reconnaissance among pharmacists, bioscientists and medical practitioners.

This essay especially focuses on the emergence and flow of the knowledge on drugs as *dravya*, and its applications in terms of pharmacognosy as described in the latest redacted versions of *Caraka* and *Suśruta Saṁhitās*. One shall note the later developments leading to the birth of the *Dravyaguṇa* as a distinct genre of medical studies under the system of classical Ayurveda and then explore the nineteenth-century renewal of interest in the Ayurvedic Materia Medica among the scientist community.

Medicinal recipes abound in all the chapters of the *Caraka*. However, for the purposes of this presentation, those related to the *rasāyana* treatment have been chosen exclusively. This is because it is necessary to relate the innate concepts of *rasa* and *rasāyana* underlying the ideas of *rasāyana* treatment and the making of drugs. I propose to discuss the ingredients in these select recipes, and try and explore the modern references to the uses of these ingredients by the nineteenth century compilers of the texts on Indian indigenous system of treatment recorded by Western scientists, as well as Indian vaidyas, and then go on find new understanding of these ingredients towards the end of the nineteenth century.

The concept of drugs in Ayurveda may be traced to the core concept of *dravya*. This is described with great clarity in the *Caraka Saṁhitā*. The theme is developed from one level of connotative philosophy to the next, revealing the foundation of Ayurveda in contemporary physical theory nurtured within the domain of the Nyāya-Vaiśeṣika and Śāṅkhya schools. I shall trace the different junctures of this development of the concept of *dravya* with its inherent properties and qualities from the concept of *padārtha*, derived finally from *bhūta*—or Matter in philosophy. Further, the evolution of the idea of *dravya* as drug, viz., *deha* or body, underpins the entire logic behind the drugs in operation in the body of animals as remedies.

The idea of *dravya* is discussed in *Caraka* '*Sūtrasthāna*'[5] in the following way:

> The five elements, along with self, mind, time and space are denoted as *dravya* (substances). *Dravya* with sense organ is sentient, while that without *cetanā* (sense organs) is insentient. This passage, therefore, talks about elements, life and the two fundamental physical dimensions as substance or *dravya*. Further clarifications of the compositions of *dravya* have been discussed in an earlier *śloka*. It has been related that, whereas similarity of all *dravya* is always the cause of increase, dissimilarity amongst the particles of *dravya* cause decrease. Both affect the final composition by their application. Similarity brings unity, while dissimilarity causes diversity. Again, similarity proposes similar purpose (or action), while dissimilarity has the opposite effect and action.[6] The innate idea in this *śloka* is that the similarity or dissimilarity of basic matter creates the different forms in nature.

Next I have definitive explanations on *dravya* and its properties or *guṇa*.

Samavāya is that quality of the *dravya* that gives it inherence. It is the inseparableness of the five *bhūtas*, that is *pṛthvī* or earth, *ap* or water, *tejam* or fire, *vāyu* or air, *ākāśa* or space/ether, etc. This is eternal because no *dravya* is devoid of *guṇa* or property.[7]

More illustrative is the next *śloka* which defines the relation of *dravya* and *guṇa*.[8] The explanation is put quite clearly. *Dravya* (substance including drugs) is said to be that substance, in which actions and properties, or *guṇa* are located and which is the material cause of its effect. *Guṇa* (property) is related with *dravya* in terms of *samavāyī* or inherence, is devoid of action, and is the inherent (*samavāyī*) cause of the effect. That is to say that *dravya* with its inherent *guṇa* or property is the active principle in which the *guṇa* remains inherent and inactive, and acts only through the *dravya*. Thus, the idea that *dravya* is the channel through which the telling effects of *guṇa* might be had. The causative factor in conjunction and disjunction located in *dravya* does the performance and this action is *karma*. This is, therefore, the visible or felt cause or the action.

Now, having explained the concepts of *dravya, guṇa* and their relation, as well as their action in *kārya* or *karma*, the *Caraka Saṁhitā* turned the discussion towards drugs as *dravya*. In the next few *ślokas*, the actions of *dravya* as drugs on the body have been explored.[9] The text now enters into the discussions on *dhātusāmyakriyā*, the declared and sole purpose of the compendium. This has been described as the good effect of drugs which brings about equilibrium of mind and body, causing nourishment. That naturally leads to the definition of diseases. The next few lines describe that loss of *dhātusāmya* or equilibrium leads to *doṣa* in bodily humours, which were seen as imbalances in *vāyu, pitta* and *kapha*, the three major bodily functions and clinical properties. There was the fourth one, the *doṣa* in the mind or mental imbalance, caused due to loss of equilibrium in mental conditions: *sattva, rajas* and *tamas*.

The effects of drugs were discussed next.[10] The discussion began by claiming that curable disorders get remitted by uses of drugs having opposite properties administered with due consideration of place, dose and time. Curiously enough, the text categorically laid down here that treatment of incurable diseases was not advised. With these premises set in order, the *Saṁhitā* goes deeper into the discussions on drugs and their actions. This begins with reference to *rasa*, which is defined as the essence of *dravya*—covering all substances including the body which is to be treated, and not the essence of drugs alone. It is quite clearly put down here that *rasa* as the essence was the actual element for treatment.[11]

The concept of *rasa* is extremely significant in understanding the philosophy of treatment in Ayurveda. *Rasa* was understood as the object of *rasa* or taste. Its material substance (*dravya*) is basically made up of the particles of the two *bhūtas*—*ap* and *pṛthvī*. In manifestation and differentiation of *rasa*, the other three *bhūtas*, viz., *ākāśa*, etc., are the causative factors. This concept probably reflects the fact that to the practising physicians the actual natural substances with which both drugs and animal bodies were constituted appeared to originate in water and earth. But that these basic constituents constantly reacted with the other *bhūtas* was also gauged, and it was roughly understood that the final manifestations of the varied animate and inanimate objects in nature were due to these reactions.

Moreover, the *rasas* themselves were said to form different combinations through conjunctions with each other and the average multiplication of these combinations were calculated to be sixty-four in number. Thus, although there were six basic *rasas*, there were sixty-four combined forms of *rasas*.[12] The discussion on drugs per se begins with categories. Drugs are said to be of three types according to the uses to which they are put. Some are pacifiers of *doṣa* or abnormalities in body and mind, some vitiate *dhātu,* and yet some are to be taken to maintain normal health. Significantly, the term for drugs is also *dravya,* thereby implying a clear understanding of the connectivity of all matter, constituting the natural substances from which the drugs were extracted, the bodies of animals and humans, and the whole of nature and the environment. This was the guiding philosophy, nurtured from the contemporary Śāṅkhya and Vaiśeṣika philosophies, which were foundational to the Ayurveda concept of treatment.

This connectivity is further reiterated when the categories of drugs (*dravya*) are discussed. Drugs are said to be of three types, according to the source of their origin, viz., (1) those of plant origin, (2) those of animal origin, and (3) those of earth origin. Then, the details of the sources and extracts of drugs have been discussed.

These ideas, probably reflecting a long term collection of tested results with different types of ingredients, were the main database for the future works on Ayurvedic medicine. The *Suśruta Saṁhita* reflects this, but adds on not only quantitatively but also qualitatively in dwelling on more sophisticated processes of drug extraction, in closer and more minute identification of natural substances as sources of medicine, and in more intricate uses of drugs for different treatments, as well as minute segregation of the extracts for different purposes of treatment.

The understanding of the medicinal properties of the natural substances had also gone much deeper and this is reflected in the categorization of drug sources. The following descriptions will be provided according to the tone and language of the original texts, in translation, in order to throw light on the contemporary chain of thoughts and the tone of directives as preserved in the texts through several redactions. Brief reviews of the history of these transitions through redactions, of both the *Caraka* and the *Suśruta Saṁhitā,* have been discussed by the present author in another article. [13]

The *Suśruta* defines diseases[14] in the following manner:

> The *Puruṣa* (body and mind) is the receptacle of many types of ailments. That which proves a source of torment or pain to him/her is denominated as a disease. There are different types of diseases, such as traumatic or of extraneous origin (*āgantuka*), that which evolves from the internal body (*śarīra*), mental (*manasā*) and natura (*svabhāvika*).

The diseases may be alleviated through *saṁśodhana* (cleansing) and *saṁśamana* (pacification of the deranged bodily humours), and regimen of diet and conduct.[15]

The next few lines declare that[16] food is the principal factor of the drug and therapeutic. By food, however, is meant anything that is edible. Nevertheless, the diet is a very big concern in Ayurveda treatment.

Food is what materially contributes to the strength, complexion and vitality of animated beings. Food consists of six different tastes (*rasas*), which are inherent (in substances). These substances which are called *oṣadhi,* may be divided into two classes—mobile and immobile. The immobile *oṣadhi* may be grouped under four heads: *vanaspatis*, *vṛkṣa, virudhas* and *oṣadhis*.

Trees bearing fruit and not flowering are *vanaspati*. Those that bear both fruit and flowers are *vṛkṣa*. Shrubs and creepers that trail on ground are *virudha*. Plants which die on ripening of the fruits are *oṣadhi,* such as cereals.

The mobile *oṣadhi* or animates are divided in classes such as viviparous, the oviparous and sweat-begotten, and those that are born of decomposed vegetable matter: *Jangamah khalvapi cetanāvidha jarāyūja, aṇḍaja, svedaja, oudbhijjaḥ*.[17]

Going into the details of identified drugs it is found that the different parts of plants, viz., leaves, flowers, fruits, roots, bulbs, the expressed juice and milky or resinous sections of plants, etc., were obtained from the vegetable world, as was the case with animal sources too. The skin, nails, wool, blood, flesh, fat, marrow and bones were procured from the animal sources.

Metals and minerals, such as gold, silver, gems, and earth minerals, such as realgar or *manaḥśilā,* as well as pearls, clay and *kapālas* (bones), etc., were included in the list of the earthly substances. The inclusion of the *kapālas* indicates that these were fossilized forms and not fresh cut bones, which would then fall under the animal-source category. The transformation in the property of bone due to long exposure in nature was understood and therefore listed under earth category.

The *Suśruta* adds a further clause to healing and this is the factor of natural environment. According to this text, natural phenomena, like gale, windfall, shade, moonshine, darkness, heat, cold and rain, and temporal settings, like day, night and fortnight, should be deemed as the works of eternal time, which, by virtue of their natural effects, contribute to the accumulation, augmentation, pacification or diminution of the deranged bodily humours. In fact, the temporal paradigm was important to observe, as it was seen to affect the properties of natural elements which constituted the sources of drugs, as well as the animal body which was the object of treatment. Chapter VI in *Sūtrasthāna* is on seasons, and here it is clearly mentioned how seasons affect the properties of waters and vegetables and, indirectly, animal life. This philosophy lends a holistic blend to Ayurveda. Finally the definition of disease and drugs is given:

> The term *vyādhi*, disease, signifies all distempers incidental to the several or combined action of the three deranged bodily humours—*vāyu* (wind), *pitta* (bile), and *kapha* (phlegm) and blood. The term *ouṣadha* medicine signifies drugs and their virtues (*guṇa*), tastes (*rasa*), potency (*vīrya*), inherent efficacy (*prabhāva*) and reactionary properties (*vipāka*). The discussion goes on to provide the entire purview of medical operations. The concept of *kriyā* denotes operations, including the use of appliances, such processes as surgical operations and injections falling under the section *cheddāni*, and emulsive measures and lubrications, etc., under the *snehādini* section fall under

this scope. The term 'time' signifies all opportune moments for medical operations and uses of appliances. All these required medicinal preparations and they have been discussed next, including pre-operative processes. Different stages of preparatory measures, training and education required by the aspiring physicians have been painstakingly listed.[18]

The prime importance of the knowledge of drugs and their uses is clarified in warnings to the aspiring physicians. A whole chapter is devoted to instructions for the budding physicians, and clear injunctions were included for proper training. The tone is categorical. The paragraph runs: 'even a panacea or a medicine of ambrosial virtues administered by an ignorant or untrained physician will prove positively baneful as a drought of poison.'[19] The final responsibility of the physician with regard to the uses of drugs is clearly referred in the chapter especially constituted of discussions on the natural resources and natures of different drugs in the *Dravya Saṁgrahaṇīya Adhyāya*.[20] It was expected that an intelligent physician (*matimānabhiṣag*) should prepare plasters (*lepana*), decoctions (*kaṣāya*), medicated oils and emulsions, like medicated clarified butter (*tailam* like *ghátas)* and potions (*sarpinṣipānakān*) according to the exigencies of each individual case. These drugs may be used in all the seasons of the year and should be stored in a room protected from smoke, blasts of cold, wind and rain. Thus, potentially speaking, the classical text hints at the shelf life possibility of the prepared drugs. Not only the final decoction, but mixtures made out of the primary preparations are also indicated for use. Therefore, it was found that it was advised in the text that the groups enumerated above should be therapeutically used according to the nature of the deranged humours involved in each individual case. Only two, three or four drugs of the some medicinal group; or a similar number of drugs chosen from different groups; or a group of medicinal drugs in its entirety; or in combination with another, should be used according to the indications of particular cases, as the physician in his discretion, would determine to be the right decoction.[21] While the warning comes across as directive to rigorous training and experience, the *śloka* also throws light on the different forms of medicines prepared at the time of specific treatment, which is extremely important from the readers' perspective.

The most important and illuminating discussions on the principles of medicines, properties of ingredients, comparative evaluation of properties, the essences of medicines, and their processes of working in remission of diseases are discussed in the three chapters entiltled *Dravya-Rasa-Guṇa-Vīrya-Vipāka-Vijñānīya-Adhyāya*, *Dravya-Viśeṣa-Vijñānīya-Adhyāya* and *Rasa-Viśeṣa-Vijñānīya-Adhyāya*.[22] The text of the *Suśruta Saṁhitā* is very methodical in explaining these matters.

A summary of the ideas may be put as follows:[23] Drug here is plainly termed as *dravya* or substance. It is defined to have both a definite and a continuous existence (the time factor). There is a certain consistence in *dravyaguṇa,* or properties of drugs, and therefore, while the drugs in the form of ripe and unripe fruits would have different characteristics, they both were said to contain certain similar medicinal properties. The drug was to be regarded as real and invariable (*nitya*), but the caution was put that its attributes were transitory and accidental at best. This idea indicates the uncertainty arising out of the lack of tools of scientific analysis at the time, and the awareness of the practitioners and guides themselves about the hypothetical nature of pre-modern Ayurveda Materia Medica may be located precisely here. However, it is experience in clinical form that had provided the foundation of faith in Ayurveda Materia Medica. By clinical here I refer to the practice concerned with or based on actual observation and treatment of disease in patients rather than experimentation or theory. Thus, in spite of anxieties about the transitory or accidental nature of the attributes of the drugs, it is specified in the text that: whatever, the uncertain nature of drugs, the real character of the drug is not destroyed despite processing, whether it is powdered or formed into a paste. This unchanging value of the medicinal property, not closely scrutinized, however, was known to be constant due to the theory of *bhūtas* developed in Indian philosophy. Processing would involve chemical change, but that was not fully understood. The concept that the medicinal property lay in the essence or *rasa*, however, was helpful, for it clarified the concept that despite physical changes the inherent medicinal essence remained the same. A drug or substance, thus, according to classical Ayurveda, does not lose its generic character.

This chapter also explains that while describing the recipes it is the name of the actual natural substance that has been mentioned and not the principal *rasa* which it is constituted of. This is an important epistemic aspect to take note of, since the nomenclature of the drug substances would have profound role in the dissemination of knowledge concerning Materia Medica and cognition of drugs per se among the contemporary practitioners of Ayurveda and among the latter-day physicians too in the subsequent times. This is again the aspect that would be completely changed once Western science takes over, as one shall note at the end of this essay. In many cases one finds that the text mentions only some parts of the actual plant as being used because it is the specific property of that part that contains the *rasa* or essence required for making the drug. That clarifies the knowledge possessed by the Ayurveda expert concerning the different properties, and efficacies of the different parts of a plant. In all these one gets the idea that the substance or *dravya,* which was the natural source of drugs, was considered the most important element in drug preparation. This also makes it obvious that the physician-cum-druggist was required to know the utmost about his/her ingredient. In fact, one may probe deeper into a debate concerning the primacy of the elements in the order of efficacious action in a prepared drug. The matter is complicated and fine, and reveals the deep contemplation on the part of the master of Ayurveda regarding the workings of the drugs.

The *Suśruta Sūtrasthāna śloka* talks about the relative importance of the actual base substance, *dravya* and its essential attributes in the actual activation of the drug.[24] An elaborate discussion follows, which actually enlarges upon the idea of the internal dynamics of the medicinal properties of the ingredients in a comparative-relative serialization of the attributes. These attributes were weighed on the scale of importance as active agents. The first is *dravya* itself as the substance which forms the drug (or therapeutic food). Next is *rasa* or the essence of the drug, and *rasa* here is identified as the essence of both drugs and food and not specifically medicine (one shall see the expansion of this discussion in the latter-day literature on *dravya*, especially from the time Cakrapāṇidatta composed the *Dravyaguṇasaṁgraha* as a special discipline). Next is *vīrya* or the potency of the substance. The characteristics of potency are described as—purgative, emetic, cathartic, pacifying, astringent, appetising, pressing, liquefying, constructive, tonic, aphrodisiac, inflammatory, absorbing, caustic, bursting, intoxicating, soporific, killing, or antitoxic. The third attribute evaluated in this scale is *vipāka,* i.e. the digestive reaction. The explanation that was given was that all ingested food, properly or improperly digested in the stomach, proves wholesome or otherwise to the body. The *Suśruta* clearly indicated that there were several schools of thought among the physicians in applying medicines regarding the exact catalyst which made a drug efficacious in the body to mitigate diseases. Different schools held different elements or attributes to be the primary cause of effective therapeutic action. The total idea in engaging in these minute discussions was to gauge the exact juncture at which the medicine assumes its therapeutic potency.

The *śloka* finally laid down that it was the *dravya,* the substance from which the drug was derived, which was the most important aspect of the study of medicines, thereby representing the school of thought to which the *Suśruta* adhered. The explanation was that the making of the drug from the substance itself necessarily implied action or potency, i.e. *vīrya* and attributes or *guṇa*, which were both inherent in the *dravya* itself. The next *ślokas*[25] provided the definition of the digestive process as it was understood, where the breakdown of the partaken substance into particles or *bhūta*s has been understood to set in motion the metabolic process and enhance the therapeutic action. But the argument put forward in favour of *dravya* was that without the substance that was being digested the question of *vipāka* would not arise. One sentence clarifies this idea; it states that *vipāka* or the digestive reaction is impossible without drug potency and there is no *vīrya* or potency without *rasa* (essence/ taste) and no *rasa* without *dravya* or substance. Therefore, substance is the greatest of all—*pāko nāsti vinā vīryād vīryam nāsti vinā rasāt raso nāsti vinā dravyād dravyam śreṣṭhamataḥ smṛtam.*[26] The *dravya* is the principal cause of the *guṇa* which were inherent in it, and *guṇa* was intimately associated with the substances in a *samavāyi karaṇa* or cause effect relation. The rationale of the working principle of the natural ingredient, the properties that the drug was made of, was thus analysed, explained and defined. The concepts, thus, reveal a budding convergence of ideas regarding the essence of substances, processes of manufacturing and intake of medicine as per the metabolic process of the patient concerned, and the characteristics of the properties of the drug ingredients, their variability and action. All of these were admittedly at a stage where deeper analyses were impossible and the physicians were dependent rather on observation of the efficacy of the drugs in clinical processes.

The *Suśruta* chapter on *Dravya-Viśeṣa-Vijñānīya-Adhyāya* described the categories of drugs.[27] The drugs were described as derived from the *bhūtas* and are placed in categories of *bhūtas—Prārthiva, Āpya, Taijasa, Vāyavīya* and *Ākāśīya*. The combination of factors in treatment by medicine was next enumerated: *kāla* was the period of action; *karma* was physiological action, potency of the drug was *vīrya*, the body or receptacle of drug was *adhikarṇa*, the agency through which drug worked or mode of its working was *upāya,* and lastly the result was *phala*.[28] The vagueness of some deeper areas of cognition regarding the workings of drugs had made way for *śāstric* and spiritual interpretations, and its impact over the practising physician is available in some *ślokas* in the *Sūtrasthāna*.

The *ślokas* described:

> inscrutable and unthinkable are the virtues of drugs which are above all rules of syllogism (*amimāṁsya*) (*acintya*). That is the reason why drugs have been recorded in the scriptures (*āgamenaupāyaujyāni*), which are well known by their own virtue. These have been observed from direct observation of results and efficacy. The efficacy of these medicines recorded in scriptures (*āgamena*), should never be tested (it is sacrilegious). These have been observed through generations and are instinctively pronounced as beneficial. A thousand arguments of causal nature (logic) cannot refute their efficacy, which is inherent. Their attributes are above the proof of effectiveness carried out by the *ambaṣṭha* and other classes of physicians. Hence, the physician who is intelligent should rest his faith in the drugs mentioned in the scriptures and not argue or introduce his own logic.[29]

Indirectly, this refers to the practice of a class of physicians, outside the sanctified orbit of the traditionals, who took constant recourse to different kinds of new medicinal preparations and the tussle between the established order and these new innovators. The days before the *Caraka* and *Suśruta*, when every new innovation was openly admitted and added to the list to be later compiled, were gradually passing out. The already-compiled list of drugs in these two texts (redacted definitely by the seventh century CE) were getting rigidified into normative and textual (*śāstric*) culture sanctified by appropriated traditions mooted through long lists of revered names of legendary sages and gods. On the other hand, the risk of quacks was also evidently potent and hence the time-tested documentations in the scriptures were generally regarded as dependable and taught to the budding physicians with great deal of caution. The concern was as much for human safety as for the close control over a significant occupational discipline. One might observe in this, a resonance with the latter-day Western physicians' attempts at regulating the practices of the apothecaries, Paracelsians and Helmontians or the barber-surgeons, since the sixteenth century, etc.[30]

This takes the readers to the matter of the origin of the concept of a separate discipline of Materia Medica. The distinct separation of the chapters on medicinal substances began in the *Caraka* with the different forms of drugs, initial introduction to their preparations, etc., which were discussed separately in this early text. The *Caraka* categorizes the processes and the final forms of drugs in the chapter on evacuative-*virecana*.[31] By *virecana*, the Ayurveda master was actually referring to the extracts of identified natural sources of medicines. The changes that took place in the concept and understanding of Ayurveda are very clear from how this particular term was later taken only in the sense of purgative drugs by latter-day practitioners. Most modern treatises and books on Ayurveda follow this narrow sense of the term.[32] Priya Vrat Sharma, on the other hand, takes the term only to mean one of the ways of treatment of diseases.[33] There are many such diversions that took place over the centuries of Ayurveda practices in ideas, connotations, knowledge and cognition, which had graduated into qualitative differences, playing a large role in how Ayurveda came to be practised and referred to in the nineteenth and twentieth centuries—the period that made great changes in the application and appreciation of the system.

However, coming back to the discussion on drugs—their sources and preparations, the *Caraka* concept starts with extracts from natural sources, especially plant sources which have been understood as evacuatives or extracts from these sources.

Six hundred evacuatives, all extracts from plant sources have been put in categories, the categorization being guided by the uses of the extracts for particular group of ailments, including diseases, promotion of health and organic deformations. The categories reveal exhaustive observation of plant sources and cognition of the different aspects of extractions. First, the five locations of *virecana* (evacuatives) in a plant source have been enlisted, i.e. latex, root, bark, leaf, flower and fruit. Next, the five sources of evacuatives have been enumerated in terms of *rasa* or essences: *madhura* (sweet), *amla* (sour), *kaṭu* (pungent), *tikta* (bitter) and *kaṣāya* (astringent)—all understood in terms of *kaṣāya*, which actually refers not to *rasa* as essence, but to the extracted form as essence of a particular natural ingredient. Then one gets the reference to the forms and processes of drug preparation. The five types of extract preparations were described as: juice, paste, decoction, cold infusion and hot infusion.

'Juice expressed out of a *dravya* by mechanical pressure is *swarasa*. Drug ground with some liquid is *kalka* (paste). The preparation of drug by boiling *dravya* on fire and then cooled down is called *śīta* (*kwātha*). When a *dravya* is kept in hot water for the whole night, the extract obtained from it is also known as *śīta* (cold infusion). *Phāṇṭa* (hot infusion) is the preparation in which *dravya* is put in hot water for a while and gently sifted.' Their potency is in the following order: *swarasa, kalka*, first form of *śīta*, second form of *śīta* and lastly, *phāṇṭa*. It is also mentioned that different strengths of extractions were used depending on the strength of the disease and the patient. Five hundred general sources have been enumerated in this chapter following this detailing.[34] Thus, one may not be wrong in concluding that the necessity for explaining the origin, identification, nature and extraction, as well as preparations of drugs were considered as a whole unit and a distinctive part of the study of Ayurveda and thus put in a separate chapter. I have already referred above to the basic concepts regarding drugs in the *Suśruta*. But what remains to be noted is more significantly, the addition to the knowledge of drugs in distinction to what is found in the earlier text of *Caraka*. The later compendium of *Suśruta* devotes more detailed chapters on preparations of different forms of medicines.[35] The new forms of preparations included were *sneha,* oil prepared from seeds of plants and animal extracts, of three strengths—*mádu, madhyama* and *khara*; *sveda* (fomentation) of four types—*tāpa sveda* (direct application of heat), *uṣma sveda* (fomentation), *upanāh sveda* (poultice), and *drava sveda* (application of heated liquid); *vamana-virecana* (here the term is used in the sense of medicines which induce purgation in the patient) or emetics and purgatives, *taila* or linctuses, *dhūma* or fumes, and *nāsya* or snuffs to be inhaled. As is evident from this description, the forms of medicine and the method of treatment were as yet tackled together in these two classical texts. Yet, these discussions throw light on the many kinds of preparations that were conceived of and prepared for different methods of treatment. A snuff, a fumigating dust, a liquid or emulsion, or a paste were all the different varieties used for different types of treatments. Moreover, going by specific preparations, one finds that the *Suśruta* goes quite elaborate over the processes of extracting, and making of alkaline substances and acids which indicate deep processing of ingredients for different kinds of medicines, both for internal and external uses. It seems drug making had progressed a lot since the times of the *Caraka*.

Post-*Suśruta* History

One has to remember, however, as pointed out at the beginning of this essay that the versions now available to the readers in editions are actually derived from the redacted forms of original compositions. The current form of the *Caraka Saṁhitā* is derived from Dṛḍhbala's late fifth or early sixth century CE redaction[36] and the *Suśruta* which was first edited by Nagarjuna before the sixth century CE which was then redacted by Cakrapāṇidatta in a compilation named *Bhānumati* in eleventh century CE, as well as by Dalhana in the twelfth century CE—the last being the more popular. The knowledge and the system expressed in these two classics, however, may actually cover the cognitive paradigm of the fifth–sixth centuries CE at the latest. Therefore, one needs to look at the texts composed beyond that juncture to observe the changes or otherwise if any, in the knowledge and approach to the concept and practices of drug making.

That takes us to the next classic, the last of the Bṛhattrayī-Vāgbhaṭa's *Aṣṭāṅgahṛidaya*, of the early seventh century CE.[37] However, as regards novel ideas regarding medicinal ingredients, processes of drug preparation, or even the philosophy of therapeutics, there is hardly any new addition to be found which go beyond what one finds in the *Suśruta*. The only novel concept that strikes one is exemplified by the new categorization of the substances according the predominance of the type of *rasa*. The concept was definitely guided by the Buddhist Vaibhāṣika atomic theory, as well as the compilation of the ideas floating in contemporary Nyāya and Vaiśeṣika schools in the works of Nyāya expert, Gautama,[38] which came by the first century CE. His work was popularized further by Vātsāyana's *Nyāyabhāṣya* which belonged to the *c.*450–500 CE according to Potter[39] and Udyotakara, who dates around the mid-seventh century CE according to Eric Frauwallner, and 550–610 CE according to Potter.[40] The Vaiśeṣika exponents like the influential thinker Prasastapāda, dated *c.*550–600 CE, according to Frauwallner,[41] Udayana, dated to the tenth century CE[42] and Sridhara around *c.*950–1000 CE according to Karl Potter.[43] These latter thinkers provided substance to the already proposed concept of the correlations between the natural ingredients for medicines, the body of the patient, and the bodily processes.

The *Aṣṭāṅgahṛidaya* reiterates on the lines of the *Suśruta* that of all the properties of drugs it was *dravya* or substance that was primary and that all *dravya*—animate and inanimate, were constituted of *pañcabhūta*. The different permutations and combinations produce different forms of substances. Thus, due to various combinations all *dravya* are constituted of different *rasa* and *anurasa*. *Guṇa* was explained similarly on the traditions of the *Caraka* and the *Suśruta*. The new concept elaborated upon was concerning the basic *rasa* of different substances. Thus, one finds categories of dravya substances divided according to the prime *rasa* they were constituted of, e.g. *pārthiva dravya, āpya dravya, āgneya dravya, vāyavya dravya, nābhasya dravya*.[44] Without going into the details of the concept, it is quite clear that distinct categorization probably facilitated the cognizance and learning of the properties of the substances used by the Ayurveda physician and trainee. It is also true that the follow up discussions reveal formalization of the previous knowledge, but little improvement and expansion. The concept of the processes of the activation of substances in the body's metabolism was elaborated and clarified wonderfully probably reflecting the contemporary developments in the Indian philosophical schools, especially as noted in Vācaspati's *Bhāṣya* on Patañjalī *Yogasūtra* (300 and 500 CE), whose composition dates from *c.*650–850 CE according to the brilliant analysis of James Haughton Woods.[45] The other concept of *prabhāva* was clarified—the impact of the substance on the body which renders it in some cases more, and in other instances, less active.[46] A major difference, however, was noted in nomenclature of the medicinal plant species, which seems to have become less Sanskritic and more oriented towards vernacularization. The reason for this is not clear. However, this was a sure sign of the popular usage of the directives in the text and a wider dissemination of the discipline of Ayurveda in the post *Suśruta* times. In the meantime, as D.N. Ray had pointed out, surgery had receded to the background and hence the discussions on drug preparations did not highlight on acid and alkali preparations, which was an important subject matter in the *Suśruta*.

So far as medical literature is concerned, the more popularly known texts that followed in the subsequent times were the *Mādhavanidāna* of the eighth century and *Śārṅgadharasaṁhitā* of possibly the eleventh–twelfth centuries, both works continuing in the tradition of the *Caraka*. The *Nidāna* actually became a major text for students of Ayurveda, as is apparent from its repeated references in later texts and the format that was followed. Chakrapāṇi had followed the *Nidāna* to some extent in his *Cakradattasaṁgraha*. But that was not all, the main departure made in the design of discussions on the discipline of medicine was struck off by Mādhavakara in the eighth century, when he composed a distinct text on *dravya*—the *Dravyaguṇa*, which is not available in the original at present. Priya Vrat Sharma refers to the manuscript studied by him as Madhavakāra's *Dravyasangraha,* but Meulenbeld is sceptical about the authorship of this particular manuscript.[47] There were two later authors of the same name in this field, one who composed the *Bhāvasvabhāva,* the text which is sometimes known also as *Dravyaguṇasaṁgraha,* and the other who composed the *Dravyaguṇratnamālā,* none tallying with the original Mādhavakara's work. However, popularization of this trend was the work of Cakrapāṇidatta. He had composed the new editions of both the *Caraka* and *Suśruta*, which became popular. But introducing the study of *Dravya* as a distinct discipline with full force in the late eleventh century CE with the *Dravyaguṇasaṁgraha*, Cakrapāṇidatta showed the way to the evolution of drug-related food habits and also helped in the intensification of the study of medicinal substances as distinct from the general science of treatment including *Śarīrasthāna*, *Cikitsāsthāna,* etc. The study of *dravya* assumed the proportions of a distinct branch of study following his scholarly contribution towards it, shaping it into the science of medicinal substances or therapeutics, in the form of food especially. The most significant addition found in this compendium is the concept of *adravya* as opposed to *dravya*, thereby posing a binary concept of substances in terms of their uses as medicine. Thus, *dravya* in Cakrapāṇidatta's *Dravyaguṇasaṁgraha* is expressly used to mean only substances medicinal, and this clearly marks the tone of the text as a compendium on Materia Medica.

Cakrapāṇidatta, in fact, begins with references to Kanāda—the Vaiśeṣika exponent and the school of Śānkhya.[48] In the commentary Śivadāsasena, who belonged to the early sixteenth century, also included an allusion to the schools of Nyāya and Mīmāmsā, which were used to reveal the methodology of categorization. It is significant that in medieval Bengal these two later schools of Indian Philosophy had gained popularity among the intellectuals and pedagogues, and that these had deeply impacted the genre in which Śivadāsasena wrote his commentary. The concept of *pañcabhūta* and its manifestations have been discussed in detail in the original text, but enlarged upon by Śivadāsasena. This text by Śivadāsasena carries the flavour of early medieval conceptions, and the medicinal sources, especially food therapeutics listed in the compendium, throw light on regional plants and crops and the dietary pattern. There is, thus, a whole new angle that was brought into the fold of Cikitsāśāstra. The contribution by Cakrapāṇidatta in rendering the *Dravyagūṇa* into a separate discipline was more important since he was a noted authority on the subject in his own days and in later times, and had also composed commentaries on both the *Caraka*, that is, the Āyurvedadīpikā, and the *Suśruta*, which was entitled: the *Bhānumatī*. Both of these were popular among the vaidya community and continued to be consulted down to the eighteenth century. The distinction of the *Dravyaguṇasaṁgraha* thus made by the exponent on classical Ayurveda had a tremendous impact which was illustrated in the numerous *Dravya* texts that were composed in the subsequent times and a resultant birth of a new genre. The net result was that for the first time in the *Dravyaguṇasaṁgraha* of Cakrapāṇidatta one can find certain new ideas regarding medicinal materials, departing from the classical trend set by the *Caraka* and the *Suśruta*. This departure was probably possible only due to the fact that in this work Cakrapāṇidatta was conceiving a new area and the conception of food as therapeutic, always dealt with as a part of medicinal ingredient in the classical texts, received a wider treatment. Many new ingredients, included in local diets in the eleventh century found their way into the discussions on *dravya*. The *Dravyaguṇasaṁgraha* in fact adds local edibles, e.g.—*nārikela*, leafy vegetables or *śāka* of six new types, and a number of regional vegetables like *paṭolapatra*, leaves of water gourd, etc., in the edible therapeutics of Ayurveda. In fact, his *dravya* includes mostly food ingredients and there were references to cooking processes and making of tasty *rasa* through cooking.[49] It is also interesting to note that in prescribing the diet as therapeutic Cakrapāṇidatta had introduced a new regional angle. The most important addition was the discussion of the medicinal properties of the specific food ingredients, various different varieties of which have been categorized according to their medicinal merits and *rasa* properties. For example, the different varieties of fine rice growing in the regions, *śāli, rakta śāli, saṣṭika*, etc., have been minutely discussed as regards their property and effect on human constitution, including digestion and diseases like sexual weaknesses, diabetes, dryness and bile disorders.[50] But more than that, the exact effects of seasonal variations of crops, the soil for cultivation, etc., have been also meticulously investigated in terms of the medicinal efficacy. The orientation of this work clearly sets the tune of early medieval and subsequent times. In fact, Cakrapāṇidatta's works continued to be immensely popular and reiterated time and again through centuries along with Mādhavanidāna and Śārṅgadhara's works, and when Uday Chandra Datta wrote his work on Materia Medica in 1877 these were his principal sources.

The medieval times witnessed compositions of various natures going into the subject of Materia Medica especially and not really dwelling upon the process of treatment as such. The Rasatantra texts highlight on *dravya* to some extent, including an overwhelming reference to the metallic extracts in medicinal preparations. In fact, the Rasatantra genre introduced a new dimension to the conception of drugs, which always remained peripheral only to the more focused and serious studies on medicine and classical Ayurveda.

However, not much of epistemic change had been wrought in the concept of *dravya* since Mādhavakāra and Cakrapāṇidatta.

The major Ayurveda text of the medieval era, the *Bhāvaprakāśa* composed by Bhāvamiśra, belongs to the sixteenth century. The *Bhāvaprakāśa* is arranged mostly in the style laid down in the *Caraka* with some additional elements from the *Suśruta*. But what is important is that, as in the *Suśruta*, a large section was devoted to the discussion of sources of drugs as categories in a specific chapter.[51] However, the categories were very different and reveal the medieval, species-based divisions approach. For example, plants and animal sources were put under different categories, but in the same section. Even processed items like 'Taila varga', 'Dadhī Varga', etc., have been put in separate sections as categories. More importantly, enlarging upon the *Suśruta* regarding the discussion on processes of drug making, the *Bhāvaprakāśa* devotes separate sections on the chemical/pharmaceutical processes in the second part—*Dvitīya Bhāga*. Under this section there are chapters on: (1) 'Mānaparibhāṣā Prakaraṇa', (2) 'Bheṣaja vidhāna Prakaraṇa', (3) 'Dhātvādi śodhana māraṇa prakaraṇa', (4) 'Snehapāṇa Vidhi Prakaraṇa', (5) 'Pañcakarma Vidhi Prakaraṇa', and (6) 'Dhūma Pāṇādi Vidhi Prakaraṇa'.[52] In fact, the kind of chemical processes for drugs preparation, etc., which was scattered throughout the text of *Suśruta* were, thus, brought under single heads in the *Bhāvaprakāśa*. Not only that, this sixteenth century text added on a number of new ingredients, as well as preparations and the new disease, *Phiraṅgaroga* introduced by the Portuguese. Bhāvamiśra had, like Cakrapāṇidatta also authored a work focused on Materia Medica—*Gūṇaratnamālā*.[53] The tradition of specific compositions of drugs and Materia Medica had thus made a hesitant, but definite start.

Although the long time-gap between Cakrapāṇidatta's eleventh-century *Dravyaguṇasaṁgraha* and Bhāvamiśra's sixteenth-century *Bhāvaprakāśa* or *Gūṇaratnamālā* remains to be explained, one does have a direction. There is at least one text that was intermediate between these two landmarks and that is *Śārṅgadharasaṁhitā* of eleventh–thirteenth century. This was most definitely much later than Cakrapāṇidatta.[54] This text contains some significant and detailed accounts of calcination and preparations based on various metals, and may be held to be a precursor of the *Bhāvaprakāśa* in providing formulae and applications of chemistry in drug processing, i.e. pharmacy.

The *Bhāvaprakāśa* may in this sense be called a full compendium on Materia Medica and pharmacy which would have been a blue print for the Ayurveda practitioners and adapted to the ambiance of the more scientific analyses of the seventeenth and eighteenth centuries. The *Nighaṇṭubhāga* of the text commences with the *Harītakyādi Varga*. Each of the ingredients has been mentioned with its variations, if available, followed by analysis of its properties, contraindications, and tests of qualities, as well as modes of uses. Interestingly enough, a number of ingredients were added which were actually adopted from Arabic Pharmacology and Arabic soil. For example, the *Harītakyādi Varga* itself contains the species named *Pārasīka Vacā-Khurāsāni Vaca*.[55] The botanical species for this ingredient has been identified as Iris germanica Linn or Paris polyphylla Sm.[56] Another completely new ingredient included was *Samudra Pheṇa*,[57] which has been identified as Cuttle fish bone[58] or shell (as the note suggests), and one notes that it contains calcium carbonate. It was understood that the bone or shell loosens from the body of the organism when it dies and floats above on the surface of the sea, is brought to the shore by waves, and hence the name *Samudra Pheṇa*.

Bhāvamiśra clearly declares in the *Mānaparibhāṣā Prakaraṇa* that in composing this part, he was following the guidelines laid down in the *Caraka*. But what strikes as the foremost contribution is that this chapter consists of some details on measurements of ingredients for medicinal preparations. The actual chemical or pharmacological procedure starts from the chapter entitled 'Bheṣaja vidhāna Prakaraṇa' of the *Pūrva Khaṇḍa*. But as far as the preparations are concerned they do not reveal much advancement on the processes detailed in the *Suśruta*. The main processes mentioned comprise drying the herbs (in some cases), soaking in water for a day and using the water as *rasa* preparation, or using the extract after boiling and reduction. Water of soaked rice is mentioned. Details of *hima nirmāṇa* or cold infusion and *mantha nirmāṇa* or churned infusion processes have been described as have been the processes of preparing *Kalka, churṇa,* and *anupāna*. However, a few new processes with their specific nomenclature are found to have been introduced, including *Bhāvanā, puṭapāka, uṣṇodaka, Prakṣepa Pramāṇa, and Guṇikā nirmāṇa* with details.[59] *Snehapāka parikṣā* or tests for proper cooking of fatty substances were important. Medicated fats of three kinds are mentioned: *mádu, madhya* and *khara*. *Āsava* or *ariṣṭa* preparations have been detailed. But the most profound change was brought in by including a special chapter on 'Dhātvādi śodhana māraṇa prakaraṇa' related specifically to metals and minerals. Interestingly enough, apart from the *Rasatantra* texts like the *Rasārṇava, Rasaratnasamuccaya,* etc., which date between the eleventh and the fourteenth centuries, the *Bhāvaprakāśa* is the only medical text that dwells on the furnaces and apparatus connected to the chemical and preparatory processes. The chemical process might have been largely adopted from the contemporary mining, metallurgical and other agro-industries, like wine making, oil milling, etc. But, it is clear from the descriptions that the *Rasatantra* genre had come closer to medical practices during this time. However, the application and processing of ingredients into drugs is what makes this all the more important in the history of pharmacy in India. *Bhāvaprakāśa*, thus, does stand out after the *Suśruta,* Cakrapāṇidatta's *Dravyaguṇasaṁgraha* and the *Śārṅgadharasaṁhitā*, to be a landmark composition reflecting major developments. In fact, the most revered, as well as popular of the pedagogic handbooks in the late nineteenth century on Ayurvedic Materia Medica, written by U.C. Dutt, derived its information mostly from the three works described above, i.e. Cakrapāṇidatta's *Cikitsāsaṁgraha*, the *Śārṅgadharasaṁhitā* and the *Bhāvaprakāśa*. This was entitled *The Materia Medica of the Hindus*.[60] The other text which dates later, but was often quoted from by U.C. Dutt is the *Bhaiṣajyaratnāvalī* of Govindadāsa. The work most probably belonged to the seventeenth–eighteenth centuries. Binodlal Sen, who also modified the work of U.C. Dutt and published it in 1877, had edited and first published the text of *Bhaiṣajyaratnāvalī* in 1798, *śakābda* (1872 CE).[61] He mentioned that the text was composed more than a 100 years ago. This statement would place the *Bhaiṣajyaratnāvalī* in the mid-eighteenth century.

The *Bhaiṣajyaratnāvalī* appears to be the last great text compiling all previous information Ayurveda Materia Medica and as the name suggests it is focused on *dravya* alone like Cakrapāni's *Dravyaguṇasaṁgraha.* According to Sen, the text included information from the alchemical texts like *Sārakaumudī, Rasendracintāmaṇi,* and *Rasendrasārasaṁgraha,* as also from the medical compilations of Cakrapāṇidatta. He also mentioned that it contains the names and properties of all drugs generally used by the Rāḍha (Bengal) School of medicine.[62] The published edited text is interesting because, the editor has not only inserted the original Sanskrit *ślokas* of the *Bhaiṣajyaratnāvalī* and their translations, but also included additional information and directions based on the nineteenth-century practices as observed by Binondlal Sen himself, a practising Ayurveda vaidya. Not only that, the information from *Bhaiṣajyaratnāvalī* has been corroborated with the original sources of Cakrapāṇidatta, Śārṅgadhara and Bhāvamiśra. Thus, one does get three tiers of information which may illuminate a history of adoptions of recipes and philosophical leanings in drug efficacy, and applications and clinical practices. This was the state of indigenous research on Materia Medica in the eighteenth century, whereby one witnesses the gradual evolution of the awareness of the fact that the study of the drugs, their sources, preparations, etc., required special focus. So far as the indigenous efforts at the theoretical reckoning of Auyrveda Materia Medica and especially drug recipe were concerned, *Bhaiṣajyaratnāvalī* marks the end of the medieval era, and yet, the edition of the text by Binodlal Sen also signified a bridge created between the late medieval Sanskrit-text-based *śāstra* tradition and the rising awareness of the colonized vaidya community of the importance of documentation of the classical theory, as well as contemporary adaptations and practices. Binodlal was indeed aware of the new turn taken in the works of trained experts in Western medicine, like U.C. Dutt, while editing Dutt's *Materia Medica.* But before I turn to Indian medical experts' efforts at rehabilitating indigenous Materia Medica within the episteme of Western medicine, let me review how the whole idea of revamping the indigenous knowledge with the Western analytic tools came to dawn on the medical personnel and officialdom working in nineteenth-century India.

In the next leg one must turn to the observation of foreign sources, which were gradually building up in number and significance. The dissemination of Indian knowledge of herbal sources of medicine had begun when the volumes compiled by European physicians and botanists came to be composed. The landmarks included the works of Garcia da Orta,[63] the Portuguese Jew physician, Christofori Acosta,[64] the Spanish botanist who was a captive in Africa,

Asia and China and drew many of his information from Orta and Hendrik Adriaan van Rheede tot Draakenstein, the Dutch Governor of Cochin.[65] These works had travelled to near contemporary Europe too. One must note that the composition of *Bhaiṣajyaratnāvalī* itself was temporally close to the investigations in the medicinal flora of the country undertaken by these foreign physicians, enthusiasts, and much later by trained botanists like Roxburgh,[66] followed by Nathaniel Wallich[67] and others.

Garcia da Orta's pioneering work *Coloquios dos simples e drogas e cousas medicinais da India* was published in 1563 in Goa. It is quite likely that this publication did not create a ripple to the shores of India's indigenous researches and compositions on Ayurveda Material Medica, which remained strictly on the path of Sanskrit text tradition. However, the late seventeenth century 12 volume magnum opus compiled under the initiative of Hendrik Adriaan van Rheede tot Draakenstein, the Dutch Governor of Cochin, (*Hortus Malabaricus*) was a major affair involving the participation of local experts, like the famous Malabar physician Itty Achuden and a host of Konkani brahmins. This might have had more of an impact at least on the regional efforts at restoring and maintaining the traditional knowledge. There is no evidence to venture upon this issue at present. But the descriptions in both Orta's and Rheede's works reveal the participation of a non-*śāstric* and grassroots level indigenous knowledge tradition. They had closely interacted with the foreign researchers in the sixteenth–seventeenth centuries, although van Rheede's team did include the local *śāstric* experts too.[68] This indeed provides with a new evidence for an alternate dimension to the knowledge and practices of indigenous drug use among the people in different locales of the country at the time. The participation by local grassroots people in knowledge accumulation by the Portuguese and the Dutch in the sixteenth–seventeenth centuries, for the first time since Cakrapāṇidatta's efforts at including new ingredients and sources from local uses in the region of Bengal, refers to local knowledge and local nomenclature on the ingredients, especially plants, that were carefully documented by Orta and Rheede. In fact, the whole exercise of data collection in van Rheede's project had involved taking cognizance about the local names of the plants in vernacular language, often even the colloquial names. Thus, the way to an interface with the grassroots level of knowledge on regional flora and herbal medicine was opened up. Although the voluminous project seemed to have left almost no impact on the cultivation of indigenous Materia Medica among the Indian practitioners, especially the traditional ones, the exchange throws light on how even in the sixteenth–seventeenth centuries, a parallel grassroots segment of knowledge had grown. The Sanskrit treatise writers in the medieval times, however, were more open to the Unani system, as I have already discussed. Perhaps, the commentaries and additions found in *Śārṅgadhara Saṁhitā, Bhāvaprakāśa* and much later Binodlal Sen's edition of *Vaishajya Ratnavali* (transcription of the spelling used by the author in this edition) also reflect this fact. The big leap in categorization and concepts was made in terms of the inclusions from Arabic medicine that was quite popular in India among the Islamic community, as well as among the mass of the people. While *Bhāvaprakāśa* provides allusions and hints towards this, Orta and Rheede's works were more steeped in Arabic science. At this juncture, one might note the fact and keep it in store for future reference that Arabic medicine had made a way into popular and bazaar medicine scenario at least in practice since the sixteenth–seventeenth centuries, and that this indicates both the readiness of the people to accept new systems, as well as the apparent similarity between the two systems, Ayurvedic-Siddha and the Unani-hekimi to the people, which had led to the reception of the latter systems as indigenous to Indian shores.

The attention of the foreign researchers of the times was mostly drawn towards the botanical sources of drugs, the largest repository of indigenous medicine. This was the period when worldwide effort was noticeably inclined towards the study of plants. Since the primary element in classical Ayurvedic Materia Medica constituted of botanical elements, therefore, it was the history of botany that one has to follow in order to understand the fate of indigenous *Dravya* in a rapidly European-dominated scene of scientific endeavour. Botany was emerging as a discipline and the discipline was closely connected to researches on medicine. On the Indian scene a start was definitely made by Garcia da Orta and van Rheede tot Drakenstein, the Dutch Governor of Malabar in the second half of the seventeenth century. Both explored the indigenous knowledge base to penetrate into the natural plant resources in India in the sixteenth–seventeenth centuries, and both had established the first officially compiled exhaustive lists of these plants from their sources of investigation which had made their way into the European culture of flora in Latin. A huge inventory of botanical raw material for drugs was created and in so doing they introduced for the first time foreign names for these plants. In most cases, however, they were latinized versions of the local vernacular names. But their efforts at nomenclature marked the start of the process of dislodging the Sanskrit names for the plant, which were part and parcel of Ayurvedic repertoire. Orta's work was translated into Latin as early as 1567 by Charles d'Ecluse or Clusius, the famous botanist.[69] Acosta's work was also translated into Latin along with that of Orta by Clusius and presented in an abridged volume.[70] However, so far as the epistemology related variously to drug cognition, reconnaissance and preparation was concerned there was not much difference that could be discerned in ideas and practices between the indigenous and foreign endeavours at the time. The picture would undergo a sea change shortly thereafter. Garcia da Orta's work gained rapid popularity among the contemporary botanists and physicians in Europe, a community of intellectuals who were regaining their interest in the subject and reinventing the significance of Galen's works. Rheede was equally popular among the contemporaries. The publication and circulation of the *Hortus* in Europe drew attention of the botanists and physicians alike towards Holland, which became the centre of researches on tropical plants, medicinal herbs being an integral and important part. In fact, Linnaeus himself drew information and depended on illustrations of rare plants from the East provided in Rheede's volumes for his final binomial referral in his *Species Plantarum.*[71] What was important was the rapid progress made in botany between the sixteenth and the eighteenth centuries, including development of plant systematics and genealogy with Carl V. Linné and A.L. de Jussieu[72] to plant physiology with Stephen Hales[73] and plant metabolism with Joseph Priestly.[74] These progresses were foundational to the study of plants for their chemical compositions and finally the integration of pharmaceutical researches with chemical analyses and botany. Not only that, between the sixteenth and the eighteenth centuries, plants from different parts of the world, including the dried Indian plants collected by the Europeans, were getting analysed in laboratories. Illustrations, detailing the parts of the plants had already been included in the *Hortus Malabaricus.* The dried plant samples along with their illustrations came to be stored in museums and herbariums in Europe. Special corners for hothouse plants from the tropics were set up in botanic gardens, like the Kew Gardens in London. By the eighteenth century, polynomial and binomial nomenclature had been imposed, with the names of the European discoverers of the species getting the stamp of scientific approval, thereby completing the process of appropriation of a vital resource of the indigenous medicine. Thus, the crucial centuries, seventeenth, eighteenth and the nineteenth, witnessed the gradual changes in the West, especially in the emergence of new disciplines and old disciplines getting reinforced by the new. The waves of these changes repeatedly flooded the local initiatives of the European researchers in India. However, it had not yet affected the traditional practitioners' world in India till the late nineteenth century. In the meantime, the European scientists had already geared up for deeper incursions into the world of plants, including medicinal plants. From the mid-eighteenth century, the British efforts were noticeable in the field of investigations in this direction at a time when huge steps had been made towards botanical chemistry, materials science and medical science in the West. Naturally this marked off a new and qualitative advancement in scientific knowledge, which came to converge at the temporal point when the British were dominating the scene in India. The works of British officers and scholars henceforth would be qualified by the scientific episteme that had emerged in the West. The popularity of what Tournefort had initiated, i.e. collection of plant species as samples from foreign lands,[75] had extended to include the colonized territories, and the exotic plants from Asia, Africa and the Americas found their way to the herbariums of scientists and finally to botanical institutions like the Kew Gardens in London. The efforts at documenting the data and collection, as well as analyses of plant resources both from the interests of medical science and botany had converged under the big umbrella of the colonial state of Britain. The Kew Gardens, under the enthusiastic supervision of Joseph Banks, had begun to collect, document and analyse the Indian indigenous plants with great vigour, and it is within this set up that William Roxburgh, followed by Nathaniel Wallich and Francis Hamilton Buchanan founded the modern Western edifice of botany in India, thoroughly changing the possibilities of researches into the medicinal plants, thereby affecting the fate of Ayurveda as a discipline. On all counts, the developments in the botanical format, especially in nomenclature and categorization of species families made giant changes in the Westerners' approach to the indigenous sources of drugs, which were primarily botanical extracts in nature. This was evident in the works of Roxburgh, Wallich and Buchanan Hamilton—all using Linnéan systematics and Hales' analytic criteria of plants. The following works exemplify this trend. To begin with, Roxburgh's *Plants of the Coast of Coromondel* was published in three volumes from London in the 1790s and early 1900s under the direction of Joseph Banks, who was the President of the Royal Asiatic Society from 1743 to 1820. William Roxburgh, MD, had served in the Madras Medical Service from 1776 to 1780 and was appointed superintendent of Samulcotta Botanical Garden and later to Calcutta Botanic Gardens. Roxburgh's interest in botany was apparent for a long time and he had received training under Dr Hope, the Professor of botany in Edinbrugh University. In India he eagerly joined the company of another noted European botanist and physician, Johann Gerhard Koenig and it is this connection that, with the intervention of Joseph Banks, made Roxburgh the repository of Johanne Gerhard Koenig's collection of data and documents out of which the above publication was made.[76]

Thus, the first step towards a British botanical compendium was made which was official and reckoned as a part of the colonial State's achievement. Roxburgh thenceforth would go forward with subsequent projects on botany. Roxbugh's *Flora Indica or Description of Indian Plant* was posthumously edited and printed by William Carey and published from Serampore in 1832 in two volumes. Nathaniel Wallich was appointed as superintendent in the Indian Museum. [77]

This is the juncture when the corresponding investigations conducted by Whitelaw Ainslie and John Forbes Royle on Indian Materia Medica could have formed a new blueprint for revival and revitalization of the indigenous system of pharmacy. But this trend was lost in the miasma of official negligence and overwhelming endeavour at proving the superiority of Western science, which mandated the correctness of keeping this science separated from traditional knowledge. While Ainslie and Forbes' works were supported by the modern, scientific botanical studies, the times were as yet unripe for molecular chemistry and germ theory. It was yet possible to include the traditional Materia Medica, as well as the practitioners to be integrated through training and education into the new system of categorization, documentation and analyses. But that was not to be. What happened, therefore, was that while under the guidance and scrutiny of Western scholars the scientific categorization of India's indigenous herbal sources aided in an overall rationalization of the indigenous Materia Medica, this knowledge hardly reached the actual practising vaidyas and hakims. Later on the chasm widened beyond repair, when organic chemistry was added as a part and parcel of pharmacy-related works both in the apothecary's work and training, as well as in the training of practising physicians. Unlike the pre-modern physicians in India, the modern Western physicians did not prepare drugs. These were now prepared by the apothecary on physicians' prescriptions. When the apothecary now actively prepared the drugs, they were exposed to the information supplied by the botanist, as well as the chemist. By this time, plant chemistry had been initiated as a new science especially with the extraction of active ingredients for medicinal and aromatic uses, which went hand in hand with chemistry and the development of the periodic table in late nineteenth century.[78]

This was far off from the scene of indigenous Indian practices, which was languishing without proper development of rational episteme for long since the medieval times. Without philosophical inputs and designs of enquiry Ayurveda continued to languish in the department of episteme and rational additions to perceptions of both diseases and treatment and the scope of Materia Medica as it was since the medieval times as Projit Bihari Mukharji points out. He expressly makes a case out of the concepts regarding diseases and abnormalities related to sex, which took a definite turn towards the irrational since the medieval times and had impacted the psychology of a section of Bengali middle class till the nineteenth century.[79] It was on this scene that the new Western science made its entry. One shall observe here the approach taken by the early British officiating-scholars to the indigenous Materia Medica in order to illuminate upon how closely the indigenous tradition missed riding on the bus to an early development into a full-fledged science supported by Western epistemic frame, which might have been made accessible to the indigenous physicians and chemists.

But, the early nineteenth century was a curiously bountiful time for the reconnaissance of Indian Ayurvedic Materia Medica, when a few enthusiastic European and British physicians, scientists and botanists were exposed to Indian indigenous practices of the contemporary times, whether Ayurveda, Unani, Hekimi or the Siddha variety, and they observed, documented, evaluated and adopted the more proven aspects and transferred the knowledge to the domain of Western science. Several efforts were made towards interpreting both the classical indigenous medical manuscripts, as well as the indigenous reserves of natural medicine, which were corroborated by contemporary practices.

The first notable publication by a foreign scientist is that of Whitelaw Ainslie in 1813. Ainslie was a surgeon in the British Indian army, first placed in Chingleput, Madras Presidency. He was knighted in 1835, after his retirement.[80] His compilation, *The Materia Medica of Hindoostan and Artisans and Agriculturalists Nomenclature*, was published in Madras at the Government Press.[81] There is hardly any introduction to the text which might have enlightened one with some details upon the motive/idea behind the curious title. However, the opening paragraph throws some light. Explanation of the items listed and discussed included the answer why they had been put together: This was evidently:

a catalogue, an account, of such medicines of the British Materia Medica, as are either the produce of Hindoostan, or are brought to it from Asiatic countries, and are to be met with in the bazars of populous towns; including many drugs of the Tamool, Arabian, and Persian Materia Medica; as also the names given by the natives to different articles of diet and other things necessary for the comfort of the sick, and the appellations bestowed as those materials which are employed in arts and manufacture: to which is added in the Tamool, Telingoo, Dukhanis, English and Latin Languages, another and numerous catalogue of the various productions of the vegetable kingdom, which are used as food by the inhabitants of these provinces; and concluding with an Appendix in which are contained the titles of diseases in Tamool, Dukhanie, Telingoo, and English; together with a list of Malabar, Persian, Arabic and Sanskrit Medical works; a table of doses and weights, with the various forms of prescriptions, etc., in use amongst the Indians.

The above explanation reveals several things. First, the work indicates the probable beginning of the adoption of some of the more commonly known medical recipes followed in indigenous practices by British and Western physicians, etc., and the identification process of the plants, etc., which were the major ingredients from indigenous sources. Second, the trend of gradual adoption of the scientific nomenclatures of these ingredients and substances is also marked, but the addition of the vernacular, as well as Sanskrit names indicates that this was at a nascent stage as yet, in the early nineteenth century. Ainslie was definitely writing for the both the general populace, as well as for the sophisticated readers of the scientist community in Europe. The preface reveals the approach of the British officials of the times, illuminating the conscious and deliberate addition of the colony's plants to the British Materia Medica. It is clearly explained in the preface that this was a list of articles of the British Materia Medica that could be found in the 'Bazars of Hindoosthan', with all the indigenous and Latin nomenclature added to help identifying, as well as inclusion of 'Native Materia Medica'. Thus, while the botanists took care to change the nomenclature, the British physicians like Ainslie provided the official stamp of the empire on the plant resource of the colony, affecting fundamental change in the future of the indigenous systems of medicine (Ayurvedic, Siddha and Unani) overwhelmingly dependent on this resource.

There is another significant aspect revealed in Ainslie's compendium. He includes a list of texts that according to him were circulating among the people and indigenous practitioners as classics. A glance at this, however, shows that these evidently were not classics, and were rather derived from popular writings compiled by the late medieval indigenous practitioners. It also seems that Ainslie's information regarding this was hazy, incorrect and poor as compared to the information on actual medicinal ingredients and diseases. The indication is quite clear. The textual culture appears to have been languishing, and original texts, even of the medieval times like the *Bhāvaprakāśa,* were probably much less accessed. Ainslie's list[82] of 'Sanskrit Medical Books (to be met with on Lower India)' included the *Vaidya Chintamunny* (in Sanskrit) mentioned as 'a medical work by Durmuntrie' (as referred by the popular sources accessed by

Ainslie). A footnote (by Ainslie) explains that this was probably a reference to *Durwantrie* (Dhanvantari). The next work mentioned is the *Vyādia Shāttāsloikie* (in Sanskrit) said to be by the same author on Materia Medica. Other texts include *Goṇnā Pātum* (by Durmunrie again) on natural history and the nature of different ailments; *Curmā Cāndum* (Sanskrit) on causes of diseases by Durmuntrie; the *Roga Needānum*, by the same author, on peculiar constitutions and temperaments and the diseases arising there from, and lastly, the *Vydia Sastrum* again referred to Durmunrie, described as a great work on pharmacy and Materia Medica. The haziness of Ainslie's source would be clear from the fact that he includes another text, the *Silpey Sastrum* (Śilpa Śāstra) described as a work which treats the arts and manufactures of the Hindoos in the same list. Girindranath Mukhopadhyay had enlisted the *Roga Nidāna*, *Vaidya Cintāmaṇi* and *Vaidya Prakāśa Cikitsā*, *Cikitsāsāra Sangraha,* as well as *Dhanvantari Nighaṇṭu*—a dictionary of Materia Medica, under the works reputedly of the legendary figure of Dhanvantari.[83] Meulenbeld points out that out of these, the *Nighṇṭu* seems to be an old work belonging to the eleventh century. It was a classical text and used by later compilers like Maṅkha, who had composed the *Śrikaṅṭhacarita* in 1135 or 1145 according to Winternitz.[84] These texts, as Ainslie found them in use, were all late renditions of the Ayurveda system processed through innumerable mediating textual and practised cultures. Like most of the texts in circulation, they were not manuscripts, but rather the handed down guidelines through generations, and Ainslie's sources were likely to have been much closer to practised information than classical text-based knowledge. It would not be wrong to assume that the practising vaidyas had, in most cases, lost touch with the original tradition and were relying on proven, age-old traditions. One cannot make a judgement as to the value of the information, and Ainslie's work definitely made a great headway in bringing Ayurvedic Materia Medica to light for the first time in an official compilation before the British authority. But what is important to note is that, without the theoretical basis of the classical texts, the original philosophy of Ayurveda, the concept of matter and drugs, and the working principles of these drugs with the body would also be distant and lost. H.H. Wilson had pointed this out.[85] However, it must also be admitted that Ainslie's work was only an incipient one, and the investigation carried out by him was rather inspired by pragmatism than scholastic ambitions. This would also clarify why he had not accessed more deeply into the tradition of indigenous systems. Ainslie's compendium received a lot of attention and was revised as *Materia Indica* to be published in 1826. The title of the revised edition ran: *Materia Indica or some account of those articles which are employed by the Hindoos and other eastern nations in their medicine, arts and agriculture comprising also formulae with practical observations.*[86] It reveals further, the progress of appropriation and modification that was already set in motion in the last two centuries, and this was published in two volumes, this time from London.

By comparison, J.F. Royle's *An Essay on the Antiquity of the Hindu Medicine*, published in 1836, was the labour of much erudition, and constitutes a seriously informative work. John Forbes Royle was a surgeon and a naturalist, in the service of the East India Company. He was appointed the superintendent of the Botanic Garden in Saharanpur during 1823–31. Later, he went back to England and joined the Kings College, London, as a Professor of Materia Medica in 1837. He was in-charge of East India House's correspondence relating to vegetable productions till 1836, and most importantly, he was one of the founders of the philosophical club of the Royal Society in 1847. While in India in his youth Royle was an assiduous student of nature and had studied the Indian flora in-depth, especially in the region of the Himalayan foothills. He had studied the indigenous use of different substances as medicine. Not only that, his work reveals an attempt made to study the original Indian texts on Ayurveda.[87] Royle (1799–1858) actually compiled the comparative information from all ancient traditions of medicine including Persian, Arabian, Greek and Indian. It is quite clear that his source for Indian classical literature was H.H. Wilson's famous work published in 1823.[88] Ainslie did not have access to such erudite researches. It seems, however, that such studies in Ayurveda texts had got initiated around this time. Royle refers to *Charak*, *Suśruta* and the *Kalpastanum* section meant to guide one to the pharmacopoeia of Ayurveda. He also is aware of the fact that in most cases the works on indigenous medicine available in Tamil or Telugu languages were derived from these more classical sources. Regarding previous works he refers to Dr Heyne[89] and Whitelaw Ainslie. His general approach to the content of classical Ayurvedic works, in brief, was quite critical, but positive in evaluation. He puts down his opinion that,

> In their works, therefore, we find notices in all departments of medicine; instances of which I have not time to adduce; but it may be sufficient to mention that with much fanciful Anatomy, imaginative Physiology and absurd attention to numbers, there are accounts of poisons and their antidotes; mention of the diseases of women and children; with valuable notices relating to surgery, medicine, Materia Medica and Pharmacy.[90]

Royle's profound interest in this particular area (Materia Medica) of Ayurvedic tradition is clearly spelt out in his own words. He clearly evaluated the idea of medicines in classical Ayurvedic texts and commented: '. . . we have . . . a long list of useful medicines, of which many continue to be employed in modern as in very ancient times'.[91] On the other hand, he followed Wilson in being extremely cautious and critical about the devolution of the classical practices. He cited Wilson in noting this fall in the standard of medicinal prescriptions, as well as preparations as practised by the Indian vaidyas contemporary to his time. He wrote, 'with respect to their prescriptions and works, Professor Wilson makes the valuable remark that in proportion as the work is modern, the compounds became more extravagant, and assume a more important place in the practice'.[92] However, Royle tries to defend and minimize the fault by citing the general trend of mystification of science in the late middle ages all over the Old World by commenting that, 'But India, gentleman, is not the only country where the simplicity and clearness of observers has been displaced by the obscurity and mystification of compilers.'

Royle did give full attention to the text of *Suśruta Saṁhitā* on the question of Materia Medica. After noting the various sources of medicines and categories mentioned in the *Suśruta*, Royle goes on to describe the forms of preparations as he understood them[93] and this illuminates the early nineteenth century scientists' understanding of the traditional Ayurvedic pharmaceutical principles. This is precisely the significant point or juncture where one might observe and assess the possibilities of an interface between the indigenous and the Western Materia Medica, where the practitioners of the former might have directly benefited from an internalization and integration of the episteme. The door to the possibility remained open for the next 30–40 years, at least, till the 1880s and the ascendance of the pathogenic theory of diseases,[94] further progress in biochemistry with advances in cell theory,[95] and moleculer as well as organic chemistry.[96]

On the medicinal preparations in the *Suśruta*, Royle observed: 'This work is also extremely interesting, as giving probably the earliest notices respecting botanical geography: the sites and climates where different kinds of plants grow; the soils and seasons whence, and when medicinal plants should be collected; modes of keeping medicines and their preparation; time during which they remain good; with the weights and measures to be used'. Among the rules of pharmacy, Royle mentions 'Rasaha' (*rasa*), 'or the expressed juice of fresh vegetables'; 'Kalkaha' (*kalka*), 'the powder of well-dried plants'; 'Sitaha' (*śīta*), 'cold infusions'; and 'Srutaha, Kashaim and Pandaha', as decoctions. He also states that, 'Ingredients that are added to the decoction after the boiling is over, as syrup, honey, pippaly, salts &c are called Brativapam by the Sastrum.' 'Decoction made with oil is called Tailam.' 'Some authors, it is said, prescribe decoctions made of meat.' And finally talks about 'The Leham or electuary, is composed of a strong decoction of dry powdered ingredients, and some oil, or ghee (clarified butter), and sugar or honey.'[97] While on the one hand, Royle made such attempts to treat the traditional systems of medicine (Indian, Persian, Arabian and Greek) from a scholastic historical perspective, on the other hand, he also integrated the approach with the contemporary trends in the sciences he was closely observing. What is most important is that Royle's publication gives the flavour of a philosophical approach to an epistemology of 'pharmacy' as a science. Explaining the main interest of his own and the scholars working around and with him, he stated:

> . . . we are interested in the laws of vegetable physiology, that we may be able to weigh the influence of the various stimulants of light, heat, air and moisture; the effects of soils and aspects, that we may understand something of their operations, modifying the products of plants, and be able to select our barks; woods and roots, bulbs, leaves, flowers, and fruits, at the age and season when they contain the principles which render them useful as medicines in the most abundant and efficient state; whether these be gums, fecula, or saccharine principle; milky juice or resin; fixed or volatile oil; or any of those numerous alkaloids which are so completely altering the forms of medicines, since the subtleties of modern chemistry discovered them to be secreted in nature's nicer laboratory.[98]

Royle had relied on Linnaeus' system for botanical identification of plants from South and South-East Asia, but he had also explained the ideas of Augustine de Candolle, who in his work *Principes élémentaires de botanique*, questioned the efficacy of the Linneaus system of classification of plants by reproductive principles in diagnosing and grouping plants of similar medicinal properties together. Royle referred to the opinion of Petiver[99] too in finally going with Linneaus. However, he does acknowledge the difficulties in applying that system in understanding the Indian medicinal plants, which were just beginning to be identified and classified according to the Western discipline of botany. In the meantime, in conceptualizing Materia Medica as a part of the knowledge and practice of medicine, Royle also gave equal importance to therapeutics, and this holistic approach is perhaps what drew him towards the ancient Indian classical texts more than the current practices of Ayurveda around him or even the informative texts on Arabic medicine. Once more one can observe here how this might have been a possible juncture when the Indian nomenclature at least might have been integrated with the Western system, and the Western system of classification of plant family disseminated to Ayurvedic practitioners. However, on a more official and pedagogic level the indigenous textual culture on therapeutics, especially the botanical element in it, came close to the Western endeavours at organizing the knowledge of Materia Medica, and the efforts of trained Indians were allowed to converge with traditional knowledge as one shall shortly observe.

But coming back to the work of Royle, the compendium reveals an overweighing but inevitable consideration of the Western systems of epistemology in assessing the natural data. The vast expanse of his understanding of the subject of Materia Medica dwarfed the interests in traditions, and he dealt with his vision and understanding of this newly resurrected subject in the light of burgeoning modern sciences of the late eighteenth and early nineteenth centuries by including the overlapping branches of disciplines linked closely with it. He includes chemistry, physiology (to understand physiological actions of medicines) and pathology within the broad scope of the study. Royle enumerates the various aspects necessary for a full investigation of Materia Medica. He mentions the following: natural history characters, physical properties, chemical composition, physiological effects, therapeutical uses 'as well as pharmaceuticals preparations and its literary and commercial history'.[100] From there, he passes on to the importance of collecting information about the sources of procurement of the medicinal plants from distant terrains. Pratik Chakrabarti found Royle's project to have made 'a case for an expansion and relocation of the European scientific capital', giving out a call for expansions in research territories.[101] On close observation one can see that Royle was also attempting to integrate a canopied terrain of knowledge under *Pax Brittannica*. In this context, Royle clearly talks in terms Great Britain as a 'country', meaning the colonies too. He comes to the conclusion: 'we shall be led, therefore, to a geographical inquiry into the countries where our drugs are produced'.[102] He compares America and the Old World both as such sources, and while America, extensive in land and nature, was looked upon as a veritable source which was a less complicated zone for recording the sources (because of its late discovery, etc.), the Old World was definitely of more interest. Among these too, it was Asia which was regarded as the most important region: 'Asia, therefore, especially India and its islands, must always have contributed a great proportion of those articles which we now know can only be produced in tropical climates. One general observation may, I think, be applied to the whole; which is, that a large number of the more powerful drugs are produced on mountains, or in their vicinity. . . .'[103] Now this clearly would refer to his close study of the Himalayan flora which was being conducted even as he was publishing his early volume in *An Essay on the Antiquity of Hindoo Medicine*. The volumes on flora of Himalaya and Cashmere would come out together in the year 1839, and profuse links with the studies of William Roxburgh and Nathaniel Wallich can be observed in this volume.

While, therefore, the phenomenon of nineteenth-century physicians' and scientists' interest in Indian Materia Medica was clearly indicated, it was also the fact that this interest was evidently modern and designed in Western scientific paradigm under the civilizing hand of the Western nations, and the approach to the indigenous knowledge was primarily utilitarian, seconded by the avid curiosity of scholarship in unknown area. As Mark Harrison pointed out, when cholera began to ravage Europe for the first time in 1830, opinions of Indian medical men were sought and information from traditional medicine was utilized.[104] But instances like these were exceptional proving their rare occurrences.

Soon this source of natural medicines would be rendered redundant. Pharmacy and Materia Medica were already emerging as specific disciplines under medical science in the West, and this progress had primed and honed in on the scientific examination of ingredients and preparations. This was aided by institutionalized attention and creation of educational curricula and in exchange of researched information through science journals and reports. From 1836 *The British and Foreign Medical Review* began to be published from England under the editorship of John Forbes, a physician and scientist.[105] Although short-lived (published between the years 1836 and 1847), this journal created a basis for future correspondences on research through journals. The Philadelphia College of Pharmacy was founded in the United States of America in 1822 under the University of Sciences, Philadelphia. This institution began to publish the *American Journal of Pharmacy* from 1825. This was to set the trend in the United States.[106] The Pharmaceutical Society of Great Britain was established in 1841 and the American Pharmaceutical Association was founded in 1852. These were not only to have a distant but inevitable impact on the organization of what came to be referred as 'Indian Pharmacopoeia' in the parlance of the British and Western scientists. In fact, the effect would manifest itself in the form of new ventures to be made by Indians trained in Western medicine to remodel the Ayurveda pharmacopoeia too towards the end of the nineteenth century. The official Pharmacopoeia of India was compiled by Edward John

Waring in 1868.[107] Waring had acknowledged the contribution of a host of Indians in compiling the volume. He had included a list of medical officers who had provided reports and informations, including those in employment as Army Medical officers: Roma Chuer Bose, Odoy Chund Dutt, Sudrul Huq, Gopaul Chuder Pauttuck, Unnoda Churn Custogery, Dinnonauth Doss, Tara Chund Banjoorjee, Obhoy Churn Newgee, Turruck Chunder Luhory, Bhoobun Mohun Chatterjee, Kanny Lall Dey, and Raheem Khan.[108] Two among these officers took the initiative to formulate their own researches. Rai Kanny Lall Dey Bahadur had already published his own compendium on indigenous drugs in 1867 before Waring's Pharmacopoeia was officially published.[109] He was closely followed by the 'Native Doctor' Moodeen Sheriff, who published a supplement to the official pharmacopoeia, a compendium on synonyms of the plants referred in the former. U.C. Dutt, another trained medical officer, brought out his work, *The Materia Medica of the Hindus* in 1877.[110]

In the meantime, printing of Sanskrit treatises on Ayurveda and compilations in translations of informations from important texts in the vernaculars popular in the nineteenth century were being undertaken by indigenous researchers and institutions. The *Suśruta Saṁhitā* was the first to be printed by the Asiatic Society (of Bengal) in 1835. *Śārṅgadharasaṁhitā* was published from Mirzapur in Samvat 1900 which comes to about mid-1800s. The *Bhāvaprakāśa* was published from Bombay with Hindi translation in 1855. *Caraka Saṁhitā* was published in 1868 with commentaries of Gaṅgādhara and Cakrapāṇidatta from Calcutta in 1868. In 1870, Mahendalal Sarkar's English translation of two chapters of *Caraka Saṁhitā* was published in the Calcutta Journal of Medicine.[111] Among the lexicographical work, the *Nighaṇṭu Ratnākara* was published from Bombay in 1867, and a new compilation, *Āyūrvediya Paribhāṣā* was published in Bengali from Baharampur in 1869. The next three decades actually saw a further gearing up of this trend. Reprints (second) of *Bhāvaprakāśa* were published from Calcutta in 1875, that (second) of *Suśruta Saṁhitā* from Calcutta in 1877, *Caraka* from Calcutta and Baharampur in the same year. *Mādhava Nidāna* was published for the first time in Calcutta in the year 1876, *Rasendra Cintāmaṇi* was published from Calcutta in 1878, and *Rasa Ratnākara* from Calcutta in 1879. Most interestingly, the Rasatantra texts along with *Bhāvaprakāśa* were popular at the time as these contained minute descriptions of dispersing and processing materials, and drugs making. This is illuminated by new compilations of the *Āyūrvedīya Paribhāṣā* and another work, on *Dravya*, the *Āyurvedīya Dravyavidhāna* from Calcutta in 1875. The edition of *Vaishajya Ratnavali* by Binodlal Sen came out in 1890. This flurry of publication of editions and translations of the old manuscripts on Ayurveda and Rasatantra mark a new phase of indigenous consciousness and revivalist trend. Chittabrata Palit and Brahmananda Gupta talk about the 'Ayurvedic Renaissance' under the patronage of Kaviraj Gangadhara Ray and Gangaprasad Sen around the 1870s which was strengthened not only by the revival of the ancient textual studies, but also by establishment of educational institutions imparting Ayurvedic knowledge. The All India Ayurvedic Congress was formed in 1907.[112] Kavita Sivaramakrishanan has highlighted on the gestation and garnering of this process of legitimizing the indigenous alternative medicinal practices in the nineteenth century and early twentieth-centuries Punjab.[113] She has pointed out how the framework for revival and integration of Ayurveda and Tibb practitoners was geared to the emergent nationalist frame of reference. The tradition of Ayurveda had indeed assumed a cultural response theme in the nationalist agenda, especially in the Swadeshi days with a clear focus on the establishment of indigenous Ayurvedic pharmaceuticals, which were notable in Bengal, Uttar Pradesh and Punjab, as well as in southern India.

Against this backdrop, Kanny Lall Dey, Moodeen Sheriff and U.C. Dutt seem to have attempted a bridging effort, although they were distinct from each other. These attempts, especially at new compendiums of drugs, and in case of U.C. Dutt's volume, the effort made to align the old drugs with their newly defined science, reveal the passover to a new stage, with a particular focus on practical exigencies of popularizing and reforming of the knowledge for the practising vaidyas, as well as for the exhibition of the efficacy of traditional knowledge. Fundamentally speaking, the Swadeshi enterprises on Ayurvedic pharmacy were informed and indoctrinated by modern Western science, so much so that the chemistry in processes and stages of preparation were understood by the educated intelligentsia among practicing vaidyas, many of whom were holders of medical degrees from Government institutions. U.C. Dutta, Binodlall Sen, Mahendralal Sarkar, and Madhusudan Gupta, all fall within this bracket. However, what remained subsumed was the possibility of redefining the old science in new light. The epistemic significance of classical Ayurveda remained inert under the neglect of modern science.

Notes

1. Amita Chatterjee, 'Naturalism in Classical Indian Philosophy', *Stanford Encyclopaedia of Philosophy*, The Metaphysics Research Lab, Centre for the Study of Language and Information, Stanford: Stanford University, Spring 2012 edition.
2. Brajendranath (B.N.) Seal, *The Positive Sciences of the Ancient Hindus*, Delhi: Motilal Banarsidass Publishers Pvt. Ltd., 1958; James Haughton Woods, *The Yoga-System of Patañjali*, vol. 17, Harvard: The Harvard Oriental Series, repr., Delhi: Motilal Banarsidass, 2007.
3. Kenneth G. Zysk, *Asceticism and Healing in Ancient India, Medicine in the Buddhist Monastery*, Delhi: Motilal Banarsidass Publishers Pvt. Ltd., 1998.
4. Ibid., pp. 32–3; see D.P. Chattopadhyaya, *Science and Society in Ancient India*, Calcutta: Research India Publications, 1977, pp. 29–30, 172, 260–1, 323.
5. *Caraka Saṁhitā* (henceforth *CS*), *Sūtrasthāna* (henceforth *Sūtra*), Ch. I, ślokas. 46–7. *Caraka Saṁhitā* (Text with English Translation), P.V. Sharma, Varanasi: Chaukhamba Orientalia, edition 2000 has been consulted for all references from this text.
6. *CS, Sūtra*, Ch. I, pp. 44–5.
7. Ibid., p. 50.
8. Ibid., p. 51.
9. Ibid., p. 53.

10. Ibid., p. 62.
11. Ibid., p. 64.
12. Ibid., pp. 63–6.
13. Nupur Dasgupta, 'Texts and Mentalities: Exploring an emergent discourse on body and health in some early Indian treatises', in *Revisiting Early India: Essays in Memory of D.C. Sircar*, ed. Suchandra Ghosh et al., Kolkata: R.N. Bhattacharya, 2013, pp. 219–46.
14. *Suśruta Saṁhitā* (henceforth *SS*), *Sūtrasthāna*, Ch. I, śloka 20. The particular edition consulted: *Suśruta Saṁhitā,* Text with English Translation, A Full And Comprehensive Introduction, Addition Text, Different Readings, Notes, Comparative Views, Index, Glossary And Plates, Kaviraj Kunjalal Bhishagratna, in 3 vols., vol. XXX, Varanasi: Chowkhamba Sanskrit Series, 1998.
15. Ibid., śloka 21.
16. Ibid., śloka 22.
17. Ibid., śloka 23.
18. *SS, Sūtra*, Ch. I, śloka 27.
19. *SS, Sūtra*, Ch. III, śloka 50. Translation of the text from Kaviraj Kunjalal Bhishagratna, text with English translation, 1998, op. cit., p. 28.
20. *SS, Sūtra*, Ch. XXXVIII.
21. Ibid., ślokas 39–40.
22. *SS, Sūtra*, Chs. XL, XLI and XLII.
23. *SS, Sūtra*, Ch. XL, śloka 2.
24. Ibid., ślokas 3, 4, 5–8 and 9.
25. Ibid., ślokas 10–15.
26. Ibid., śloka 15.
27. Ibid., Ch. XLI
28. Ibid., śloka, 4.
29. Ibid., ślokas. 19–21. Translation of the text from Kaviraj Kunjalal Bhishagratna, text with English translation, op. cit., 1998, p. 356.
30. Andrew Wear, *Knowledge and Practice in English Medicine, 1550–1680*, Cambridge: Cambridge University Press, 2000, pp. 11–45; Juanita G.L.A. Burnaby and Juanita G.L. Burnby, 'A Study of the English Apothecary 1660–1760', *Medical History Supplement* 3, London: Wellcome Institute for the History of Medicine, 1983.
31. *CS, Sūtra*, Ch. IV.
32. For example see the publication of Benjamn Kligler and Roberta A. Lee, *Integrative Medicine: Principles of Practice*, New York: McGraw Hill Companies, 2004, pp. 234, 236.
33. He states that, conceptually Ayurvedic treatment consists of *śodhana* (purification of the body by eliminating *mala*), followed by *śamana* (pacification of vitiated *doṣas*). For *śodhana*, five measures are employed which are collectively known as Pañcakarma. They are vamana (emesis), virecana (purgation), āsthāpana (non-unctuous enema), anuvāsana (unctuous enema) and śirovirecana (head-evacuation or snuffing). Discussions in Priyavrat Sharma, *Essentials of Ayurveda*: *Sodasangahrdayam*, 2nd edn., Delhi: Motilal Banarsidass, 1998, p. lv.
34. *CS, Sūtra*, Ch. IV.
35. *SS, Cikitsā,* Chs. XXXI–XL.
36. See, G.J. Meulenbeld, Appendix Two, from *The Mādhavanidāna with 'Madhukośa', the Commentary by Vijayarakṣita and Śrikaṇṭhadatta*, Leiden: E.J. Brill, 1974, Delhi edn., 2008, pp. 412–13.
37. Meulenbeld, op. cit., pp. 423–4.
38. It has not been possible to assign the exact date to the thinker, as Karl Potter points out in *Indian Metaphysics and Epistemology: the Tradition of Nyāya-Vaiśeṣika up to Gaṅgeśa*,

part I, Delhi: Motilal Banarsidass Pvt. Ltd., 1977, p. 9. But according to most other scholars, he belongs definitely to the first century CE, as pointed out by Bruno D'Amore, 'Secondary School Students' Mathematical Argumentation and Indian Logic (Nyaya)', in the *Journal For the Learning of Mathematics*, vol. 25, no. 2, July 2005, pp. 26–32.

39. Potter, op. cit., p. 9.
40. Eric Frauwallner, *History of Indian philosophy*, vol. II, The Nature-philosophical schools and the Vaisesika system; Eric Frauwallner, *The System of the Jaina: The Materialism*, Delhi, 1st edn., 1973; repr., Motilal Banarsidass, 1993, p. 8; Potter, op. cit., Delhi, 1977, p. 9.
41. Potter, op. cit., p. 9.
42. B.N. Seal, op. cit., pp. 92–123.
43. Potter, op. cit., p. 10.
44. *Aṣṭāṅgahṛdaya* (henceforth *AH*), *Sūtrasthāna*, Ch. X, pp. 25–6. Upendranath Sen and Debendranath Sen, *Aṣṭāṅgahṛdaya, Maharṣi Vāgbhaṭa*, Bengali translation, 2 vols., Kolkata: Deepāyan, first published, 1937; repr., *Srāban* 1407 (Bengali year), has been consulted for all references from this text.
45. James Haughton Woods, *Yoga System of Patanjali*, 1914, repr., Cambridge, Massachusetts: Harvard University Press, repr., Delhi: Motilal Banarsidass, 2007, Introduction, pp. xx–xxi, xiii–xix.
46. *AH, Sūtra*, Ch. X, pp. 30–1.
47. G.J. Meulenbeld, *The Mādhavanidāna with 'Madhukośa'*, Introduction, translation and notes, the commentary by Vijayarakṣita and Śrikanṭhadatta, Leiden: E.J. Brill, 1974; Delhi edn., 2008, p. 13.
48. *Cakrapāṇidatta, Dravyaguṇasaṁgraha, Śloka* I. Two editions have been consulted for this text: (1) *Cakrapāṇidatta, Dravyaguṇasaṁgraha, with commentary by Śivadāsasena*, edited by Jivananda Vidyasagara Bhattacharya, Calcutta: Siddhesvara Printer, 1897; edition collected from Sanskrit Sahitya Parishad Library; and (2) *Dravya Gooṇa Sangraha (A Sanskrit System of Materia Medica)* by *Chakrapāni Datta with Commentary by Shivadās Sen*, ed. Vaidya Jādavjī Tricumjī Ācharyā, with Hindi commentary by Vaidya Chandrakānt Sonāre, Jaikrishnadas Ayurveda Series, no. 85, Varanasi: Chaukhamba Orientalia, repr., 2006.
49. *Dravyaguṇasaṁgraha, Māṣādivarga*, p. 28.
50. Ibid., *Dhānyavarga*, pp. 12–14.
51. *Bhāvaprakāśa, Miśraka* Prakaraṇa; The edition consulted for this text: *Bhāvaprakāśa of Bhāvamiśra*, Text, English Translation, Notes, appendices and Index, K.R. Srikantha Murthy, 2nd edn., 2 vols., Varanasi: Chaukhamba Krisnadas Academy, 2001.
52. Ibid., *Dvitīya Bhāga*, part II, Chs. I–VIII.
53. This is referred in J. Eggeling, Catalogue of the Sanskrit Manuscripts in the Library of the India Office, part V, no. 2751, 96b, folio, 130, London, 1896, p. 981.
54. For most of the discussion on dates of the works cited in the paper, I have consulted not only the editors' comments on the works that are in print and have been consulted by me, but also G.J. Meulenbeld's discussion in the Appendix 2, of his edition on 'Mādhavanidāna'.
55. *Bhāvaprakāśa* of Bhāvamiśra, op. cit., Pūrva Khaṇḍa, Prathama Bhāga, Harītakyādi Varga, *śloka* 104.
56. *Bhāvaprakāśa* of Bhāvamiśra, ed. and tr. Prof. K.R. Srikantha Murthy, vol. I, Varanasi: Chaukhamba Krishnadas Academy, 2001, p. 175.
57. *Bhāvaprakāśa, śloka*, pp. 118–19.
58. K.R. Srikantha Murthy, op. cit., p. 178.
59. Pūrvakhaṇḍa-Dvitīyabhāga, Bheṣaja Vidhāna Prakaraṇa, *śloka*, 8, 25 are especially indicated here.

60. U.C. Dutt, *The Materia Medica of the Hindus*, with a glossary of Indian Plants by George King, Additions and Alterations by Kaviraj Binodlal Sen and Ashutosh Sen, 1877; repr., Delhi: Mittal Publications, 1989.
61. Bhaiṣajyaratnāvalī (transcription from original Sanskrit word)/Consulted edition of the text: *Vaishajya Ratnavali* (the spelling referred in the edition by Binodlal Sen), enlarged, improved and published with a Bengali translation by Kaviraj Binodlal Sen, first pub., Calcutta, Ayurveda yantra Sri Madhusudan Bandyopadhyay pub., 1798 śakābda (1872 CE), 3rd edn., 1296, Bengali year (1890 CE).
62. Ibid., 'Introduction', p. 4.
63. Garcia da Orta, *Coloquios dos simples e drogas e cousas medicinais da India,* volume consulted: *Colloquies on the Simples and Drugs of India By Garcia Da Orta*, new ed. (Lisbon, 1895) edited and annotated by Conde De Ficalho, translated with an introduction and index by Sir Clements Markham, London: Henry Sotheran & Co., MCMXIII, 1913 in 2 vols. The work was first published from Goa in 1563 by Johannes de Andem.
64. Christofori Acosta, *Tractado Delas Drogas, y medicinas de las Indias Orientales,* con fus Platas debuxadas albuio por Christoual Acosta medico y cirujano que las vio ocularmente, En Burgos, por Martin de Victoria, 1578.
65. Hendrik van Rheede tot Draakestein (1678–1703) (in Latin), *Hortus Indicus Malabaricus*, Latin version consulted, *Horti Malabarici, adornata Henricum van Rhede tot Draakestein et Johannem Caeserium et Theodorum, Janson ab Almeloveen and Joannes Commelinus,* sumptibus, Joannis van Someren et Haeredum Joannis van Dyck, Henrici & Viduae Theodori Boom, Amstelaedami, 1686, pars Prima, Preface, 20 April 1675.
66. William Roxburg, *Hortus Bengalensis or a Catalogue of the Plants growing in the Honourable East India company's Botanic Garden at Calcutta,* Calcutta: Mission Press, 1814, Introduction, p. v.
67. Nathaniel Wallich, *Plantae Asiaticae Rariores*, vol. I, London: Treuttel & Wurtz, Treuttel Jun. & Richter, 1830.
68. Garcia Da Orta, op. cit., Introduction, pp. viii–ix; van Rheede tot Draakestein, op. cit., Alia Prefaetio ad Lectorem, see the handwritten acclamation by Ranga Bhatta, Vinayaka Pandit and Appu Bhat in Sanskrit script., Pars Prima; Further discussion in Richard Grove, *Green Imperialism: Colonial Expansion, Tropical Island Edens and the Origins of Environmetalism*, Delhi: Oxford University Press, 1995, pp. 80–1.
69. Grove, op. cit., pp. 77–8.
70. Caroli Clusii Atrebatis, opera X, *Hispanico sermone Latinus, in Epitomen contractus, and quibusdam notis illustratus* (Christofori Acosta, Medici et Chirurgi, Aromatum et Medicamentorum in Orientali India Nascentium, Liber: Plurimum Lucis Adserens iis quae Doctore Garcia de Orta in hoc genere scripta sunt), Antwerp, 1582.
71. N.C. Majumdar and D.N. Guha Bakshi, A Few Linnaean Specific Names Typified by the Illustrations in Rheede's Hortus Indicus Malabaricus, *Taxon*, vol. 28, no. 4, August 1979, pp. 353–4; William T. Steam and Carl Linnaeus' 'Acquaintance with Tropical Plants', *Taxon*, vol. 37, no. 3, August 1988, pp. 776–81.
72. Julius Von Sachs, *History of Botany (1530–1860),* authorized translation by Henry E.F. Garnsey, revised by Isaac Bayley Balfour, second Impression, London: Clarendon Press, 1906.
73. Stephen Hales, *Vegetable Staticks, or an Account of some Statical Experiments on the sap in Vegetables*, London: W. & J. Innys, 1727. Also see Francis Darwin, 'Stephen Hales 1677– 1761', in *Makers of British Botany, A Collection of Biographies by Living Botanists*, ed. Francis Wall Oliver, Cambridge: Cambridge University Press, 1913, p. 65.
74. Joseph Priestly, *Experiments and Observations Related to Various Branches of Natural Philosophy*, London: J. Johnson, 1779, section XXVIII, pp. 298–304; sections XXX–XXXII, pp. 320–9.

75. Julius Von Sachs, op. cit., p. 76, fn 1.
76. William Roxburgh, M.D., Preface, *Plants of the Coromondel Selected from drawings and descriptions presented to the Hon. Court of Directors of the East India Company*, published by their order under the Direction of Sir Joseph Banks, BART, P.R.S., vol. I, London: W. Bulmer & Co., George Nicol, Bookseller to His Majesty, Pall Mall, 1795.
77. N. Wallich, *Numerical List of Dried Specimens of Plants in the Museum of the Honble East India Company which have been supplied by Wallich, superintendent of Botanic Garden, Calcutta*, London (s.n.), handwritten document, from http://www.biodiversitylibrary.org/permissions, accessed on 15 February 2010; Wallich, op. cit.; For general discussions see Desmond Ray, *European Discovery of Indian flora*, Oxford, Royal Botanic Gardens: Oxford University Press, 1992; repr., Delhi: Oxford University Press, 1994.
78. J. David Phillipson, 'Phytochemistry and medicinal plants', *Phytochemistry*, vol. 56, 2001, pp. 237–43; Development of the cinchona extract from cinchona plant by the French scientists, Caventou and Pelletier; see R.C. Burrell, 'Phytochemistry. What it is and how it has developed', *J. Chem. Educ.*, vol. 14, no. 11, 1937, p. 520; E.R. Scerri, *The Periodic Table: Its Story and Its Significance*; New York: Oxford University Press, 2007, Chs. 3 and 4, pp 63–123.
79. Projit Bihari Mukharji, *Nationalizing the Body, The Medical Market, Print and Daktari Medicine*, London and New York: Anthem Press, 2011, pp. 228–47.
80. See *The Gentleman's Magazine*, vol. 159, 1835, p. 87; D.V. Subba Reddy, 'Dr Whitelaw Ainslie and his contribution to Materia Medica and history of medicine in India', *Bulletin of the Institute of History of Medicine*, vol. 2, no. 1, Hyderabad, 1972, pp. 35–51.
81. Whitelaw Ainslie, *Materia Medica of Hindoostan and Artisan's and Agriculturalist's Nomenclature*, published by the Special Permission of the Government of Madras, printed at the Government Press, 1813, inner cover page.
82. Ibid., pp. 290–1.
83. G. Mukhopadhaya, *History of Indian Medicine*, Calcutta: University of Calcutta, 1922; repr., New Delhi: Munshiram Manoharlal, vol. II, 2003, pp. 328–30.
84. Meulenbeld, op. cit., Delhi edn., p. 413.
85. H.H. Wilson, 'On the Medical and Surgical Sciences of the Hindus' (first published in *The Oriental Magazine*, vol. 1, Calcutta, February 1823, pp. 207–12, 349–56), reprinted in *Works by the Late Horace Haymen Wilson*, vol. III, *Essays Analytical, Critical and Philosophical on Subjects Connected with Sanskrit Literature*, Collected and edited by Dr Reinhold Rost, vol. I, London: Trübner & Co., 1864, p. 270.
86. Whitelaw Ainslie, *Materia Medica; Or, some Account of Those Articles which are Employed by the Hindoos and other Eastern Nations in their Medicine, Arts and Agriculture*, vol. I, London: Longman, Rees, Orme, Brown and Green, 1826.
87. J.F. Royle, *An Essay on the Antiquity of Hindoo Medicine including an Introductory Lecture to the Course of Materia Medica*, London: Wm. H. Allen & Co., 1837.
88. Wilson, op. cit., pp. 269–76, 380–92.
89. Benjamin Heyne, *Tracts historical and statistical on India; with journals of several tours through various parts of the peninsula; also, an account of Sumatra, in a series of letters*, London: Black, Parry & Co., 1814, Tract VI, Trans of some Indian Books, I: Kalpastanum, II: Treatise on Medicine, pp. 125–71. Cited in J.F. Royle, op. cit., p. 48.
90. Royle, op. cit., pp. 48–9.
91. Ibid., p. 52. Quotation from H.H. Wilson in Royle.
92. Ibid., pp. 53–5.
93. This began from the 1870s–80s in earnest. Joseph Lister went on to develop applications of the pathogenic theory in surgery from 1870s; Robert Koch's Postulates were published in 1890. See Ann Lamont, 'Joseph Lister: Father of Modern Surgery', *Creation*,

vol. 14, no. 2, March 1992, pp. 48–51; T.D. Brock, *Robert Koch: A life in medicine and bacteriology*, Washington, DC: American Society of Microbiology Press, 1999.

94. Joseph Stuart Fruton, *Proteins, Enzymes, Genes: The Interplay of Chemistry and Biology*, New Haven, Connecticut: Yale University Press, 1999, Ch. 4; William Coleman, *Biology in the Nineteenth Century, Problems of Form, Function and Transformation,* first pub. by New York: John Wiley & Sons, 1971; repr., Cambridge: Press Syndicate of the University of Cambridge, 1977, pp. 5–7, 12–15, and Ch. II.
95. John Dalton's theory gained ground only towards the beginning of the twentieth century with Jean Perin's experiment. Jean Perin, *Atoms,* authorized translation by D. LI. Hammick, New York: D. van Nostrand Co., 1916.
96. Royle, 1837, op. cit., pp. 54–5.
97. Ibid., p. 3.
98. Ibid.
99. James Petiver was an apothecary and a Fellow of the Royal Society ([vide James Petiver, 'An Account of Some Indian Plants, etc. with Their Names, Descriptions and Vertues, Philosophical Transactions (1683–1775)'], vol. 20, 1698, pp. 313–35.
100. Royle, op. cit., p. 23.
101. Pratik Chakrabarti, *Materials and Medicine, Trade, conquest and therapeutics in the eighteenth century,* Manchester and New York: Manchester University Press, 2010, p. 133.
102. Royle, op. cit., p. 24.
103. J.F. Royle, *Illustrations of the Botany and Other Branches of Natural History of the Himalayan Mountains and of the Flora of Cashmere*, 2 vols., London: W.H. Allen & Co., 1839.
104. Mark Harrison, 'Tropical Medicine in Nineteenth Century India', *British Journal for the History of Science*, vol. 25, no. 3, September 1992, pp. 299, 318–20.
105. P.J. Bishop, 'The Life and Writings of Sir John Forbes (1787–1861)', *Tubercle*, vol. 42, 1961, p. 255; William Alexander Greenhill, 'Forbes, John (1787–1861)', *Dictionary of National Biography*, 1885–1900, vol. 19, pp. 405–7; E.A. Parkes, 'Sir John Forbes, M.D., D.C.L., F.R.S.', in Memorium, *The British and Foreign Medico-Chirurgical Review,* vol. xxix, January–April 1862, pp. 271–82.
106. William Frederick Norwood, 'American Medical Education From the Revolutionary War to the Civil War', *History of Medical Education Series,* June 1957, vol. 32, no. 6, pp. 433–47; Glenn Sonendecker, ed., *Kremers and Urdang's History of Pharmacy*, Madison: American Institute of the History of Pharmacy, 1976; repr. pb. edn., 1986, Chs. 14 and 15; Joseph. W. England, ed., *The First Century of the Philadelphia College of Pharmacy 1821–1921*, Philadelphia: Philadelphia College of Pharmacy and Science, 1922.
107. Edward John Waring, *Pharmacopoeia of India*, India Office, London: W.H. Allen & Co., 1868, p. xiii.
108. Kanny Lall Dey, *Indigenous Drugs of India or Short Descriptive Notices of the Medicines Both Vegetable and Mineral in Common Use Among the Natives of India*, Calcutta: Thacker & Spink, 2nd edn., 1867.
109. Moodeen Sheriff, *Supplement to the Pharmacopoeia of India, or a Catalogue of Indian Synonyms of the Medicinal Plants, Products, Inorganic and Organic Substances Included in that Work with Explanatory and Descriptive Remarks, and C. in Fourteen Languages*, Madras: Government Gazette Press, 1869.
110. Udoy Chand Dutt, *The Materia Medica of the Hindus Compiled from Sanskrit Medical Works*, Calcutta: Thacker & Spink, 1877.
111. For some details see Gurdip Singh and P.D. Joshi, 'Impact of European Science and Technology on the Development of Modern Ayurveda During 19th Century', *Indian Journal of History of Science*, vol. 17, no. 2, 1982, pp. 313–25.

112. Chittabrata Palit, 'Ayurveda in Colonial Bengal: Survival and Revival', in *Ancient System of Rasayana, Suvarnatantra—A Treatise on Alchemy/Rasayana*, ed. Chittabrata Palit and Nupur Dasgupta, Delhi: Kalpaz Publications, 2009, pp. 147–60; Brahmananda Gupta, 'Indigenous Medicine in the Nineteenth-Twentieth Century Bengal', in *Asian Medical Systems: A Comparative Study*, ed. Charles Leslie, Delhi: Motilal Banarsidass, 1998, pp. 368–78.
113. Kavita Sivaramakrishnan, *Old Potions, New Bottles, Recasting Indigenous Medicine in Colonial Punjab (1850–1945), New Perspectives in South Asian History Series 12*, Hyderabad: Orient Longman, 2005, pp. 1850–945.

8

Revisiting an Indigenous Medical Practice

The *Tikadars* in Colonial Bengal

Arabinda Samanta

Admittedly, scholars of colonial medicine have not paid adequate attention to the role of indigenous medical practice. 'It is remarkable', observes Irfan Habib, 'that the practice of smallpox inoculation that was being followed extensively by "primitive practitioners" in the eighteenth century from Turkey to Bengal seems to have been totally ignored in contemporary Unani and Ayurvedic text.'[1] Nevertheless, the practice persisted, and it continued with remarkable tenacity till the advent of Jennerian vaccination that dislodged it from colonial Bengal. The present essay would arguably seek to explore how smallpox epidemics in colonial Bengal was intervened by indigenous practice of inoculation/variolation by the *tikadars* and how the disease was interpreted, understood and constructed in the context of people's collective imagination and cultural tradition.

Antiquity and Incidence

Smallpox had all along been a general disease in India. People did die from it, and even many of those who recovered, carried marks of the disease with them as pits on the face and sometimes even the loss of the eyes, and such other defects. In order to diminish the evils of smallpox, inoculation or *tika* was resorted to in parts of India. Matter was taken from a person who was ill of smallpox and inserted under the skin of a healthy person. People who were, thus, 'inoculated' did get smallpox but in a much milder form than it came of itself. But inoculation/variolation was not without danger. Sometimes, a very severe attack followed and the person used to die of it. Again, inoculation kept up the disease.[2]

The incidence of smallpox in India was great and uniform from year to year ever since its presumably first historically recorded virulence in Assam in 1574.[3]

Stavorinus, a Dutch naval commander in Chinsura, recorded an incidence of severe type of smallpox in Bengal in 1770, which he argued, spread among persons of all ages and killed people in great numbers.[4] Holwell wrote in 1767 about the prevalence of smallpox in Bengal where every seventh year without any respite smallpox raged epidemically during the months of March, April and May, until the annual returning rains, around the middle of June, put a stop to its fury.[5]

However, references to a disease called *masurika*, a kind of pulse similar to the kind of eruptions during the disease, in early medical compilations suggest that it was much an ancient affliction among the people of India. *Basanta Roga* or smallpox was also known as *paproga, shitalika, shitala, gunri*, and *guli*.[6] Even *masurika* was of nine varieties: *bataja, pittaja, slesmaja, tridosaja, batapittaja, bataslesmaja, pittaslesmaja, raktaja, and charmaja*.[7] The term *small pokkes*, meaning pockets and bags, was introduced in India in the fifteenth century. Due to its prevalence during spring, the ailment was also known in eastern India as the *Basanta Roga* or the spring disease.[8] *Basanta Rwitu*, being a season of festivities facilitating social mobility, helped transmit the disease in all directions. Moreover, the political disintegration of the mighty Mughals facilitating the British acquisition of power, the recurring Maratha raids resulting in displacement of population, the severe drought of 1769 and the consequent famine of 1770, might have favoured its dissemination.[9] Admittedly, therefore, smallpox was a scourge of India, responsible for more victims than all other diseases combined, outstripping even cholera and plague in its tenacity and malignancy.[10]

The Disease Deity and the *Tikadar*

What exactly was the nature of socio-religious observances associated with the propitiation of smallpox through inoculation? From very early times, one knows, there existed in India the worship of a goddess of smallpox, Shitala, and among certain castes it is still a rule to take no precaution whatever against the disease, a visitation of it in their households being regarded as a sign that they are favoured by the Goddess. Smallpox was a direct intrusion of the Goddess into the body of her victim. She expressed her presence in the patient's body in the form of fever.[11] If worshipped, it was believed, she would prevent the disease, but if provoked, the patient would be perished.

But if familiarity with this dreaded disease evoked its ritualization, believes David Arnold, it prompted attempts at medical control as well.[12] For more than half a century after the introduction of vaccination in 1802, nearly all the inhabitants in some parts of India were wedded to the practice of *tika* or smallpox inoculation, and many thousands of Brahmin inoculators, having great influence with the people, were violent opponents of vaccination.[13] This was so, partly because of the religious inhibitions and partly because of the large expenses involved, which had made it extremely difficult for the Bengalis to employ skilled medical agencies in the actual work of vaccinating and for many years the only vaccinators who could be obtained were generally illiterate and very ignorant. The purdah system which led to the lack of female vaccinators also posed serious problem.[14]

There was, however, certain kind of rumours spread among the urban poor. During the summer of 1878, for instance, when smallpox had broken out in Lahore, John Campbell Oman was told by one of his servants that 'the Sarkar had given orders that the native women should be vaccinated, not as usual, on the arm but on the breast'.[15] From time to time, indeed, prejudices arose and rumours were spread in rural areas, which on account of the credulity of the people resulted in a serious halt to the progress of vaccination. A very early prejudice against vaccination arose because vaccine disease came from the cow, an animal highly revered by the Hindus. One of the rumours causing most difficulty in early years was to the effect that the object of vaccination was to set the 'government mark' upon the people who would afterwards be sent as coolies to other British possessions. Another rumour that floated was that the 'government mark' was a means of obtaining a census of the people with a view to imposing a new capitation tax.[16] It was a ploy of introducing plague; it was a well-calculated attempt at proselytization; it was intended to sacrifice the vaccinated people for ensuring construction of a bridge or railway embankment.[17] Much more incredulous rumours were afloat for many years.

The trade of *tikadars*, therefore, flourished. It was noted that in 1850 there was at least one *tikadar* for every 8 or 10 groups of houses, and that in Calcutta town alone the names and addresses of 68 inoculators were known in that year. From 1848 to 1867 attempts were made by various civil surgeons to estimate the extent to which smallpox inoculation was practised in Bengal. From an examination of more than 35,000 people in those years, it appears that over 81 per cent had been inoculated.

How was the feat performed? At least two accounts of the mode in which the operation was performed by the professional inoculators of comparatively older times in India are available: one by R. Coult in 1731, and the other by J.Z. Holwell in 1767. Francis Buchanan has also elaborated information on the practice and its practitioners.[18] All of them did concur that inoculation consisted of matters originally taken from the pus of smallpox pustules with a thick needle, but disagree on the process of administration. While Coult argued that the pus was taken from a patient when the pox came to maturity, Holwell believed that it was taken from persons who contracted it in a milder form from the inoculation itself and was then preserved in cotton within a rag for a year. Buchanan says it was only taken from pustules of those who had contracted the ailment 'naturally', and kept cotton for no more than three days. Again, while Coult believed that punctures were made with a needle, impregnated with the pus, the *tika* was laid on the upper arm, Holwell argued that the incisions were made on the outside of the arm by a barber's instrument for cutting nails, and the variolous matter was secured by placing it in a moistened cotton-wad put on the cut for hours. Buchanan corroborated Holwell that first the incisions were made and then the variolous matter soaked in the cotton was rubbed on them.[19]

There is again little agreement in the contemporary evidences about who the inoculators were. Holwell says, 'inoculation is performed in Hindoostan by a particular tribe of Brahmins', who came on regular tours from Brindaban, Allahabad, Banaras, and 'arrive commonly in the Bengal provinces early in February'.[20] Buchanan believes that the inoculators were 'of both religions (i.e. Hindus and Muslims) and of all castes'. *Tikadars* or mark-makers also hailed from marginalized caste groups such as *napits* or barbers, *malis* or gardeners, cultivators, garland-makers, *tanty* or weavers, *koomars* or potters.

Both Holwell and Buchanan believed the success rate to be high. To Holwell, it was 'a miracle to hear that one in a million fails of receiving the infection' from the inoculation. Buchanan testifies that when smallpox struck Diaper as an epidemic, it could take as its tolls only one of a hundred of those inoculated. J.Z. Holwell, however, gives a detailed story of how the feat was performed:

> The inhabitants of Bengal, knowing the usual time when the inoculating Brahmins annually return, observe strictly the regimen enjoined, whether they determine to be inoculated or not; this preparation consists only in abstaining for a month from fish, milk, ghee. . . . When the Brahmins begin to inoculate, they pass from house to house and operate at the door, refusing to inoculate any one who has not, on a strict scrutiny, duly observed the preparatory course enjoined them. They inoculate indifferently on any part, but left to their choice, they prefer the outside of the arm midway between the wrist and elbow, and shoulders for the females. Previous to the operation, the operator takes a piece of cloth in his hand and with it gives a dry friction upon the part intended for inoculation, for the space of eight or ten minutes; then, with a small instrument, he wounds by many slight touches, about the size of a silver groat, just making the smallest appearance of blood. Then opening a linen double rag (which he always keeps in a cloth round his waist) he takes from thence a small pledgit of cotton charged with the variolous matter, which he moistens with two or three drops of the Ganges water, and applies it to the wound, fixing it on with a slight bandage, and ordering it to remain on for six hours without being moved; then the bandage to be taken off, and the pledged to remain until it falls off itself. The cotton, which he preserves in a double calico rag, is saturated with matter from the inoculated pustules of the preceding year; for they never inoculate neither with fresh matter, nor with matter from the disease caught in the natural way, however distinct and mild the species. Early in the morning succeeding the operation, four *collons* of cold water are ordered to be thrown over the patient from the head downwards, and to be repeated every morning and evening until the fever comes on, which usually is about the close of the sixth day from the inoculation; then to desist until the appearance of the eruption (about three days) and then to pursue the cold bathing, as before, through the course of the disease, and until the scabs of the pustules drop off. They are ordered to open all pustules with a sharp pointed thorn as soon as they begin to change their colour, and whilst the matter continues in a fluid state. Confinement to the house is absolutely forbid, and the inoculated are ordered to be exposed to every air

that blows; and the utmost indulgence they are allowed, when the fever comes on, is to be laid upon a mat at the door. But in fact the eruption fever is generally so inconsiderable and trifling as very seldom to require this indulgence. . . . Their regime is ordered to consist of all the refrigerating things the climate and season produce. . . . These instructions being given, and an injunction laid on the patient to make a thanksgiving *poojah* or offering to the goddess on their recovery, the operator takes his fees, which from the poor is a pun of cowries, equal to about one penny sterling, and goes on to another door, down one side of the street and up on the other; and is thus employed from morning till night, inoculating sometimes eight or ten in a house.[21]

It can also be seen from the contemporary accounts that the operation was carried out with great care, and there can be no doubt that in those comparatively olden times a high degree of knowledge about the procedure necessary for success had been attended. In this connection, certain other important details regarding the practice that was carried out during that period are worth mentioning: first, infants at breast were not inoculated, but children above one year of age were considered old enough for the operation. Second, the rules to which, in accordance with ancient custom, everyone desiring inoculation had to conform were not only arduous in themselves but interfered greatly with daily work and business. The restrictions included abstinence for a month prior to inoculation from milk, fish and *ghee*. In addition, for 21 days after the operation, no member of an inoculated household was permitted to have contact with the outside world, and no person from another village was permitted to enter a house containing inoculated patients. Each time, if either of these rules was infringed, the guilty person was regarded as 'unclean', and was required to bathe and to put on different clothes. Third, the early professional inoculators freely acknowledged the infectiousness of the disease set up by inoculation and the elaborate code of rules to which the people in inoculated villages had to conform, bears abundant testimony to this. Therefore, no inoculation was allowed in a village unless nearly all the unprotected people were willing to have the operation performed; all the inoculation in a village were done on the same day; women who were pregnant and others who could not arrange to be inoculated on the date fixed had to leave the village until the danger of infection was past. The clothes of all inoculated persons were kept for 21 days and then washed on a fixed day separately from those of unprotected people; no barber was allowed to ply his trade in any house where inoculated persons resided; bathing in public tanks were not permitted until the eruption had disappeared. Finally, the fatality attending the operation, depending as it did very greatly on the skill and care of the operator, was probably very low at the period to which I am referring. This is evidenced by Holwell himself, and much later by the observations of Bedford who saw 79 inoculations performed without a death, and Wise reported that in Chittagong the mortality attending the operation was only 0.5 per cent.[22]

One can see then that in olden days when all the rules enumerated above were strictly adhered to, and when only the professional Brahmin inoculators performed the operation, the measure proved a real blessing to the inhabitants of certain parts of India, especially Bengal. One must also remember that the conditions of certain parts of India, where the operation was general, were very favourable to the success of the measure. The great bulk of the inhabitants of Bengal, Assam and Burma lived in small villages, hamlets, each house being some distance from the next, and each village, hamlet a mile, or more from neighbouring ones. Under such conditions, and with the strict rules of segregation in force, the danger of spreading the disease set up by inoculators was not great.

Unfortunately, there remains still another side of the story. With the increasing belief in the efficacy of the measure, the demand for inoculators became greater than the supply and the price charged for the operation rose. In 1850, a usual fee was four *annas* and some rice for the operation on a boy and two *annas* and some rice for a girl.[23] Other writers of the same period say that the lowest fee taken for puncturing was Rs. 2 or Rs. 3 and the highest being Rs. 16 and a shawl. As time went by, the work of inoculation was undertaken by Hindus of low castes or people who were not only exceedingly ignorant but who did not have the necessary influence to make the people conform to the rules for preventing the spread of the disease. The result was that around the middle of the nineteenth century many epidemics were definitely traced to the operations of inoculators. In 1831, Dr Cameron stated: 'It is now well ascertained that inoculation is the great means by which smallpox is kept in existence in Calcutta', and in 1844 the Superintendent of Vaccination reported, 'Smallpox is annually introduced into Calcutta by a set of inoculators, numbering about 30, to the great endangerment of the public health'.[24]

By 1850, it was ascertained that in Bengal their number had risen to 68. It appears that 42 of them were permanent inhabitants of Calcutta, residing chiefly in the northern or native part of the town. They were principally of low Hindu castes or trades, such as those of *maulee, tanty*, *koomar*, and *napit*, from which they derived their principal livelihood during nine months of the year, practising as they did their profession only during the other three. It appears that very poor people used to pay about Rs. 2 to the *tikadars* for two, three, four, or even five children at once in a group or family, which was the custom. The middle class people paid from Rs. 3, Rs. 4 to Rs. 10 to the operator for a similar party, and much more to the Brahmins for the performance of pooja or worship, the most expensive part of which was the *gaun* or canticle to be sung for several successive days in the honour of Goddess Sitala.[25] When the operator was a Brahmin himself, or rich enough to possess an idol of the goddess, the pooja was performed at the nearest shrine of the deity, the fees were in that case paid to the officiating priest there.[26]

At that time, the *tikadars* increased their income largely by treating cases of smallpox so that it was to their pecuniary advantage when an epidemic broke out. Indeed, it was said that when they reached a village, where, in consequence of the absence of smallpox, the people were reluctant to be inoculated, it was not an unusual custom for them to throw pieces of cotton soaked in smallpox matter in places where children played, knowing fully well that if they could set up an epidemic of smallpox, the people would flock to them for inoculation. No one would, therefore, be surprised to read that in the practice of inoculators of this period the mortality attending the operation was often very high. Thus, the civil surgeon of Serampore reported in 1850 that one inoculator admitted, having operated upon 400 individuals of whom 200 died during the season.[27] It was stated publicly in the *Bhaskar*, a reputed Bengali newspaper, that in the villages of Sonatikoree in Hooghly district nearly 1,000 boys and girls were inoculated sometime before 1850 of whom 300 died. Again, in the village of Caderpore, among 100 children who were inoculated, more than 20 cases had terminated fatally.[28]

Many in Bengal, therefore, sought to prohibit the practice of inoculation since it supposedly led to the outbreak of smallpox epidemics if the rules of inoculation were not strictly adhered to. Some of the *bhadraloks* in Calcutta including Pundit Modusoodan Gupta, Coomar Kally Kissen Ray, Issurchunder Singh, G. Naylor, Sub-Assistant Surgeon of the Gurranhattah Dispensary, and many other civil surgeons believed that inoculation was more often than not fatal.[29]

Apart from the practice of *tika* in a supposedly 'para-medical' form, epidemic smallpox also evoked 'treatment' of religious intervention. The usual treatment followed by the Indians was essentially 'cooling' and expectant. One of the benignant divinities of the Hindu pantheon, variously named *Sitala,* Bhawani, etc., was specially the guardian of those affected by smallpox. At her shrines, prayers were generally offered and vows made by the relatives of the afflicted. Duncan Stewart tells us that he happened to possess a 'curious' ancient gold coin of about half an inch square, which he believed represented Goddess Sitala in her usual attire.[30] Goddess Sitala is seated naked upon an ass bedecked with flowers and jewels. She holds in one hand a broom, representative of the duty of cleanliness. Resting on the left hip and supported by that arm is a large water jar indicative of the necessity of ablution and coolness. On her head she carries a winnowing sheaf or fan to be used as a ventilator. Medals of the same description of gold or silver were, in fact, very commonly worn by people as amulets. However, it appears that the essential duties of observance of cooling, cleanliness and proper ablution enjoined on the worshippers of Sitala were very much neglected for the more supposed important ones of priest craft, incantation ceremonies and propitiatory offerings.

Contemporary Bengali dignitaries too expressed an almost similar opinion. Baboo Russomoy Dutta, for instance, argued that there was hardly any medical treatment; the recovery was more relied on the superstitious belief, on the mercy of Sitala than on any medical treatment. A passage in the prayer usually offered to Sitala runs: 'No charms or medicines exist for the wicked disease.' The usual mode of treatment, as evidenced by Dutta, was as follows.[31] In the first stage of five days, when the patient was labouring under fever, he was almost starved; dry sweets or sugar candy (*batassa*) only was given for food, and some ingredients, *jaree* and *panchan*, were administered as medicines. In the second stage after five days, when the fever went off, food was given, milk and rice, rice and *moog jurie*, and milk *mooky* after the eleventh day. On the seventh day, cold water was sprinkled over the body, and on the ninth day a thin poultice made of turmeric, linseed meal, and milk was applied over the pustules. On the twelfth day, the diet was restricted and confined to thin *chapatee* or bread, *moog jurie* and fried potatoes, *potol* and *katchkala* grain, and that too in small quantity. This continued up to the fifteenth day when generally the patient was expected to recover.

Constructing the Epidemic

These were evidently the discourses of the literati. But the moot question is what was the popular approach to health in Bengal as evidenced by the outbreak of smallpox in the early nineteenth century? The focus was arguably not on microbes, vectors, antigens and antibiotics, but on right conduct, over-indulgence, sin, and the intervention of demons and deities.[32] There had existed a popular belief, industriously supported by succeeding generations, that the observance of this practice by Hindus at some point of life was a religious duty, and its neglect was criminal or at least disreputable.

The Committee on Smallpox Inoculation, 1850, instituted a most searching enquiry on this matter. It submitted several questions on smallpox inoculation to different pundits. First, is there in the holy *Shastras* any distinct commandment enjoining *tika* as a religious duty, or recommending it as a commendable act? Second, what religious or other observances are enjoined on those who are attacked by smallpox? Third, is the omission to be inoculated considered a sin, or disreputable? Fourth, is there in this world any penalty for the omission or punishment in the next, and if so, how may it be atoned for? Fifth, supposing it is proved that the vaccine disease is really a modified form or variety of the smallpox, should not all the religious ceremonies observed hitherto in cases of common smallpox be attended to after vaccination by good Hindus?[33]

The replies to these questions received from the pundits of Nadia, from those of the Banaras College and of the Sanskrit College of Calcutta, as also from the pundits of the Court of Sudder Dewanny Adalat indicate that they were quite unanimous in declaring that although certain religious observances were proper or incumbent on all persons being Hindu who contracted smallpox in any form, either casually or by *tika*, yet there was no sort of obligation, moral or religious, imposed by Hindu laws upon anyone to subject himself or his children to the disease by practising inoculation. They further argued that neither penalty nor reproach was attached to its omission.[34]

The replies of the Banaras pundits in these regards are nevertheless instructive and can be reproduced here. They argued:

> There is no reference to inoculation in the Holy Books, but if the practice be calculated to save life, it must deserve to be praised. . . . On the appearance of smallpox, the Goddess Sitala is to be worshipped by recitation of praises and feeding of Brahmans. . . .

As neither praise nor blame is assigned to the practice of inoculation in the Shastras, so neither in the practice in common life regarded either with approval or disapproval. . . . In consequence of the absence in the Shastras of any injunction as regards inoculation, of course there is no penalty with reference to it. . . . If it is ascertained that there is no essential difference between the ordinary smallpox and the pustular disease which follows vaccination, of course the ceremonies proper in the one case are proper in the other.[35]

Nevertheless, the pundits differed. A more guarded reply to the same queries was that of the Sanskrit College Professors and Pundits, which runs thus: 'In case of *modified smallpox* in a person who has been punctured in the English manner, the worship of Sitala may be performed with all the usual formalities, she being the guardian Deity of Smallpox Disease; such religious observances are necessary.'[36] However, the most definite answer was from the Pundit of the Sudder Dewanny Adalat in Calcutta:

The Vaccine Disease is in reality a modification or variety of smallpox; such being the case virtuous Hindoos when vaccinated, should with veneration, faith and purity, observe the same religious ceremonies mentioned in my answer to the fourth question as they do when attacked with smallpox.[37]

It was necessary, they argued, for those who were naturally attacked with smallpox to live in secluded, pure, cool, and pleasant rooms, free from impure things, such as remnants of food, etc., and to keep themselves clean. It was also necessary for them to hang leaves of *neem* trees (Melia azadirachta) around the rooms; to worship Sitala Devi according to their ability, with devotion, faith, and purity; to repeat her name frequently; to make *homa*, to present offerings, to give alms, to perform *sustian* or propitiatory rites for the averting of evil, to adore Brahmins, to worship cows, to worship Shambhu and Gauri, and to cause faithful Brahmins to sing hymns to Sitala. All these were necessarily to be done by the patient for the alleviation of the pain of smallpox.[38]

Nevertheless, indigenous practitioners and informed literati in Bengal were more often than not in favour of vaccination. In 1857, one Ramnarayan Vidyaratna Bhattacharyya, in fact, wrote a treatise on vaccination arguing that the Western method of vaccination was more rational and effective.[39] Bhattacharyya was further corroborated by Haradhan Vidyaratna Kaviraja who in 1868 observed that inoculation had almost ceased to be practised in Bengal and that the Bengalis should go in for vaccination for their own interest.[40]

Generally speaking, the prevalent attitude of the people in Bengal towards vaccination was one of passive acceptance of the prophylactic.[41] But in nearly every village there were certain families who habitually refused vaccination either openly or by covertly hiding away their children from the vaccinators. This was not so much due to the vaccination itself as to the use of human vaccinifers. What the villagers seemed to object was having to pay for the operation and using some of their children as vaccinifers. For this attended by the problems of carrying their children to the neighbouring villages which entailed severe discomfort to the parents.[42] Moreover, their principal objection was that it was done without puja or any kind of sacrificial offering.[43]

There were, however, many doubts even among the educated Bengalis about the effectiveness of the method of vaccination. 'Many people', writes a Bengali medical journal in 1894:

> are taking vaccinations for fear of smallpox, in some cases this is yielding results, in some cases the vaccines are being rejected by the body, and in others, those who are being vaccinated are falling prey to pox as soon as they are vaccinated. However, *those who have not yet got themselves vaccinated should better not take it now, for quite a few people have succumbed to smallpox after taking the vaccine meant to prevent it*'. [emphasis added][44]

Nevertheless, the objection to vaccination can indeed be explained in four ways: first, the very great prejudices of the indigenous people from the highest to the lowest to adopt anything contrary to or deviating from the established customs of their ancestors; second, the inoculators were principally Brahmins of high caste, who enveloped in 'mystery' the process of inoculation, bringing in religion to their profession, i.e. Sitala must be propitiated, puja should be performed and offerings made; third, to get vaccinated with lymph drawn from cow was to the Hindus nothing less than eating beef;[45] four, the Hindus were impressed with a belief that *Basanta* or smallpox was above all medical care, for the native medical works prescribed no remedy for it, and that a patient was entirely at the mercy of Sitala, whom they considered it their duty to propitiate by worship and various offerings, the *tikadars* acting in the capacity both of doctors and priests on such occasions.[46] The Hindus who most resisted vaccination were the higher and better off classes, viz., Brahmins, Marwaris, Rajputs and Baniahs. Among the Muslims, the Ferazis gave most trouble and there was a growing feeling of opposition.[47] They successfully withstood every attempt, whether by the Sanitary Department or local officials, to introduce vaccination among them.[48] As years rolled on, some progress undoubtedly occurred in the popularizing of vaccination, as the people came to regard it as the government *dustur* or order to have the operation performed. To a certain extent, they then seemed to appreciate its benefit.

The therapeutic as practised by the *tikadars* might relate to Leslie's category of 'learned magico-religious curing'.[49] 'Most Indians', argues Leslie, 'resort frequently to magical and religious therapy, and practitioners range from illiterate villagers to sophisticated urban literati.' Supernatural curing has had an edge with folk and popular culture, but at higher levels of learning the ideas associated with supernatural curing certainly commands a prestige that sets them apart. This, Leslie believes, raises an interesting problem of historical sociology. The classical medical texts are neither always secular nor without magic, but the indigenous medicine was associated with magico-religious elements presumably to draw much wider clientele. A problem for historians would be to identify the processes through which the relatively secular and rational medicine of the texts was transformed into the magico-religious forms of indigenous medicine.

Notes

1. Irfan Habib, *Medieval India: The Study of a Civilization*, New Delhi: National Book Trust, 2008, p. 201.
2. B.J. Vyas, *Notes on Sanitary Primer*, Ahmedabad, 1886, pp. 19–20, Oriental and India Office Collection (hereafter OIOC), British Library (hereafter BL), London.
3. E.A. Gait, *A History of Assam*, Calcutta: Thacker, Spink & Co., 1906, p. 100.
4. *Voyages to the East Indies*, cited in *Extracts from Records of Past Epidemics in India*, National Archives of India (hereafter NAI), New Delhi, 1912, pp. 153–4.
5. J.Z. Holwell, *An Account of the Manner of Inoculating for the Smallpox in the East Indies*, London, 1767, repr. in Dharmapal, *Indian Science and Technology in the Eighteenth Century: Some Contemporary European Accounts*, Delhi: Impex India, 1971, p. 144.
6. Vidyaratna Haradhan Kaviraja, *Basanta Roger Nidan O Chikitsa*, Calcutta, 1868, p. vi, VT/1343, OIOC, BL, London.
7. Ibid., p. 1.
8. Kabita Roy, 'Smallpox and the Introduction of Vaccination in Colonial Bengal', in *Explorations in History: Essays in the Honour of Prof. Chittabrata Palit*, ed. Abhijit Dutta et al., Kolkata, 2003, p. 106.
9. Ibid.
10. *Annual Report upon Vaccination in the North-Western Provinces, 1866–7*, p. 4. S.P. James, *Smallpox and Vaccination in British India*, Calcutta, 1909.
11. Lawrence A. Babb, *The Divine Hierarchy: Popular Hinduism in Central India*, London, 1975, p. 277.
12. David Arnold, 'Smallpox and Colonial Medicine in Nineteenth-Century India', in *Imperial Medicine and Indigenous Societies*, ed. David Arnold, Manchester and New York, 1988, p. 49.
13. James, op. cit., p. vi.
14. *The Indian Medical Records*, vol. LII, February 1932, p. 42.
15. Oman John Campbell, *Cults, Customs and Superstitions of India*, Delhi, 1972.
16. James, op. cit., p. vii.
17. Ibid.
18. *An Account of the District of Purnea in 1809–10*, Patna, 1928, p. 187; *An account of the District of Bhagalpur in 1810–11*, Patna, 1939, p. 173. See also Montgomery Martin, *The History, Antiquities, Topography and Statistics of Eastern India*, vol. II, London: W.H. Allen and Co., 1838, pp. 690–1.
19. For a much detailed account see Irfan Habib, 'Inside and outside the system: Change and innovation in medical and surgical practice in Mughal India', in *Paper From The Aligarh Historians Society*, ed. Irfan Habib, Indian History Congress, Millennium Session, Calcutta University, 2–4 January 2001, pp. 5–8.
20. James, op. cit., p. 7
21. Cited in James, op. cit., pp. 7–8.
22. Ibid., p. 10.
23. Ibid.
24. Ibid., p. 11.
25. *Report of the Smallpox Commissioners appointed by Government with an Appendix, Calcutta, 1 July 1850*, Calcutta, 1850, p. 36, NAI, New Delhi.
26. Ibid.

27. *Report of the Smallpox Commissioners appointed by the Government for the purpose of enquiring by what means the extension of smallpox can be prevented or rendered less destructive*, Calcutta, 1850.
28. *Report of the Smallpox Commissioners appointed by Government with an Appendix, Calcutta, 1 July 1850*, Calcutta, 1850, p. 35, NAI, New Delhi.
29. *Report of the Smallpox Commissioners, 1850*, vol. XXXII, pp. 32–3.
30. Duncan Stewart, *Report on Smallpox in Calcutta, 1833–4, 1837–8, 1843–4* and *Vaccination in Bengal from 1827 to 1844*, Calcutta, 1844, V/27/857/2, OIOC, BL, London, p. 48.
31. Ibid., pp. 49–50.
32. *Report of the Smallpox Commissioners, 1850*, p. 5.
33. Ibid., pp. 5–6.
34. Ibid., p. 29.
35. Ibid., p. 30.
36. Ibid., p. 31.
37. Ibid.
38. Ibid., Appendix, p. xxii.
39. Vidyaratna Ramnarayan Bhattacharyya, *Gobij Proyog*, Calcutta, 1857.
40. Kaviraja Vidyaratna Haradhan, *Basanta Roger Nidan O Chikitsa*, Calcutta, 1868.
41. W.H. Gregg, *First Triennial Report of the Sanitary Commissioner for Bengal on the Working of the Vaccination Department in Bengal during the three years 1887–8, 1888–9, and 1889–90*, Calcutta, 1890, p. 9, NAI, New Delhi.
42. Ibid., p. 9.
43. From A. Halliday, Superintending Surgeon, Benaras, to Duncan Stewart, 6 November 1841. Vide Stewart's Report, op. cit., p. iii.
44. *Chikitsak-O-Samalochak*, Phalgun (February–March), BS 1301 (1894).
45. From W. Findon, Superintending Surgeon, Barrackpur, 20 November 1841. Vide Stewart's Report, op. cit., p. vi.
46. Reply of Baboo Ramchunder Mullick, Chore Bagan, Calcutta. *Report of the Smallpox Commissioners, appointed by Government, with an Appendix, Calcutta 1 July 1850*, Calcutta, 1850, Appendix, p. xxii.
47. Gregg, op. cit., p. 9.
48. H.J. Dyson, *Second Triennial Report of the Sanitary Commissioner for Bengal on the Working of the Vaccination Department in Bengal during the three years 1890–1, 1891–2 and 1892–3*, Calcutta, 1893, p. 16, NAI, New Delhi.
49. Charles Leslie, 'Ambiguities of Revivalism in Modern India', in *Asian Medical Systems: A Comparative Study*, ed. Charles Leslie, Delhi, 1998, p. 360.

9

Healing in an Indigenous Context

Leaves from the Journal of Dr Martin Honigberger in the Punjab

Chhanda Chatterjee

Healing from diseases and afflictions in pre-modern societies had long been a contested terrain between religion and science. Popular response to the art of healing had not been far different in these respects in European and non-European societies. While European science and technology made very rapid strides in respect of armaments and consumer goods, so far as medical science was concerned, it was still groping in the dark till the middle of the nineteenth century. Thus, while evidence for the progress of medical treatment is quite abundant for the colonial period,[1] the state of health and medicine before the advent of the Europeans is not very well documented. An interesting light is thrown on the state of progress in European medicine, the application of such knowledge in a pre-modern state and the response of the people to such medicine in the memoirs of Dr John Martin Honigberger, who had visited Punjab during the reign of Maharaja Ranjit Singh (1799–1839).

Honigberger had come to Punjab towards the middle of Ranjit Singh's rule in the 1820s, when the Maharaja embarked on a lavish programme of modernizing the state. The wealth and fame of the state attracted many fortune seekers to Punjab. While several military adventurers came to train the Sikh army, the frequent maladies suffered by the monarch from the intemperance indulged in him,[2] required the services of European doctors like Streel, Murray, Carmichael Smyth and Honigberger. Of these long array of medical practitioners, Honigberger alone left his memoirs in two volumes—*Thirty-five Years in the East Adventures, Discoveries, Experiments and Historical Sketches Relating to Punjab and Cashmere, in Connection with Medicine, Botany and Pharmacy* (London, 1852). As the title suggests, the author has not only left a narrative of long case histories, but adds an account of the various useful herbs available in Punjab and Kashmir and the various ways in which they could be made useful for medical treatment.

Honigberger did not have a high opinion of the medical treatment administered by the local hakims (medical practitioners) based on Unani medicine learnt from Greece, Egypt and Arabia and derived from two Persian works—*Tohfat-ul Khani* and *Tohfat-ul Mominin.* Nor did he have a very high opinion of the indigenous or Hindu form of medicine, which he called 'a defective medical science, which is found in the old manuscripts' and in which he could detect nothing but 'extravagances and superstitions . . . to which the Hindus add astrology'.[3] At the same time, he was aware of the pitfalls of allopathic medicine in wide currency in contemporary Europe. He did not forget to mention that allopathic remedies operated so violently that if the doses administered, were not very nicely adjusted to the disease, or a mistake occurred (which too often happened), the impact on the patient could be fatal. Honigberger quoted the Heidelberg Clinical Annal in this context that 'more individuals perish through the interference of physicians than are saved by their assistance'.[4]

Honigberger's concerns were shared by other contemporaries like Lord Bacon. Lord Bacon did not deny the physician's capability of recognizing the general symptoms of a disease. However, he doubted their ability to apply the right kind of medicine and was apprehensive of 'the addition, diminution or alteration of medicines in the most arbitrary manner'.[5]

The general fear of the hazards of wrong diagnosis and the consequent suffering is also reflected in Peter Frank's *System of Medical Police*, who found it 'strange that the government should interfere only in time of epidemics and against charlatans, whilst it takes no notice of the thousands who are daily sacrificed in their solitary chambers'. To combat the risks to life from ill-informed medical practitioners, Peter Frank went to the extreme length of demanding state intervention in such matters. 'Governments should determine either to banish all physicians and their art,' he laid down very clearly, 'or take measures to render men's lives more secure than they are at present'.[6]

Honigberger came to India from his native country Transylvania, by way of Levant, Egypt, Arabia and Persia. He resided in Punjab for several years and returned again to Transylvania a few years after the annexation of Punjab by the British through Afghanistan, Bukhara and Russia. He continued his medical practice and medical experiments in these countries, which in those times were little known to the Europeans and left a history of the common diseases and the remedies applied to those diseases.

Honigberger had his motto that 'Nothing brings man neare to God than man's helping his fellow creatures.' With this noble aim in mind, he proceeded to the examination of the various systems of the day and to the experimenting on the quality of numerous medicines, whether known or unknown to practitioners. 'It is no easy matter to eradicate systems which have been deeply rooted for centuries,' was the opinion of Dr Honigberger. 'Accurately expressed, my system can scarcely be called a new one', and he went on to elaborate, 'it is more properly, a medium between two extremes, a system grounded on experiments, which I advisedly adopted, and which success impelled me to pursue.' Thus, Honigberger based his treatment on observation of many years and tried to follow a middle course.

During Maharaja Ranjit Singh's times, the *Dar-ush shifa* or hospital was looked after by the two brothers—Faqir Aziz-ud-Din and Fakir Nur-ud-Din, Ansari Arabs from the desert, who had learnt the art of a barber and had secured the confidence of the Maharaja by healing him of some ailments.[7] After the first Sikh War in 1845–6, the English Resident ordered a public hospital to be erected in the city. The common diseases treated in this hospital were inflammation, fever, cholera, and serpent bite. Jail patients often died of severe wounds, marasmus or dysentery from the grimy briny water of the wells.

Honigberger recounted the treatment of several diseases by him partly in accordance with the prevalent practice of the times and partly by experimenting with his own remedies. In July 1831, he read an article on the treatment of hydrophobia from the bite of a jackal in a public assembly at Calcutta. He would cauterize the bitten portion and try to excite the puss and use stimulants to ensure that there was a copious flow. He would also try to get the venom out by making the fellow urinate through the application of a pill made up of a compound of mercury and the extract of tobacco. A tincture of cantharides in an emulsion of bitter almond was to be repeatedly given to excite a slight degree of dysuria. This was the novel method tried by Honigberger to treat hydrophobia resulting from jackal bites.[8]

At other times *Nux vomica* was applied on the enlarged bitten part. One grain of *Nux vomica* was also given for internal consumption with carbonate soda. This resulted in an evacuation which relieved the patient of the affliction.

Honigberger also mentioned cases of plastic surgery being practised locally which could compare favourably with those done in Europe. One learns from his *Memoirs* that such operations were performed by the Hindus even in ancient antiquity when noses could be restored from the skin of one's forehead. As the forehead remained hidden under the turban, the scar on one's forehead was not exposed. Honigberger witnessed one such restoration of the nose of one Akali having been performed on the mountains. The ears, noses and hands of this Nihang or Akali had been cut off by the orders of Maharaja Ranjit Singh by way of punishment. In contemporary Europe, such nose replacements from the enticle of one's arms had been heard of to cure ulceration in the nose.[9]

Another novel treatment mentioned by Honigberger was his cure for diabetes through the application of milk sugar. Raja Hira Singh, the son of the Minister Dhian Singh, had been afflicted by the disease and Honigberger was consulted by Maharaja Ranjit Singh along with five other physicians. None of them had ever heard of milk sugar earlier. So Honigberger prepared white and fine crystallized milk sugar, which was not sweet unlike cane sugar, and cured

Raja Hira Singh of his diabetes. Similarly, unknown in Punjab were coffee, morphine and cantharides. Cantharidine's use for blistering was unknown to the native physicians of the Punjab.[10]

Honigberger had also cured a case of external misapplication of mercury by an Army General (probably Court), while he was in Amritsar in the summer. The General's stomach and intestines were affected, which disturbed the function of digestion and caused a violent purging with burning of the arms. Bleeding with leeches brought some remission in his diarrhoea, but an intermittent fever lasting from three to seven days continued. The patient was taken to a cooler place at Deenanagar. In spite of that, the intermittent fever continued for three months. The patient became weaker and began to complain of a burning in the region of the heart. Applying leeches could not be tried for long as the patient would fall into a swoon. He later became delirious, with his eyes open and feet cold. Honigberger then applied three blisters, one on the nape of the neck and the other two on the calves of his legs and he was given Honigberger's favourite (opium, camphor, ipecac cuanha and tartar emetic) and he was saved. At the same night an eruption appeared, consisting of many thousand pustules, principally on the neck, shoulders and groins. From that moment, the disease visibly diminished and the patient recovered entirely in a few weeks.

Smallpox was a raging malady in early nineteenth century Punjab. The Maharaja himself had been a victim of the deadly disease in his early childhood, which left its imprint on the Maharaja's face by taking away one of his eyes. While Honigberger was on his way back to Transylvania, General Ventura wanted him to vaccinate his daughter Victorine. But Madame Ventura insisted that before getting her daughter vaccinated, the vaccination be tried on the local children. Honigberger paid one rupee each to some poor children and vaccinated them. But the rumour spread that the Sahib would cut the *moomiai* from their arm and all of them disappeared. When at last, the *Kotwal* succeeded in finding out one boy, more vaccinating material could be prepared from him and Victorine was vaccinated. This encouraged many people to be vaccinated of their own free will.[11] Honigberger mentions in course of his sojourn in Afghanistan and Bukhara that smallpox was also prevalent in those areas also. He tried to inoculate cows with venomous matter taken from smallpox and turn cow pox venom into a remedy.

Honigberger also tried his hand in surgery and cured the Amir of Bukhara of a gastro-bilious fever by extracting a stone from his udder about the size of a hen's egg with 25 points apple stalks. He was also cured of spasmodic and periodic asthma.

In Lebanon, Honigberger practised another surgery on a child and removed a stone from the urinary tract of the child. This was an interesting case of psychosomatic disease. The boy was being suckled by his mother when she was very upset to hear that her husband had lost all the money taken to buy some oxen in a fit of intoxication. The impact of the lady's anxieties on the boy was that he ceased to pass urine since then. Later, urine had to be passed through suction and the stoppage came back periodically. However, it was cured after the removal of the stone.

Honigberger also cured people of Guinea worm, which used to hide in the hollow of the person's knee. When the worm appeared and was pulled, it broke and the knee became inflamed and swollen. After accumulation of matter, Honigberger made an incision and there was a flow from the wound. The fluid was allowed to come out for several days and wax oil was applied to the swollen parts. Thus, it was healed in several days.

Oil distilled from wax (cerelaeum) was employed by the native physicians of the East in various diseases, especially in paralysis, contractions, swellings, wounds, itching, impotence, colds and cholera morbus. It was necessary that the massaging be made in the rays of the sun. Wax oil also proved to be very effective in case of severe swelling of the testicles, which was the consequence of an external injury.

Honigberger also reported interesting ways of treating the cholera morbus. After massaging the patient with wax oil in the sun, the patient was made to drink hot broth. Hot bricks were enveloped in rugs and applied to the soles of the feet. They were then covered with woollen sheets over the head, to produce perspiration. In Bukhara, Honigberger experienced the treatment of cholera in a novel manner. The remedy was called 'Turcoman-Sudorific remedy' by him and was cheap and simple. It was applied when nothing else could be found. They procured a quantity of wheat bran, sifted it seven times and washed it superficially almost a similar number of times. It was then rubbed into water with fingers and strained. The strained water was simmered until it was reduced to one half, to which they added some garlic and almond oil and it was often drunk lukewarm. The garlic served to drive away the evil spirits according to the physicians of Bukhara.

The close association of religion with the art of healing in the psyche of the people of the East was recorded by Honigberger in an unusual practice followed during the outbreak of the cholera epidemic in Bukhara. To get rid of cholera, Bukharians took out a procession and took it to the middle of the city, where a new horse hide was procured and buried. As horse-meat formed a staple diet of the Bukharians, that might have been at the root of the odd practice.

Use of animal hides in the act of healing was also heard of in Afghanistan. Honigberger noted that a peculiar method of curing nervous fevers was to envelop the patient in the skin of a newly filled animal (goat or sheep) in which he broke into perspiration. He was left in that state for the whole night. He was also made to drink a decoction of bran. However, the drinking of bran was considered to be a mild remedy and was not generally in use.

Honigberger had also gone through an outbreak of plague while passing through Palee in Rajasthan and was himself affected by it. He thought plague was a disease peculiar to India and similar to that in Egypt and Turkey. It was accompanied by carbuncles, buboes and bleeding of the nose. It was highly infectious and only one in twenty survived. When Honigberger reached plague-affected Palee, he found the shops and bazaars closed and the greater part of the inhabitants had died. When he himself got affected by it, he took Strychnos Faba St. Ignatic.

In 1838, after the visit of Lord Auckland, Maharaja Ranjit Singh became very sick and Honigberger treated him with Tinctura dulcamara, 3 dilutions for three days. It was administered to him in the usual potion of wine and opium that the Maharaja used to take. The medicine restored the Maharaja for a few days. But his constitution had already been undermined by severe intemperance and he was suffering from a paralytic stroke as he had lost his ability to speak. Thus, Honigberger's remedies could not restore him to good health and the Maharaja ultimately succumbed to his disease in 1839.

Honigberger's diaries contain an interesting account of the diseases widely prevalent in the region running from the Punjab farther to the north-west in Afghanistan, Bukhara, Lebanon and Turkey and refer to the remedies applied to those diseases in those regions. He did not believe in making a sharp break from the prevalent way of treating those diseases. He merely experimented with a few new herbs found in Punjab and Kashmir and tried some new drugs like morphine, tobacco, coffee and arsenic not so commonly used in those days. Although an European himself and alert of the Delphic Oracle about knowing one's anatomy, he denounced the violent methods of allopathic medicine. Hahnemann's doctrine of *similia similibus curantor* appealed to him more. He, thus, blended the eastern techniques of treatment with herbs and portions made from herbs with Hahnemann's remedies along with his knowledge of allopathic medicine, anatomy and surgery. It, thus, formed a bridge between the ancient and the modern. Honigberger's memoirs stand as a testimony to the prevalent medical practice of his times. Maharaja Ranjit Singh had tried to introduce the fresh air of new science and technology in a pre-modern state. Men like Honigberger tried to accommodate the new values in a traditional society with great patience and an open mind.

Notes

1. The state of health and medicine in colonial India has received attention in influential works in recent times. Some of the major titles are David Arnold, *Colonializing the Body: State Medicine and Epidemic Disease in Nineteenth-Century India*, Berkley, 1993; Mark Harrison, *Public Health in British India: Anglo-Indian Preventive Medicine 1859–1914*, Cambridge, 1994; Sanjoy Bhattacharya, Mark Harrison, and Michael Warboys, *Fractured States: Smallpox, Public Health and Vaccination Policy in British India, 1800–1947*, Hyderabad: New Perspectives in South Asian History, 2005; Anil Kumar, *Medicine and the Raj: British Medical Policy 1835–1911*, New Delhi, 1998; Andrew Cunningham, and Bridie Andrews, *Western Medicine as Contested Knowledge*, Manchester, 1997.
2. Khushwant Singh, *Ranjit Singh: Maharaja of the Punjab, 1780–1839*, London: George Allen & Unwin, 1962.
3. John Martin Honigberger, *Thirty Five Years in the East: Adventures, Discoveries, Experiments and Historical Sketches Relating to the Punjab and Cashmere, in Connection with Medicine, Botany, Pharmacy*, London, 1852.

4. Heidelberg Clinical Annal, vol. V, part 3.
5. Quoted in Honigberger.
6. Peter Frank, *System of Medical Police*, vol. I, quoted by Honigberger.
7. In former days, minor surgical operations were trusted to the care of the barbers. It was not at all unprecedented for a barber to gain recognition as a practitioner of the art of healing. See Major Carmichael Smyth, *History of the Reigning Family of Lahore*, Calcutta, 1847; Fakir Syed Waheed-ud-din, *The Real Ranjit Singh*, Patiala, 2001.
8. Honigberger, op. cit., p. 47.
9. Ibid., p. 48.
10. Ibid., p. 49.
11. For the continued menace of the smallpox even beyond the colonial period see Sanjoy Bhattacharya, *Expunging Variola: The Control and Eradication of Smallpox in India, 1947–77*, Hyderabad, 2006.

10

Clinical and Ergometric Evaluation of Terminalia Arjuna in Chronic Angina Pectoris

Arunangshu Ganguly & Anil Bharani

Coronary artery disease is rightly called the enigma of the modern world. The advent of industrialization has aggravated the possibilities of this disease. It has emerged as a major killer worldwide as also the principal disease of the bread earners in the family leading to wide ranging social impact. It causes more deaths in the world than many groups of diseases comprising of 30 per cent deaths in male and 25 per cent deaths in female in Western population.[1] In Indian population, the incidence is quite high 65.4 and 47.8 per 1,000 males and females respectively. In Indian rural population, the prevalence was found to be 22.8 and 17.3 per 1,000 males and females respectively.[2]

The coronary artery disease may manifest clinically as angina stable or unstable, myocardial infarction and sudden cardiac death. The treatment approaches of myocardial ischemia are multidimensional. The first approach aims at improving blood supply to the myocardium either pharmacologically by drugs like nitrates[3] or mechanically by coronary angioplasty or CABG.[4]

The second approach aims to limit oxygen requirements of the myocardial cells either by decreasing the preload (nitrates, diuretics) or after load (arterial vasodilators) and also by decreasing myocardial contractility and heart rate (like beta blockers).[5]

Besides these two principal modalities the drugs that decrease platelet adhesiveness like aspirin and clopidogrel, the drugs that help in plaque stabilization like statins have revolutionized the management of ischemic heart disease. There are a few drugs acting at cellular level to prevent them from toxic effects of ischemia like trimetazidine, ranolazine. Trimetazidine does not have vasodilator effect.[6] It decreases intracellular acidosis;[7] preserves cellular energy potential;[8] normalizes ion transport[9] and limits free radical activity.[10]

Terminalia arjuna, about which I have discussed below, acts by many of the above modalities. The possible modes of action include:

1. Facilitatory role in production of vasodilatory prostaglandins (PGE2).[11]
2. Negative chronotropism.[12]
3. Prolongation of prothrombin and euglobin lysis time.[13]
4. Decreasing the serum cholesterol.[14]

This study was intended to prove antianginal efficacy Terminalia arjuna in chronic stable angina including clinical and ECG evaluation.

Chronic Stable Angina

Chronic Stable Angina is defined as a discomfort in chest and adjacent areas associated with myocardial ischemia but not necrosis. Discomfort is described often not as pain but rather unpleasant sensation like pressing, squeezing, contraction, burning, and the like. The symptom should be present and remain stable for 12 weeks.

The ideal anti-anginal drug would include among its properties the ability to control symptoms, improve exercise performance, reduce or eliminate ischemia ECG changes, improve longevity, and have no side effects.

Nitrates, beta blockers, and non-dihydropyridine calcium channel blockers are the conventionally used drugs. Nitrates act by vasodilatation thereby reducing the myocardial oxygen demand and also dilate the epicardial coronary arteries.[15] Beta blockers decrease heart rate and hence decrease myocardial oxygen demand and contractility caused by adrenergic activity.[16] Calcium channel blockers are coronary vasodilators that produce dose dependant decrease of myocardial oxygen demand, contractility and arterial pressure. But being potential large vessel dilatory, they can cause reflex tachycardia increasing cardiac work. The free radical scavengers protects intracellular homeostasis, optimize myocardial uptake of residual oxygen and substrate supplies ensuring long term protection of myocardium against dreadful effects of myocardial ischaemia.[17]

Terminalia Arjuna and its Review of Literature

Terminalia arjuna is an important medicinal plant described in Indian medical system of Ayurveda. Its bark extract has been used in a variety of cardiovascular disorders including chest pain akin to present day description of chronic angina pectoris from very ancient time in India. It belongs to the family of Combitraceae and found on the banks of river mainly in the sub-Himalayan regions as well as Madhya Pradesh and Deccan Plateau. The trees of Terminalia arjuna are generally 20–30 metres in height with huge trunk and horizontally spreading branches.The various parts of the plant have been used in a variety of medicinal preparations as is found described in ancient

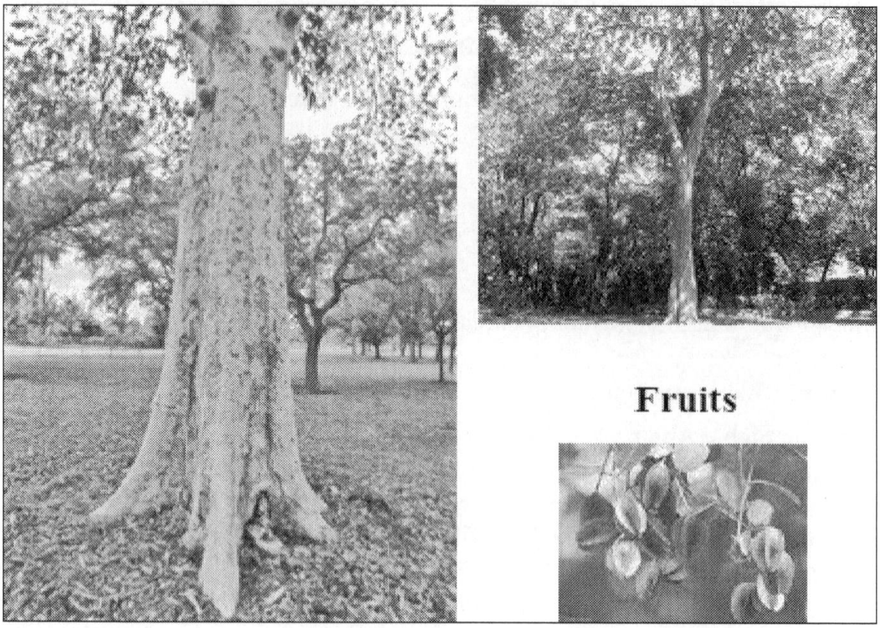

Fig. 10.1: Tree of Terminalia Arjuna

Indian literature. The stem bark has been used most frequently in various forms, viz., dried powder and decoctions, etc. Due to its medical use, efforts are continuously made since 1930s to isolate various active principles present in different parts of the plant. Consequently, many triterpenes belonging to oleanoic acid series, flavones and glycosides have been isolated by various workers.

Agarwal and Dutt isolated a compound Arjuna ($C_{26}H_3O_3$ mp 192°) from benzene extract of the bark. They characterized it as an acid.[18] From alcoholic extract of Terminalia arjuna bark, they isolated an amorphous red colouring matter (mp 132°)—called Arjunetin.They considered it to be a lactone.[19]

King et al., carried on ether extraction of Terminalia arjuna heartwood that brought out a tripene carboxylic acid—arjunolic acid ($C_{30}H_{48}O_s$, mp 337°–40°, [α] y ^{9}D + 63.5).[20] Besides that oleanoic acid, β sitosterol ($C_{29}H_{50}O$, mp 136–7 [α] °D–35°) and ellagic acid also obtained.[21] In their later work King et al., showed the structure of arjunolic acid as 2α3β23-trihydroxyolean-12–en-28-oic acid by chemical transfusion of arjunolic acid and by comparison with known compounds, viz., hederagenin and terminolic acid.[22]

Other workers like Row and Rao separated a complex saponin, an amorphous powder along with arjunolic acid, β sitosterol, and leucodelphin. The sugar moiety of saponin was diglucoside.[23] Row et al., also synthesized arjunolic acid starting from hederagenin.[24] Again Row, Murty, Rao Sastry isolated a triterpenes monocarboxylic acid called arjunic acid ($C_{30}H_{48}O_5.H_2O$ mp 335°[α] D +20) containing 19αOH group from alcoholic extract of the bark. Later on, Rao also isolated arjunetin from alcoholic extract of Terminalia arjuna bark.[25] They found it to be an ester glucoside of arjunic acid.[26] The Japanese isolators have isolated newer triterpenes which were arjungenin and arjunglucoside I, II, and III.[27] Besides, the works of many others suggested the presence of calcium magnesium silica in significant quantities.

Therefore, the constituents so far extracted are:

From Stem Bark

Arjunin

Arjunic acid

Arjunetin

Minerals: Calcium 3133µg/gm; magnesium 4000µg/gm; zinc 119µg/gm; copper 19µg/gm

Others: tannins, oxalic acid, essential oils, colouring matter

From Root Bark

Arjunoside I	[arjunic acid—3-0-β-D (+) galactoside]
Arjunoside II	[arjunic acid—3-0-β-D (+) glucopyranosyl–α-L(-)2 deoxy rhamnoside]
Arjunoside III	[arjunic acid—28–β–D (+) glucopyranoside]
Arjunoside IV	[3-0-α-L (-) rhamnoside of arjunic acid]
Terminic acid	[3β,13β dihydroxy–lup 20 (29)–en–28–oic acid]

From Heartwood

Arjunolic acid	[$C_{30}H_{48}O_5$]
β Sitosterol	[$C_{29}H_{50}O$]
Ellagic acid	
Saponin of Arjunolic acid	[$C_{42}H_{68}O_5$]
Haemodelphinidin	[$C_{15}H_{14}O_8.1H_2O$]
Terminic acid	

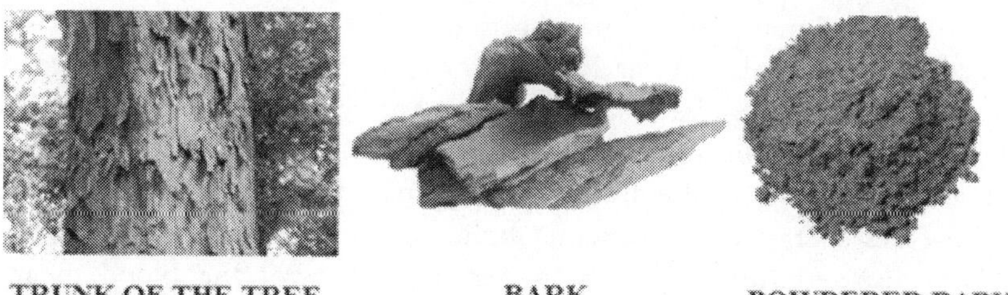

Fig. 10.2: Useful parts of Terminalia Arjuna

From Fruits

Arjunone	[5,7,2′4′-tetramethoxyflavone]
Cerasidin	[2,4,4′6′-tetramethoxychalcone]
Others	β sitosterol; ellagic acid; friedelin; methyl oleanate

Pharmacological Studies

The initial mention of Terminalia arjuna as 'Hridaya', a drug which strengthens the heart was interpreted as if the drug has cardiotonic action. It was conceived that it improved rate and force of contraction.

Ghosal (1909) first studied the crude bark powder in frog and rabbit heart. He found the drug to be cardiac stimulant.[28] Chopra and Ghosh (1929) studied its effect on experimental animal and it reportedly produced persistent rise in blood pressure.[29] Contrary to these observations Singh et al. (1982) noted a dose dependant decrease in BP and heart rate in cat and dog following intravenous administration of aqueous extract of the drug. These workers also noted similar hypotensive and bradycardic response when drug was injected into lateral cerebral ventricle and vertebral artery. The dose, in this case, was significantly lower. The bradycardic effect of lower dose was abolished by bilateral vagotomy. However, large doses would still induce bradycardic changes. The hypotensive action would still be observed in bilaterally vagotomized animals suggesting presence of central effects.[30] Chopra et al. (1958) demonstrated increase of heart rate and contractility.[31] Caius et al. reported presence of diuretic properties.[32] Regarding the effects on prothrombin time also there are conflicting reports in experimental animals. Gupta et al. (1976) did not notice any alteration in prothrombin time[33] whereas Chaturvedi (1973) found prolongation of prothrombin time and also euglobin lysis time.[34] Dwivedi et al. (1987) found that Terminalia arjuna pretreatment cause increase in PGE2 activity in ischemic rabbits. When Terminalia arjuna pretreated rabbits were challenged with isoproterenol, they required higher dosage of isoproterenol for induction of ischemia compared to controls. The ECG changes suggestive of myocardial ischemia appeared at a relatively later stage in drug pretreated animals. In addition, it prevented appearance of ventricular arrhythmias following isoproterenol infusion. The histopathological changes were less pronounced in Terminalia arjuna pretreated ischaemic rabbits.[35] Recently, it has been demonstrated that crude powder aqueous and alcoholic extracts exert a negative chronotropic action on isolated spontaneously beaten atrium. The crude powder has been found to be most effective in this regard. The negative chronotropic and inotropic property of the drug may ultimately prove to be cardioprotective as it conserves energy and lowers metabolic demand of the heart. Dwivedi et al. (1988) also reported a decrease in serum cholesterol and blood sugar in experimental animals after three months of drug pretreatment.[36]

So the criteria that establish its usefulness in ischemic heart diseases are:

1. Decreasing heart rate,
2. Increasing production of vasodilatory prostaglandins (PGE),

3. Inhibitory action on prothrombin time, and
4. Cholesterol lowering effects.

Initial clinical studies were concluded by Vagbhatta (*c.*AD sixth century); Chakradutta (eleventh century AD); and Bhawa Mishra (*c.*AD 1550).[37] Vagbhatta in *Astang Hridayam Samhita* advocated its use in cardiac disorders but no specific group was mentioned.[38] Chakradutta used it with success in relieving pain and burning sensation of chest thought to be of cardiac origin.[39] However, the subsequent works were directed at its cardiotonic properties. Chaturvedi (1973) tried alcoholic decoction of bark in stable cases of IHD and found that prolonged use of this drug brings a sense of well being and ECG improvement along with increase of euglobin lysis time and prothrombin time.[40] Dwivedi et al. (1989) also tried 500 mg. of crude extract in 30 stable angina patients and reported alleviation of angina pain.[41]

Aims and Objectives

Aims and objectives of this study is to evaluate anti-anginal efficacy of Terminalia arjuna bark extract in chronic stable angina pectoris patients clinically and by exercise testing on treadmill system in a double blind placebo controlled study and to compare it with isosorbide mononitrate to find out drug tolerance and possible causes of side effects, if any.

Materials and Methods

The study was carried out in the cardiology department of Mahatma Gandhi Memorial (MGM) Medical College and Maharaja Yashwantrao (MY)Hospital, Indore from July 1991 to August 1992 and subsequently at The Mission Hospital, Durgapur, West Bengal between 2008 and 2009.

Case Selection

Cases were accepted consecutively for this study amongst patients attending the cardiology outdoor with angina symptoms and who were willing to undergo the trial protocol after discussion with the consultants and residents.

Patients with typical angina were chosen on the basis of history and physical examination. History was taken with special reference to: number of angina attacks per week, duration and character of angina pain, precipitating factors and relieving factors. Those patients who had stable symptoms for 12 weeks or more prior to entry into the study were considered suitable for the study. History regarding hypertension, diabetes, gout, CVA, smoking, tobacco chewing, alcohol and family history of coronary artery disease, sudden cardiac death, cerebrovascular accident, and hypertension diabetes mellitus was obtained.

Detailed clinical examination was performed in all cases. Patient with old myocardial infarction were also included in the study if they fulfilled the criteria of stable angina pectoris. The patients were explained about the study and a written consent was obtained.

Exclusion Criteria

1. Myocardial infarction—impending or acute
2. Unstable angina
3. Acute myocarditis and pericarditis
4. Known ominous coronary artery disease (left main or left main equivalent)
5. Severe aortic stenosis
6. Hypertrophic obstructive cardiomyopathy
7. Congestive cardiac failure
8. Severe uncontrolled hypertension
9. Uncontrolled cardiac arrhythmias
10. Intracardiac conduction defect greater than 1st degree and LBBB
11. Acute systemic illness and physical inability to perform TMT
12. Patients on digitalis and diuretics
13. Unwillingness to give informed consent.

Trial Design

After selection on basis of history and physical examination, the patients were subjected to a treadmill test after getting an informed consent. If positive, they were taken up for trial with informed consent.

Then, the patients who were on β blockers, diltiazem or verapamil were gradually tapered over a week. Then, a week washout period was given wherein they were stopped from taking medications except sublingual isosorbide dinitrate and aspirin was allowed to continue. A detailed note was made regarding the number of angina episodes during a routine work and number of isosorbide dinitrate tablets consumed during the preceding week. They were then subjected to a Treadmill Test [Baseline TMT; TMT—(1)]. Each patient served as his own control. They were subjected to three different drug therapies one after another lasting over one week each with adequate washout period in between two therapies. Three identical capsules were used—one containing 500 mg. dried arjuna powder; and other contained ISDN 20 mg. and third, a placebo.

The performing doctor was blind to what drugs were used. One of the investigators knew about the drugs used and he distributed the drugs to the patients. The drug key was not opened until completion of the trial. The patients were then given one of these capsules at a dose of one capsule 8 hourly at random for 7 days to be followed by treadmill testing (TMT 2). Then a week washout period was given and the second drug was given for seven days at random in the same dose of one capsule 8 hourly and another treadmill testing was performed at the end (TMT 3). It was followed by yet another weeks washout period and the patient was given third capsule to eat randomly and likewise treadmill was performed at the end of the week (TMT 4).

The patients were given counted number of isosorbide dinitrate tablets (5 mg.) and after each week number of isosorbide dinitrate tablets consumed were counted. The patients were asked to report any untoward side effects immediately.

Before they were put to treadmill, the patients were reevaluated to rule out new ischaemic events, viz., unstable angina, acute myocardial infarction, and to find out probable drug side effects. The patients with new ischaemic events or serious drug side effects were planned to discontinue from trial after breaking the drug code. The Treadmill Test reports were evaluated by independent blinded observers.

The following parameters were noted and compared during the I, II, and III stages of drug therapies:

1. Duration of exercise on treadmill.
2. Time to significant ST segment response.
3. Magnitude and morphology of ST segment shift.
4. Recovery time.
5. Double product.
6. Presence or absence of angina and significant rhythm disturbance.
7. BP response.

Work Capacity

Treadmill Test was done following standard Bruce protocol. The standard contraindications were followed and the response evaluated as per standard guidelines as normal response, uninterpretable response, and mild, moderate and strongly positive response. Clinical modifiers were also considered. Positive modifiers included significant hypotension at moderate levels of exercise; classic angina pectoris thus placing the subject in a population with a high prevailing coronary disease; development of severe typical angina with significant electrocardiographic changes; development of S3 gallop or abnormal precardial motion; development of holosystolic murmur of mitral regurgitation, development of unusually severe shortness of breath or lightheadedness. Negative modifiers included presence of LVH pr digitalis use and a sub-population with low incidence of coronary artery disease. A students 't test' was used to determine the significance of difference between therapy and baseline and placebo and baseline.

Observations

Age and Sex

Of the total 15 cases that continue in the study, 14 were males. Mean age of population in the study was 51.19±8.62. Of them, seven were hypertensive, two suffered from NIDDM and 3 persons had previous subendocardial infarction. One person was 70 years old but being physically active and desirous of better treatment for angina symptoms, he was included in the trial.

Angina Episodes

14 out of 15 patients showed a decrease in consumption of isosorbide dinitrate tablets during therapy with dried arjuna extract as compared to pretreatment period. One showed no change. During the treatment period with isosorbide dinitrate, 14 patients showed decrease in angina episodes and reduced consumption of isosorbide dinitrate tablets. One showed no change. During therapy with placebo, 10 out of 15 patients showed decrease in angina episodes; three showed increase and one showed no change as compared with baseline.

Table 10.1: Number of Angina Attacks per Week

BASELINE (B)	*ARJUN (A)*	*ISMO (I)*	*PLACEBO (P)*
3.73 ± 1.22	*1.60 ± 1.06*	*1.73 ± 1.22*	*2.73 ± 1.47*

- t A / P : B = 4.437 ($p < 0.001$)
- t I / P : B = 3.4159 ($p < 0.001$)
- t A / I = 0.6496 ($p > 0.05$)

Table 10.2: Amount of ISDN Consumed per Day (mg/day)

BASELINE (B)	*ARJUN (A)*	*ISMO (I)*	*PLACEBO (P)*
2.62 ± 0.88	*1.14 ± 0.75*	*1.19 ± 0.88*	*1.94 ± 1.06*

- t A / P : B = 4.3798 ($p < 0.001$)
- t I / P : B = 3.5674 ($p < 0.001$)
- t A / I = 0.3753

Table 10.3: Duration of Exercise on Treadmill (in minutes)

BASELINE (B)	*ARJUN (A)*	*ISMO (I)*	*PLACEBO (P)*
2.00 ± 1.51	*3.47 ± 1.30*	*3.20 ± 1.47*	*2.00 ± 1.41*

- t A / P : B = 6.2050 ($p < 0.001$)
- t I / P : B = 5.3928 ($p < 0.001$)
- t A / I = 1.0742 ($p > 0.05$)

Table 10.4: Magnitude of St Segment Depression (in mm)

BASELINE (B)	*ARJUN (A)*	*ISMO (I)*	*PLACEBO (P)*
2.58 ± 0.84	*1.72 ± 0.51*	*1.75 ± 0.53*	*2.45 ± 0.57*

- t A / P : B = 5.5015 ($p < 0.001$)
- t I / P : B = 4.8734 ($p < 0.001$)
- t A / I = 0.3229 ($p > 0.10$)

Table 10.5: Recovery Time (in min)

BASELINE (B)	*ARJUN (A)*	*ISMO (I)*	*PLACEBO (P)*
13.87 ± 2.75	*8.93 ± 2.63*	*10.27 ± 2.76*	*14.13 ± 2.19*

- t A / P : B = 7.8124 ($p < 0.001$)
- t I / P : B = 6.7247 ($p < 0.001$)
- t A / I = 2.1693 ($p < 0.05$)

$22.26\times10^3 \pm 3.70\times10^3$	$25.88\times10^3 \pm 5.10\times10^3$	$26.33\times10^3 \pm 5.07\times10^3$	$22.64\times10^3 \pm 4.74\times10^3$

- t A / P : B = 3.1597 ($p < 0.01$)
- t I / P : B = 3.6246 ($p < 0.01$)
- t A / I = 0.5379 ($p > 0.10$)

Discussion

There are various drugs which are used in the treatment of chronic stable angina like the betablockers, calcium channel blockers, the nitrates, the free radical scavengers like trimetazidine, the ranolazines and so on. The armamentarium is on the rise. Each has its own advantages and limitations. But the search for an ideal anti-anginal is still on. So newer drugs which can be used as adjuvant or replacements are being added quite often. Terminalia arjuna bark has anti-anginal properties too and this study aimed at evaluation of these properties.

Terminalia arjuna is reported to be a beneficial drug in cardiac ailments from very ancient age. In ancient literature, Vagbhatta first mentioned the use of this drug in treating heart disease about 1,400 years ago. Later, Chakradutta prescribed the use in chest pain akin to present day angina and also by Bhawa Mishra during the early medieval and medieval period. Following that, a series of animal experiments by various workers revealed various pharmacological aspects of the drug. They include central hypotensive and negative chronotropic effect,[42] positive inotropic effect and prolongation of prothrombin and euglobin lysis time,[43] increased PGE2 synthesis;[44] and diuretic effects.

Limited clinical trials carried out by Chaturvedi (1973) of Banaras Hindu University and Dwivedi et al. (1987) of Manipal University documented alleviation of chest pain with this drug in patients with chronic stable angina pectoris.[45] Chaturvedi also reported electrocardiographic improvement in these patients.

From all these observations, it has been proposed that Terminalia arjuna extract benefited ischemic heart disease patients by the following probable mechanisms: negative chronotropism; increased production of vasodilatory prostaglandins; prolongation of prothrombin time and euglobin lysis time and cholesterol lowering effects.

No ergometric study has so far been carried out in my knowledge in order to quantify its effects in stable angina pectoris other than clinical evaluation of relief from pain. The present study was carried out to assess the anti-anginal efficacy of Terminalia arjuna on ergometric and clinical parameters on human volunteers and to compare its efficacy with nitrates—the age old specific anti-anginal—the age old gold standard.

This study population comprised of 14 males and 1 female volunteer with mean age of 51.19 ± 8.62 years, of whom seven were hypertensive, two had NIDDM, 3 had suffered previous subendocardial infarction. Since the same patient population passed through all phases of study, problem of homogeneity and subjective variation did not arise. The dose in which the extract was given was 500 mg. three times a day as stated in IPC (Indian Pharmaceutical Codex) dose of crude bark was stated as 2–4 gm./a day. Since was used, alcoholic extract that was free from unwanted bark contents a dose of 1.5 gm./a day was given. Since no proper pharmacokinetic or pharmacodynamic study was available, dosage schedule was arbitrarily fixed at 500 mg. three times a day.

Effect on Angina Symptoms

The results showed a highly significant decrease in angina episode per week and also an amount of isosorbide dinitrate consumption in mg/day during therapy with Terminalia arjuna extract in comparison with placebo and pretreatment phase and matched with ISMN in its anti-anginal efficacy. This agrees with results obtained by Chaturvedi (1973) and Dwivedi et al. (1987) with alcoholic extract of Terminalia arjuna in patients with stable angina pectoris.

Effect on Exercise Duration

Terminalia arjuna was found to prolong the exercise duration on the treadmill in patients with effort angina suggesting an increase in exercise threshold and matched in efficacy with isosorbide mononitrate and it also matched with clinical benefits observed in these patients as they showed improvement in angina symptoms while continuing the normal daily activity during the Terminalia arjuna therapy.

Effect on Magnitude of ST Depression

It correlates with degree of myocardial hypoxia. The results show highly significant decrease in magnitude of ST depression on Terminalia arjuna therapy as compared with placebo and pretreatment phase and was similar to ISMN therapy. This denotes more work done with lesser ischemia suggesting an increase in ischemic threshold.

Work Capacity

Work done during treadmill can be judged from the number of METS expended, e.g. in Bruce protocol exercising up to first stage denotes a METS expenditure of 4.8 METS. The patients exhibited higher work capacity while on Terminalia arjuna therapy as compared to placebo. The increase was from 0.7 METS to 3.9 METS.

Recovery Time

There was a statistically significant faster rate of recovery from induced myocardial ischemia on treadmill as compared to placebo and pretreatment phases. There was also a statistically significant faster recovery as compared to isosorbide mononitrate. The early recovery from myocardial ischemia means curtailing of duration of induced myocardial ischemia which is substrate to ischemia based cardiac arrhythmias and ventricular dysfunction and Terminalia arjuna therapy excels over ISMN in this regard.

Double Product

The heart rate blood pressure product is an externally derived indicator of myocardial oxygen demand. It progressively increases during treadmill exercise. In chronic stable angina pectoris, this becomes fixed that is symptoms get reproduced at a fixed double product. There was a statistically significant increase in double product with Terminalia arjuna therapy as compared to placebo and pretreatment phase and matched that of ISMN.

Grading of TMT Positivity

Seven out of 15 patients showed improvement in grade of TMT positivity while on Terminalia arjuna therapy as compared to 5 out of 15 patients during ISMN therapy. There was a greater change in positivity, from moderate to severe, while on placebo therapy.

No untoward side effects were reported during therapy. Side effects depend on various factors like dose, metabolic milieu, allergy, idiosyncrasy and co-administered drugs. The absence of side effects in the study indicate that the dose of the preparation of Terminalia arjuna used in the study did not present any untoward effect. However, more data is required in this matter.

The possible mechanism has already been postulated as: increased production of vasodilatory prostaglandins; negative chronotropism; prolongation of prothrombin time and euglobin lysis time; cholesterol lowering effects and increased PGE2 synthesis.

Prostaglandins are eicosanoids produced from arachidonic acid by cyclooxygenase pathway. Pathway of various prostaglandins produced by this pathway PGE2 and PGI2 which exerts broadest physiological effects and they are potent vasodilators. PGE2 dilate arterioles, precapillary sphincter and postcapillary venules. The vasodilatation is due to direct action on vascular smooth muscle. It has also been observed that blood flow to brain, heart, and kidneys is preferentially increased by PGE2 and PGI2 if systemic blood pressure remains normal. In a study, Dwivedi et al. (1987) showed that there was an enhancement of aortic PGE2 like activity following isoproternol induced ischemia in rabbits which had been pretreated with Terminalia arjuna.[46] So by enhancing PGE2 like activity, Terminalia arjuna may cause dilatation of arterioles and postcapillary venules and thereby reducing preload and also afterload. So work done by myocardial oxygen demand decrease benefitting angina and heart failure. In addition, PGE2 produces direct vasodilatation and also preferential increase of coronary blood flow thus correcting demand supply mismatch in angina. However, drugs causing vasodilatation may also cause reflex tachycardia that may paradoxically aggravate angina. However, this was not observed during the study. This could probably be due to the central negative inotropic effect of Terminalia arjuna.

Centrally Acting Negative Chronotropism

Singh et al. reported a negative chronotropic effect on using Terminalia arjuna bark alcoholic extract in rabbits. The negative chronotropism was seen in accompaniment with hypotension even in bilaterally vagotomized animals although dosage required was higher. This suggests that the major mechanism was centrally acting negative chronotropism although partly the action may be mediated by inhibition of cardiac sympathetic pathway.[47]

Srivastava et al. demonstrated that crude powder, aqueos and alcoholic extracts of Terminalia arjuna, extract a negative chroonotropic action on spontaneously beating rat atrium.[48] This suggests that centrally acting negative chronotropism may be one of the modalities benefitting patients of ischemic heart disease. However, this is unlikely to be the only pathway as there was no bradycardic response in this study. It could be that PGE2 induced vasoldilatation and consequent reflex tachycardia may have been negated by the negative chronotropism. Again, if negative chronotropism had been the major manifestation then there would have been reduction of double product there by reducing myocardial oxygen demand. However, we did not encounter it during the study. Thereby negative chronotropism as major contributor remains a remote possibility in the dosage used in the study. However, higher dosage may encounter these effects and it may positively contribute in anti-ischemic effect.

Increased Prothrombin/Euglobin Lysis Time

Chaturvedi (1973) of Banaras Hindu University reported that on using alcoholic decoction of Terminalia arjuna bark extract there was a prolongation of prothrombin as well as euglobin lysis time.[49] However, Gupta et al. administered 5 gm/day Terminalia arjuna bark extract in powdered form for 30 days in rabbits but they found no such effect.[50] It may be possible that alcohol extract alone exhibited the property. Alcoholic extract was used in the study and this effect may also have contributed to the benefit observed in our patients.

Antioxidant Properties

In a study by Uchida et al. they had demonstrated in animal models that tannins in a plant Persimmon prolonged survival of stroke prone spontaneously hypertensive rats. To explain the mechanism, they used electron spin resonance analysis to demonstrate that tannins in Persimon plant had potent concentration dependant action on free radicals and strongly inhibited lipid peroxidation I rat brain homogenates. In the extract there was 61.73 per cent weight by weight of tannins. If tannins of persimmon can produce free radical scavenging an effect similar to it can also be expected from tannins of Terminalia arjuna. Therefore,Terminalia arjuna extract may have benefited angina by preventing toxic cellular damage by free radicals at sites of myocardial hypoxia simulating the action of an established free radical scavenging drug Trimetazidine. This, however, is speculative and requires further scientific study to prove the same.

Cholesterol lowering effects:

Tiwari et al. (1989) reported that on treating rabbits with Terminalia arjuna powder for 2 months, there was a significant decrease in serum total cholesterol compared to cholestyramine and control. Terminalia arjuna was very effective in enhancing VLDL clearance, TG, not reducing HDLc level and reducing TC/HDLc ratio more than cholestyramine proving to be a potent hypocholesteolemic agent.[51]

However, since these effects were obtained after 2 months of therapy it is likely that it is useful for prevention of ischemic heart disease rather than producing immediate therapeautic effects.

In conclusion it may be said that Terminalia arjuna is a useful drug as an antianginal agent alone or as an adjuvant to betablockers, nitrates or calcium antagonists. However, the exact mechanisms of action, pharmacokinetics and pharmacodynamics have yet to be evaluated in further ongoing studies.

Notes

1. G.A. Rose, *Chronic Diseases: Public Health in Europe*, no. 2, WHO Regional Office for Europe, Copenhagen, 1973.
2. S.G. Sarvottam and J.N. Berry, 'Prevalence of Coronary Heart Disease in an Urban Population in Northern India', *Circulation*, vol. 37, 1968, pp. 339–52; B.D. Dewan, K.C. Malhotra and S.P. Gupta, 'Epidemiological Study of Coronary Heart Disease in Rural Commuity of Haryana', *Indian Heart Journal*, vol. 26, 1974, pp. 68–78.
3. H.V. Anderson, G.S. Roubin, P.P. Leimgrucer, J.S. Douglas, S.B. King and A.R. Gruentzig, 'Primary Angiographic Success Rate of Percutaneous Transluminal Coronary Angioplasty', *American Journal of Cardiology*, vol. 56, 1985, pp. 712–17; W.S. Aronow and H.M. Chesluk, 'Evaluation of Nitroglycerin in Angina in Patients on Isosorbide Dinitrate', *Circulation*, vol. 42, issue 1, 1970, pp. 61–3.
4. B.R. Lucchesi and L.S. Whitsett, 'The Pharmacology of Beta Adrenergic Blocking Agents', *Progress in Cardiovascular Diseases*, vol. XI, no. 5, 1969, pp. 410–30.
5. P. Messner-Pellenc, 'Trimetazidine: Conclusions of Experimental and Clinical Studies', *Presse Med.*, vol. 15, no. 35, 1986, pp. 1791–3.
6. Ibid.
7. J.F. Renaud, 'Exudes Relatives an Mode di Action de al trimetazidine an nivean des systems membraniaises in charge due transport des: ons Mat,Kt,Ca++ at du proton dane le cellulae cardiaque', 1986 (unpublished results); Idem, 'Internal pH, Na +, and Ca_2 + regulation by trimetazidine during cardiac cell acidosis', *Cardiovascular Drugs and Therapy*, vol. 1, issue 6, 1988, pp. 677–86.

8. L. Rochette, M. Fitoussi and J. Bralet, 'Effects du pre-traitmente par la trimetazidine sur la metabolisme energetique du coeur isole de rat soumis a une ligature coronaire et perfuse en normoxie ou en hypoxie', *Gazette medicale de France*, vol. 91, Suppl. 26, 1984, pp. 17–21.
9. M. Nagata, I. Imumura, R. Fugono and J. Sugimoto, 'The Actions of Trimetazidine on Isolated Guinea-pig Atria', *Japan Journal of Pharmacology*, vol. 21, 1971, pp. 337–43; Y.M. Gargouil and M. Chahine, 'Effets de la trimétazidine, sur les mouvements ioniques cellulaires dans le myocarde', *Gazette Medicale de France*, vol. 91, Suppl. 26, 1984, pp. 40–7.
10. I. Maridonneau-Parini and C. Happey, 'Effect of Trimetazidine on Membrane Damage Induced by Oxygen Free Radicals in Human Red Cells', *British Journal of Clinical Pharmacology* (*BJCP*), vol. 20, issue 5, 1985, pp. 148–51.
11. S. Dwivedi, J.P.N. Chansouria, P.N. Somani and K.N. Udupa, 'Influence of Certain Indigenous Drugs on Prostaglandin E2 Like Activity in Ischaemic Rabbit Aorta', *Indian Drugs*, vol. 24, issue 8, 1987, pp. 378–82.
12. N. Singh, K.K. Kapur, S.P. Singh, K. Shankar, J.N. Sinha and R.P. Kohli, 'Mechanism of Cardiovascular Action of Terminalia Arjuna', *Planta Medica*, vol. 45, issue 6, 1982, pp. 102–4.
13. G.N. Chaturvedi, 'Study on Ischaemic Heart Disease and Its Management by Indigenous Drugs', Ph.D. Theses (Department of Kayachikitsa), Institute of Medical Sciences, BHU, 1973.
14. S. Dwivedi, J.P.N. Chansouria, P.N. Somani and K.N. Udupa, 'Cardioprotective Effects of Certain Indigenous Drug in Myocardial Ischaemia in Rabbits', *Indian Journal of Experimental Biology* (*IJEB*), vol. 26, 1998, pp. 969–75.
15. S. Yenamandra Prabhakar and S. Damodaran Kumar, 'Chemistry of Terminalia Arjuna (Roxb.) Wight & Arnot—A Review', *Plantes Medicinales et Phytotherapii*, vol. XX, issue II, pp. 30–9; S. Yenamandra Prabhakar and S. Damodaran Kumar, 'On the Ethnomedical Significance of the Arjun Tree, Terminalia Arjuna (Roxb.) Wight and Arnot', *Journal of Ethnopharmacology*, vol. 20, issue 2, 1987, pp. 173–90.
16. R.R. Agrawal and S. Dutt, 'Chemistry, Pharmacology and Therapeutic Actions of Terminalia Arjuna', *Proceedings of National Academy of Science*, vol. 6, 1936, pp. 305–8.
17. J.F. Renaud, op. cit.; L. Rochette et al., op. cit.; Nagata et al., op. cit.; Gargouil, op. cit.; Maridonneau-Parini et al., op. cit.; Dwivedi et al., op. cit.; N. Singh et al., op. cit.
18. R.R. Agrawal and S. Dutt S., op. cit.
19. F.E. King, T.J. King and J.M. Ross, 'The Chemistry of Extractives from Hardwoods. Part XVIII. The Constitution of Arjunolic Acid, a Triterpene from *Terminalia Arjuna*', *Journal of Chemical Society*, 1954, pp. 3995–4003.
20. F.E. King, T.J. King and J.M. Ross, 'The Chemistry of Extractives from Hardwoods, Part XXIII. The Isolation of a New Triterpene (Terminolic Acid) from *Terminalia Ivorensis*', *Journal of Chemical Society*, 1955, pp. 1333–7.
21. F.E. King and T.J. King, 'The Chemistry of Extractives from Hardwoods. Part XXVII. The Structure of Terminolic Acid', *Journal of Chemical Society*, 1956, pp. 4469–77.
22. F.E. King, T.J. King and J.M. Ross, 'The Isolation of a New Triterpene'; F.E. King, T.J. King and J.M. Ross, 'The Structure of Termindic Acid'.
23. L.R. Row and G.S.R. Subbarao, 'Chemistry of Terminalia Arjuna Species. Part IV, Chemical Examination of Terminiaia Arjuna Bedd; Isolation of Arjunic Acid Saponin and (+)_ leucodelphenidin', *Journal of Indian Chemical Society*, vol. 39, 1962, pp. 89–92; L. Ramchandra Row, C. Rukmini and G.S.R. Subba Rao, 'Chemistry of Terminalia Species, Part VIII, Partial Synthesis of Arjunolic Acid', *Journal of the Indian Chemical Society*, vol. 40, 1963, pp. 311–14.

24. L. Ramchandra Row, C. Rukmini and G.S.R. Subba Rao, op. cit.
25. L.R. Row, P.S. Murty, G.S.R. Subba Rao, C.S.P. Sastry and K.V.J. Rao, 'Chemical Examination of Terminalia Species, Part XII—Isolation and Structure Determination of Arjunic Acid, a new trihydroxytriterpene carboxylic acid from the Terminalia arjuna bark', *Indian Journal of Chemistry*, vol. 8, 1970a, pp. 716–21.
26. L.R. Row, P.S. Murty, G.S.R. Subbarao, C.S.P. Sastry and K.V.J. Rao, 'Chemical Evaluation of Terminalia Species. Part XIII—Isolation and Structure Determination of Arjunetin from Terminalia Arjuna', *Indian Journal of Chemistry*, vol. 8, 1970b, pp. 772–5.
27. T. Honda, T. Murae, T. Tsuyuki, T. Takahashi and M. Sawai, 'Arjungenin, Arjunglucoside I and Arjunglucoside II, a new triterpene and new triterpene glucosides from Terminalia Arjuna', *Bulletin of Chemical Society of Japan*, vol. 49, 1976, pp. 3213–18.
28. L.M. Ghoshal, *Terminalia Arjuna*, Ph.D. thesis, Calcutta: Calcutta University, 1909.
29. R.N. Chopra and S. Ghosh, 'Terminalia Arjuna: Its Chemistry, Pharmacology and Therapeutic Action', *Indian Medical Gazette*, vol. 64, 1929, pp. 70–3.
30. N. Singh, K.K. Kapur, S.P. Singh, K. Shankar, J.N. Sinha and R.P. Kohli, op. cit., pp. 102–4.
31. R.N. Chopra, I.C. Chopra, K.L. Handa and L.D. Kapur, Chopra's *Indigenous Drugs of India*, Calcutta: Dhur & Sons Pvt. Ltd., 1958, pp. 421–5.
32. J.F. Caius, K.S. Mhaskar and M. Issacs, 'A Comparative Study of the Driedbarks of the Commoner Indian Species of Genus Terminalia', *Indian Medical Research Memoirs*, vol. 16, 1930, pp. 51–75.
33. L.P. Gupta, S.P. Sen and K.N. Udupa, 'Pharmacological Studies on Terminalia Arjuna', *Journal of Research in Indian Medicine, Yoga and Homeopathy*, vol. 11, 1976, pp.16–24.
34. Chaturvedi, op. cit.
35. S. Dwivedi, P.N. Somani, J.P.N. Chansouria and K.N. Udupa, 'Influence of Certain Indigenous Drugs on PGE—Like Activity in the Ischemic Rabbit Aorta', *Indian Drugs*, vol. 24, issue 8, 1987, pp. 378–82; S. Dwivedi, P.N. Somani, J.P.N. Chansouria and K.N. Udupa, 'Cardioprotective Effects of Certain Indigenous Drugs in Myocardial Ischemia in Rabbits', *Indian Journal of Experimental Biology* (*IJEB*), vol. 26, 1988, pp. 969–75.
36. S. Dwivedi, P.N. Somani, J.P.N. Chansouria and K.N. Udupa, *Indian Journal of Explerimental Biology* (*IJEB*), vol. 26, 1988, pp. 969–75.
37. J. Vajpai, ed., *Chakradutta*, Venkateswar Press, Bombay, 1959; Shivani Ghiladiyal and Vinod Kumar Joshi, 'A Critical Review on Two Types of *Laghupanchamula*', vol. 33, no. 3, 2012, pp. 343–7.
38. Vagbhatta in Astanga Hridayan: Commentaries by Pandit Lalchandra Vaidya, Motilal Banarsidass, Varanasi, 1st edn., 1963.
39. *Chakradutta*, op. cit.
40. Chaturvedi, op. cit.
41. S. Dwivedi, J.P.N. Chansouria, P.N. Somani and K.N. Udupa, 'Effect of Terminalia Arjuna on Ischaemic Heart Disease', *Alternative Medicine*, vol. 3, issue 2, 1989, pp. 115–22.
42. N. Singh, K.K. Kapur, S.P. Singh, K. Shankar, J.N. Sinha and R.P. Kohli, op. cit. pp. 102–4.
43. S. Dwivedi, J.P.N. Chansouria, P.N. Somani and K.N. Udupa, *Indian Drugs*, pp. 378–82.
44. S. Dwivedi, J.P.N. Chansouria, P.N. Somani and K.N. Udupa, *IJEB*, loc. cit., pp. 969–75.
45. G.N. Chaturvedi, op. cit.; S. Dwivedi, J.P.N. Chansouria, P.N. Somani and K.N. Udupa, *IJEB*, op. cit., pp. 969–75.

46. S. Dwivedi, J.P.N. Chansouria, P.N. Somani and K.N. Udupa, *Indian drugs*, op. cit., pp. 378–82.
47. N. Singh, K.K. Kapur, S.P. Singh, K. Shankar, J.N. Sinha and R.P. Kohli, op. cit., pp. 102–4.
48. R.D. Srivastava, S. Dwivedi, K.K. Srinivasan and K.N. Chandrasekar, 'Cardiovascular Effects of Terminalia Species of Plants', *Indian Drugs*, vol. 29, issue 4, 1992, pp. 144–9.
49. G.N., Chaturvedi, loc. cit.; L.P. Gupta et al., loc. cit.
50. S. Uchida, H. Ohta, M. Niwa, A. Mori, G. Nonaka, I. Nishioka and M. Ozaki, 'Prolongation of Life Span of Stroke Prone Spontaneously Hypertensive Rats Ingesting Persimon Tannin', *Chemical and Pharmacological Bulletin*, vol. 38, issue 4, pp. 1049–52.
51. A.K. Tiwari, J.D. Gode and G.P. Dubey, 'A Comparative Study between Terminalia Arjuna and Cholestyramine Effect on Serum Lipids and Lipoproteins in Hypercholesterolemic Rabbits', *Indian Drugs*, vol. 26, issue 12, 1989, pp. 664–7.

11

Fundamentals of Unani Medicine, Its Growth and National Scenario in Post-Independent India

ANIS AHMAD ANSARI

THE UNANI SYSTEM OF MEDICINE, as its name suggests, owes its origin to Greece. It was the Greek philosopher-physician Hippocrates or Buqrat (460–377 BC) who freed medicine from the realm of superstition and gave it the status of science. The theoretical framework of Unani medicine is based on the teachings of Hippocrates. After Hippocrates, a number of other Greek scholars enriched the system considerably. Out of them, Claudius Galenus better known as Galen or Jalinoos (AD 131–210) was the one who stabilized its foundation. Later on, Arab and Persian physicians like Abu Bakr Mohammad bin Yahia bin Zakaria Al-Razi known as Rhazes (AD 865–925), Abu Ali al-Ḥusain ibn Abdullah ibn Sina better known as Avicenna (AD 980–1037) and many others developed it by their original research and innovations in the method of treatment.

Unani medicine got enriched by imbibing what was best in the contemporary system of traditional medicine in Egypt, Syria, Iraq, Persia, China and India. It also benefited from the native medical system in vogue at the time in various parts of Central Asia. That is why this system is known in different parts of the world, with different names such as Greeco-Arab medicine, Ionian medicine, Arab medicine, Islamic medicine, Traditional Iranian medicine, Uighur medicine, Oriental medicine, etc.

Fundamentals of Unani-tibb and Concept of Seven Natural Principles

Arkan or elements basing the concept of body and its environment, *mizaj* or the concept of temperament and *akhlat* or the concept of humour are three basic fundamentals of Unani-tibb system. Various states of the body, in health and ill health, and the reasons for which the health is lost and the lost health is restored, forms the fundamentals of Unani-tibb. The concept of body under Unani-tibb system is known as *Umore tabi'yah*, a concept primarily based on the philosophy of health and disease discussed by Avicenna in *Kulliyat al-Qanun*. *Umore tabi'yah*[1] or concept of body is based on seven natural principles which are:

1. *Arkan* (elements),
2. *Mizaj* (temperament),
3. *Akhlat* (humours),
4. *A'aza* (organs),
5. *Arwah* (spirit),
6. *Quwa* (powers), and
7. *Afa'l* (function)

Arkan or elements are four, i.e. Air, Water, Earth and Fire. These four elements denote the temperaments or in other words, Air represents hot and moist; Fire, hot and dry while Earth cold and dry but Water represents cold and moist temperament. They together form the basic component of body with its environment. *Mizaj* or temperament is the interaction between the chemical combination of four elements that produce various states and determine the temperament of an individual human being, plants or minerals. *Tabi'yah* or *tabiyat* is, in fact, a power in all living beings, and it maintains good health. It not only ensures smooth functions of body but it fights against disease during illness. Of the seven natural principles in *Umore tabi'yh*, the concept of *akhlat* or humours is most significant. *Akhlat* or humours are the fluid contents of the body residing chiefly in blood. The humour or body fluid consists of *dam* or blood, *balgham* or phlegm, *safra* or yellow bile and *sauda* or black bile. Blood also is regarded as a mixture of all four kinds of humours. Balance in *akhlat* maintains health and their imbalance invites disease. These factors are responsible for health and the loss of any one of these components may lead even to death of an individual. *A'aza* or organs of human body are composed of cell, tissues, nerves and blood vessels also. Various organs of body and health in diseased condition of each individual affect the state of health. *Arwah* or pneuma is a life force which carries of different powers, without which human body is dead. *Arwah* carry different forces/energy from vital organs of body mainly from brain, heart and liver as well as from testes of men and ovaries of women. They are considered important in the diagnosis and treatment of disease. *Quwa* denotes physique power while *afa'l* signifies proper shape and movement of various organs of body which performs various functions.[2]

Concept of Humoural Balance

Every individual is supposed to have a unique humoural constitution or *akhlat* which represents his or her state of health. Imbalance in quality or quantity of humour leads to sickness. Correct digestion and correct diet is considered responsible for humoural balance. Theory of *mizaj* or temperament is another

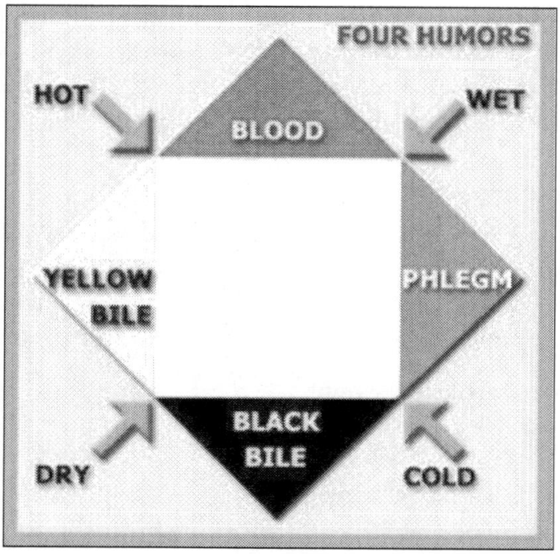

Fig. 11.1: Humoural Balance
Source: www.google/mizajinunanimedicine

vital concept in Unani. *Mizaj* denotes the tendency of a person to develop a specific disease based on morphological, physiological and psychological characteristics. Human temperament or *mizaj* is determined by the proportion in which the four humours, i.e. blood, phlegm, yellow bile and black bile, are found in an individual's body. On the basis of the proportion of humours, temperament is divided in four categories, viz., *damvi mizaj* or sanguine temperament, *safravi mizaj* or bilious temperament with yellow bile, *balghami mizaj* or phlegmatic temperament and *saudavi mizaj* or melancholic temperament. Blood predominates in sanguine temperament, proportion of bile increases in bilious temperament while yellow bile augments in phlegmatic temperament and *balgham* along with sauda or black bile swell in melancholic temperament. When a person is said to have a *haar mizaj* or hot temperament, whether naturally or unnaturally it means that *khilt dam* or sanguineous humour is dominant over other humours, in the same way, *barid mizaj* or cold temperament shows the dominance of *sauda* or black bile, *yabis mizaj* or dry temperament signifies the increase of *safra* or yellow bile, and *ratab mizaj* or moist temperament hints the raise of *balgham* or phlegm.

Principle of Six Essential Causes

Like Ayurveda, Unani medicine believes in preventive measures rather than curative. There are six basic factors which are supposed to be essential for the maintenance of good health and causation of disease. Body becomes healthy or prone to diseases due to these factors which are called *asbab-i sittah zaruriah* or six essential causes. They are: *hawa-i muhit* or atmospheric air, *makul-o-mashrub* or food and drink, *harkat-wa-sukun-i badani* or bodily movements and rest, *harkat-wa-sukun nafsania* or psychic activity and repose, *nom-o-yaqza* or sleep and wakefulness, and *istafragh-o ihtibas* or excretion of waste materials and retention of nutrients. Each and every one of these six essential factors plays significant role in maintaining health of a person.

Methods of Treatment

Diagnosis of a disease is laid great emphasis upon in Unani. Apart from the chemical analysis of different *akhlat* or humours, the Unani-tibb physicians have devised certain parameters to diagnose the *mizaj* or temperament of a patient on the basis of specific signs and symptoms. These parameters are:

1. *Malmas* or tectiles sensation,
2. *Leham wa sheham* or muscles and fats,
3. *Ashaar* or hairs of the body,
4. *Laun* or colour of the body,
5. *Hayat àl-a'za* or stature,
6. *Kaifiat al-infial* or quality or passiveness of the organs,
7. *Naum-o yaqza* or sleep or wakefulness,
8. *Afa'al al-a'za* or body functioning,
9. *Fuzlat al-badan* or excretion from the body, and
10. *Ifalat-i nafsania* or psychic reaction.

Generally, there are four methods adopted for therapy and treatement in Unani system. These four methods are:

1. *Ilaj bil-ghiza* or dieto therapy,
2. *Ilaj bil-dawa* or pharmaco therapy,
3. *Ilaj bil-yad* or surgery, and
4. *Ilaj bil-tadbeer* or regimental therapy.

Ilaj bil-ghiza or dieto therapy is the distinguished line of treatment in Unani system. It was first advocated by Buqrat (460–337 BC) and now largely taken into consideration by Unani practitioners. It is considered significant particularly in preventing deficiencies and lifestyle diseases by prescribing specific diet or by regulating the amount and quality of food. Unani lists the use of various food items used specifically in treating various diseases. In this way, food pattern and intake regulation are the fundamental approach adopted under the method of *Ilaj bil-ghiza* or dieto therapy. *Ilaj bil-dawa* or pharmaco therapy has been the main method of treatment by single or compound herbal formulations. The drugs of mineral and animal origin are also used to treat some diseases. Unani scholars have described several *tadbeer* or regimens effective for treatment of variety of humoural diseases. *Ilaj bil-yad* or surgery has been an integral part of Unani-tibb since beginning. Many surgical instruments and procedures were developed by Arab physicians. *Ilaj bil-tadbeer* or regimental therapy includes *fasad* or venesection, *hijamat* or cupping, diaphoresis, *idar-i baul* or dieresis, *hamam* or Turkish/medicated bath, *dalak* or massage, *amal-i kai* or cauterization, *is'hal* or purging, *takmeed* or fomentation, *qai* or emesis, *riyazat* or exercise and *taleeq* or leeching. In the cases of phlegmatic diseases or *amraz-i balghami* some useful *tadbeer* of regimens are: *qai* or vomiting, *is'hal* or purgation, *dalak* or massage, *riyazat* or physical exercise. While *Ilaj bil-taleeq* or leeching is prescribed useful in *saudawi* diseases. It was also considered useful in osteoarthritis. *Hijamat* or cupping is found beneficial in common arthritis and many neuromuscular disorders.[3]

Arrival and Growth of Unani Medicine in India

Unani system of medicine was introduced in India during the Sultanate rule and soon it took firm roots in the soil. The first Unani physician who came to India was Hakim Ziauddin Abdul Rafe who came to Lahore from Herat in AD 1160 during the reign of the Ghaznavid ruler Khusrow Malik (r. AD 1160–8). The Delhi Sultans as well as provincial sultans, the Khiljis, the Tughlaqs and later the Mughal Emperors provided state patronage to the scholars and even enrolled some Unani-tibb practitioners as state employees and court physicians. The system found immediate favour with the masses and soon spread all over the country even the remotest areas due to its capacity of adoption and adaption. It adopted Indian ideas and therapy as well as used indigenous drugs and herbs, and at the same time adapted itself to the Indian conditions. During the thirteenth–eighteenth centuries, Unani medicine had its heyday in India. Among host of leading Unani-tibb practitioners Abu Bakr bin Ali Usmani Kashani, Badruddin Damishqui, Sadruddin Tabib, Hakim Alauddin, Maulana Hamid Mutriz, Maulana Izzuddin Badayuni, Meh Chandra Tabib, Mian Bhu'a bin Khwas Khan, Hakim Shamsuddin Gilani, Hakim Hummam, Hakim Ali Gilani, Hakim Fathullah Gilani, Akbar Arzani and Mohammad Hashim Alvi Khan were living legends.[4]

The scholars and physicians of Unani medicine migrated to India right from the Sultanate period and a good number of them settled in India. They were earlier not aware of the known drugs of the land but in course of time they subjected Indian drugs to clinical trials. As a result of their experimentation, they added numerous native drugs to their own system. This enriched the knowledge-treasure of Unani-tibb which continued to hold an unchallenged sway for long even after the downfall of the Mughal Empire. These physicians not only treated the members of the royal family but they compiled medical anthologies recording their observations, experiments, drugs and clinical aspects. This trend continued in later periods as a result of which scores of excellent works were brought about on Unani-tibb system in India.[5] *Majmu'-i Zia'i*[6] compiled in 730 AH/AD 1329 by Zia Muhammad Masud Rashid Zangi during the reign of Muhammad bin Tughluq (r.1325–51) and *Tibb-i Firuz Shahi* was written by Firuz Shah Tughluq (r.1351–88) who was well-versed in medicine and was a bone-setter. 'Surma-i Firuz Shahi', a collyrium prepared by him became famous for curing several diseases of eye. *Rahat-ul Insan* by Ilyas bin Shahab bin Zia was also written during the time of Firuz Shah Tughluq and

Ma'dan-ul Shifa-i Tibb-i Sikandari was composed by Mian Bhu'a during the reign of Sultan Sikandar Lodi (r.1489–1517).[7] In the provincial sultanates also a number of treatises were compiled. *Tibb-i-Shahabi* (in verse) and *Shifa al-Khani* (in prose) written by Shahab bin Abdul Karim Nagori who was associated with Muzaffar Shah I (r.1407–11), the founder of the ruling dynasty in Gujarat. A third work titled *Shifa-i Mahmudi* was also produced in Gujarat by Ali bin Muhammad bin Ismail Usaili during the reign of Sultan Mahmud Beghara (r.1458–1511). Prominent Unani-tibb practitioners such as Malikul-Hukama flourished as the chief physician at the court of Sultan Nasiruddin Khalji (r.1500–10) of Malwa as is reported by Sheikh Rizqullah Mushtaqi in his well-known work *Waqi'at-i Mushtaqi*.[8] Most of these authors have largely used the Ayurvedic literature of Sanskrit also.[9]

The physicians received generous royal patronage, grants and honour from the Sultanate and Mughal rulers. This enabled them to sustain and flourish and to establish several hospitals and dispensaries in the royal capitals and other towns. *Tarikh-i Firuz Shahi* informs that there were seventy hospitals and dispensaries in Delhi during the time of Firuz Shah Tughluq.[10] Apart from Delhi, several *Darul-shifa* or hospitals were established in Malwa, Gujarat, Bidar and other provices. Medicines and even foods were supplied to the patients free of cost in these hospitals and physicians were paid salary from the government.[11]

Unani-tibb during the Mughal Period

The Mughal period is considered a golden period for the growth of Unani-tibb medical system in India. The number of Unani-tibb practitioners both royal and in public domain as well as the number of *shafa-khana* or hospitals swelled squarely during the Mughal period (1526–1800). A wide range of literature on Unani-tibb subject also came up in Arabic and Persian during this period. The series of this literature surpassed in forms and contents those produced during the Sultanate period. The Mughal rulers took keen interests in the provision of medical facilities to the public and provided all possible patronage and support to the cause of the growth of Unani-tibb in India. Yusuf bin Muḥammad Hervi (d.1543), Hakim-ul mulk Shamsuddin Gilani, Abul Fath Gilani, Shah Fathullah Shirazi, Ain-ul Mulk Shirazi, Hummam Gilani, Ali Gilani, Jalaluddin Muzaffar Ardastani, Fathullah Gilani, Muhammad Amin Gilani, Muhammad Baqar Tabrizi and several others were prominent physicians during the time of Babur, Humayun and Akbar.

Yusuf bin Muḥammad Hervi, a court physician of the first Mughal emperor Ẓahiruddin Muḥammad Babur (r.1526–30) and then of his son and successor, Humuyun (r.1530–40 and 1555–6) compiled a well-known medical dictionary titled *Baḥr al-jawaher fi ḥall loghat al-saher*. He also wrote *Jame al-fawaed*, on pathology and treatment as well as *Riaz al-adwia*, a glossary of drugs dedicated to Humayun. Several physicians were attached to the court of Jalāl-al-Din Akbar (r.1556–1605). Masiḥuddin Abul Fatḥ Gilani (d.1589), who was appointed *Ṣadr* (the head of religious affairs and land-grants) wrote a Persian commentary entitled *Fattāḥi*. Fatḥulah Gilani translated into Persian in 1593 the first book of the *Qanun*. The most extensive work was the Arabic comprehensive commentary of the *Qanun* by Ḥakim Ali Gilani (d.1609) Ayn-ul Mulk Shirazi (d.1595) who was an ophthalmologist and a poet with the pen name 'Dawāi', composed for him the *Fawaid-ul Insan* (comp. 1595).

Jahangir was well acquainted with the basics of Unani treatment. He released necessary grants from time to time for meeting the expenses on medical treatment in the public hospitals. Hakim Rukna Kashi, Hakim Sadr Shirazi alias Masih al-Zaman, Hakim Momena Shirazi and Muqarrab Khan were famous physicians in his time. A large number of works, some of them devoted to special treatments and drugs also came up during this period. *Tibb-i Abul Fath* compiled by Hakim Abul Fath Gilani (d.1589), *Sharh-i Qanun* by Ali Gilani (d.1609), *Dasturul Hunud* (*Tarjama Madan Vinod*), a dictionary of drugs and foods composed by Hakim Amanullah (d.1637) were the prominent works of the time of Jahangir and Shah Jahan. Hakim Abdullah Shirazi's (d.1648) *Tibb-i Dara Shikohi*, a medical work of encyclopaedic character also became famous. Most of these works are preserved in the public and private libraries, archives and museums in India and abroad.[12]

Eminent physicians of the time of Aurangzeb also composed several works on medicine. Abul Fatḥ Ḥeyri wrote the *Dar al-shaf-i Aurangshahi* (comp. 1670) on pathology and treatment. The work of widest circulation during this period was the *Ṭibb-i Aurangshahi* (also referred to as *Ṭibb-i Aurangzebi*) that is a general compendium on Indian medicine by Darvish Moḥammad. In the post-Aurangzeb's period, Mir Muḥammad Akbar, known as Shah Arzāni (d.1722) composed *Mofarreḥ al-qolub* which became the most diffused text on Unani medicine. He composed some other works and a treatise on *Ṭibb-i nabawi*. Alawi Khan Shirazi (d.1749) and Moḥammad Ḥusain Khan Shirazi (d.1790) were also leading Unani practitioners during the colonial period.[13]

A New Phase in Unani-tibb: Survival without Patronage

It is generally believed that Unani medicine suffered a setback and its development was hampered during the British rule because it did not gain the government patronage and support. But, since this medical system had already spread its roots in India, it enjoyed faith among the masses. It continued to be practised and got promotion even without the government patronage.

During the colonial period (1858–1947) Indian traditional medicines were called unscientific by the Western critics. As a result, a reformist approach was adopted by some traditional physicians to assimilate Western knowledge and methodology in the domain of India's indigenous medicine. A Unani medical college was established at the Aligarh Muslim University in 1927 and instead of Arabic and Persian languages, Urdu was preferred as the medium of instruction and language of the medical writings. The Niẓams of Hyderabad extended support for the cause of Unani-tibb medical studies and an imposing hospital of Unani started at Hyderabad where Hakim Kabiruddin, the most influential writer and translator of Unani medical texts into Urdu, worked till 1948. The first known history of Islamic medicine in Urdu was published in 1937 in Hyderabad by Rahber Faruqi.

Besides, the two renowned families of Unani physicians, viz., the Sharifi family of Delhi and the Azizi family of Lucknow, made commendable contribution in the promotion of Unani-tibb in north India. Hakim Abdul Majeed Khan (1833–1922) and Hakim Ajmal Khan (1868–1927) of the Sharifi family became major force for the growth and popularity of the system. Hakim Ajmal Khan who was also the personal physician of the Nawab of Rampur, advocated for the modernizing Unani-tibb. He also travelled to Europe and directed the first modern scientific analysis of a traditional simple drug, the Rauwolfia serpentina, which had been used by Avicenna in the treatment of mania. Because of this experiment, the alkaloids were named after him as ajmaline and ajmalinine. The British later recognized and appreciated his skill and endeavour in the field of Unani-tibb. He established Madrasah Tibbia Zanana (Women Tibbia College) in 1909 and it was inaugurated by Sir Louis Dean, the British Governor of Punjab. Ajmal Khan was also an important figure on the political and cultural scene. He strongly supported the idea of unity among Hindus and Muslims and had close contacts with Mahatma Gandhi who attended the opening ceremony of Ajmal Khan's new medical college, named Hindustani Dawakhana in Delhi in 1921. The Azizi family took their name from Hakim Abdul Aziz (1855–1911), who in 1902 opened the family school called Takmil-ul-Ṭibb at Lucknow. The most important among the later physicians of this family was Abdul Laṭif Falsafi (1900–70), who also taught at the Unani college of Aligarh and contributed several works and articles in Urdu on Unani-tibb.[14] Besides, the Majeedi family of Delhi, especially Hakim Abdul Hameed (1908–99) made valuable contributions towards modernization of Unani drug industry. He also established an Institute of History of Medicine and Medical Research (IHMMR) in Delhi that now has the status of a Deemed University under the Jamia Hamdard and played a significant role in the advancement of Unani medicine.[15]

Promotion of Unani Medicine in Post-Independent India

Promotion of India's indigenous medical systems like Ayurveda, Unani, Siddha and Homoeopathy received a new impetus after the country's independence. In 1969, the Government of India established the Central Council for Research in Indian Medicine and Homoeopathy (CCRIMH) with the objective to develop scientific research in different branches of the Indian systems of medicine, viz., Ayurveda, Unani, Siddha, Yoga, Naturopathy and Homoeopathy. Research activities in these systems continued under the aegis of the CCRIMH until 1978 when it was split into four separate research councils for further growth of these systems in consonance with the basic philosophy of the respective healing system. Later, the Indian Parliament passed the Indian Medicine Central Council Act, 1970 in order to streamline and regulate the education, research and practices in Indian systems of medicine, i.e. Ayurveda, Unani, Siddha, Yoga, Naturopathy and Homoeopathy. Under this Act, the Government of India set up the Central Council of Indian Medicine (CCIM) in 1970.

In 1995, the Government of India also setup a full-fledged Department of Indian Systems of Medicine & Homoeopathy (ISM&H) under the Union Ministry of Health and Family Welfare to further boost the development of Unani and other Indian systems of medicine. The Department of ISM&H was later renamed as Department of Ayurveda, Yoga, Unani, Siddha and Homoeopathy (AYUSH). Subsequent to this Unani system of medicine, its recognized practitioners, hospitals as well as educational and research institutions formed an integral part of the National Health Care Delivery System. The Government of India has been providing regular financial and other support for the promotion and development of Unani medicine at par with other indigenous medical systems for the purpose of providing medical facilities to the larger proportion of the masses not only in urban but rural areas too. India is today the world leader so far as the growth of Unani medicine is concerned.

Public Healthcare and Unani-tibb

Unani-tibb system of medicine is encouragingly becoming popular among the masses in recent decades. The practitioners of Unani medicine are now scattered all over the country. They form an integral part of the National Healthcare Delivery Structure. According to official figures available, there were around 44,000 registered Unani practitioners in the country in 2007. Out of them, 21,597 were institutionally qualified and 21,511 non-institutionally qualified physicians. Eighteen states run Unani hospitals with dispensaries and the total number of hospitals functioning in different states of the country was 312. While the total bed strength in these hospitals together was 5,128 and the total number of Unani dispensaries was 958. Besides, eight dispensaries were functioning under the Central Government Health Scheme (CGHS). Out of these eight dispensaries, two were located in Andhra Pradesh, one each in Uttar Pradesh and West Bengal while four were operative in Delhi.[16] These numbers and figures have now swelled.

Educational and Research Institutions on Unani-tibb

Education, research and training in Unani is monitored by the Central Council of Indian Medicine, a statutory body set up by the Act of Parliament known as Indian Medicine Central Council Act, 1970. At present, there are forty recognized colleges of Unani medicine in the country. These colleges provide education and training facilities in the system. These colleges have a total admission capacity of about 1,800 students per year for undergraduate courses. Some of these colleges are government institutions. However, most colleges have been set up by voluntary organizations. All these colleges and educational institutions are affiliated to different universities. Curriculum of these have been framed and prescribed by the Central Council of Indian Medicines.

Apart from undergraduation, there are facilities for postgraduate education and research too. Postgraduate teaching is offered in the subjects, like *Ilmul advia* or Pharmacology, *Moalejat* or Medicine, *Kulliyat* or Basic Principles, *Hifzan-i sehat* or Hygiene, *Tashreeh* or Anatomy, *Jarrahat* or Surgery and *Qabala wa Amraz-i niswan* or Gynaecology at Ajmal Khan Tibbia College, Aligarh Muslim University, Aligarh. Government Nizamiah Tibbi College, Hyderabad offers postgraduation in *Moalejat* (Medicine), *Amraz-i niswan* (Gynaecology) and *Amraz-i Atfal* (Paedriatics). Ayurvedic and Unani Tibbi College in Karol Bagh, New Delhi has also started postgraduation in *Moalejat* (Medicine) and *Ilmul advia* (Pharmacology), *Hifzan-i Sehat* (Hygiene) and *Jarrahat* (Surgery).

In 1984, the National Institute of Unani Medicine was set up in Bangalore by the Ministry of Health and Family Welfare, Government of India for offering postgraduate education in all disciplines of Unani medicine and overall growth of Unani medicine and research in the country.[17]

Central Council for Research in Unani Medicine (CCRUM), started functioning under Ministry of Health and Family Welfare, Department of AYUSH, New Delhi from 1978. It has 23 centres in the different parts of the country. CCRUM has made some commendable achievements in clinical research in Unani. The area chosen for research include clinical research, drug research, survey and cultivation of medicinal plants, research on fundamentals of Unani, literary research and family welfare research programme. The clinical research programme of the Council aims at critical appraisal of the theory of pathogenesis, symptomatology, clinical methods of diagnosis and prognosis, principles, lines and methods of treatment enunciated in the classical texts of Unani system of medicine. Some of its achievements are as follows:

Diseases undertaken for clinical studies: 30
Drugs formulation undertaken for screening: 120
Formulations undertaken for extensive clinical trials: 55
Single/compound Unani drugs studied
for their pharmacological action and safety evaluation: 100
Formulations/drugs developed for various diseases: 30
Formulation decoded and studies published: 12
Formulations filed for grant of patent rights: 8

The disease in which clinical trials have been undertaken and taken a lead include *Bars* (Vitiligo), *Nar-e-Farsi* (Eczema), *Dausadaf* (Psoriasus), *Iltehab-e-Kabid* (Infective Hepatitis), *Hasat-ul-Kulliya wa Masana* (Urolithiasis), *Qarah-e-Medda wa Asna-e-Ashri* (Duodenal Ulcer), *Ishal-e-Muzmin* (Chronic Diarrhoea), *Ishal-e-Aftal* (Infantile Diarrhoea), *Deedan-e-Ama* (Helminthiasis), *Humma-e-Ijamia* (Malaria), *Zusantaria Mevi* (Amoebic Dysentry), *Kala Azar* (Leishmaniasis), *Dual Feel* (Filariasis), *Ziabetus Sukkari* (Diabetes Mellitus), *Waja-ul-Mafasil* (Rheumatoid Arthritis), *Iltehab-e-Tajaweef-e-Anf* (Sinusitis), *Zeeq-un-Nafas* (Bronchial Asthma), *Sailanur Rahem* (Leucorrhoea) and *Kasrat-e-Shahmuddam* (Hyperlipidemia).

Apart from clinical/pharmacological and photochemical research, CCRUM translated and published 25 classical books, 60 manuscripts and 24 important manuscripts have been digitalized.

CCRUM has made several strides also in single and compound drug standardization and formation of Unani pharmacopoeial standards as per the latest methods and requirements. Thousands of specimens and plant species from different forest divisions throughout the country are collected and preserved. Further, the Council significantly contributed in literary research, Traditional Knowledge Digital Library (TKDL) Unani and Extramural Research Projects. CCRUM has been granted 8 patents by Indian patent office and more than 30 applications for patents are in pipeline.

Licensed Unani Pharmacies Drug Control System

It is notable that there are about 550 licensed Unani pharmacies in different parts of the country. Besides, Indian Medicine Pharmaceuticals Corporation Ltd. (IMPCL) which is a Government of India undertaking, is one of the major manufacturer of Unani drugs.

The manufacturing of Unani drug is regulated and controlled by Drugs and Cosmetic Act, 1940. Rules are framed and amended under this Act from time to time. There is a permanent Unani Pharmacopoeia Committee (UPC) under the Ministry of Health and Family Welfare, Government of India, which consists of experts in Unani medicine, chemists, botanists and pharmacologists. The Unani Pharmacopoeia Committee of India has published 6 volumes (298 monographs of single drugs), and 2 volumes (100 monographs of compound drugs) and 5 volumes of National Formulary of Unani Medicine (consisting of 1228 formulations).

Centres of Unani in Overseas Countries

It is significant that the Unani system of medicine and its education is available in the countries like Bangladesh, Sri Lanka, Iran, Saudi Arabia, UAE, Kuwait, UK, China and in South Africa. An undergraduate course of five years in Unani medicine recognized by Dhaka University in Bangladesh is in force. Similar courses are run in Pakistan and Sri Lanka too. In Iran, practice in traditional medicine is allowed and controlled by Traditional Medicine and Materia Medica Research Centre (TMRC) established at Shaheed Beheshti Medical University, Tehran, Iran. A degree course—Bachelor of Unani-tibb Medicine (BUTM)—is conducted by the University of the Western Cape Town in South Africa and after one year of internship, one could get registered as practitioner in Unani medicine. A diploma course in eastern medicine is offered at Mohsin Institute of Tibb at Leicester in UK. An undergraduate course in Uighur medicine (Greeco-Arab medicine) at Xinjiang Uighur Medical College & Research Centre at West Beijing Road, Khotan City, Xinjiang, China is also popular course in medicine. Table 11.1 reveals the present status of Unani medicine in Pakistan, Bangladesh and Sri Lanka.[18]

Table 11.1: Present Status of Unani Medicine

Countries	*Total number of Unani hospitals*	*Total number of beds in Unani hospitals*	*Total number of dispensaries*	*Total number of pharmacies*	*Total number of registered Unani practitioners*
Pakistan	57	260	360	95	52,600
Bangladesh	1	100	–	–	2,230
Sri Lanka	1	100	230	2	Not available

Conclusion

To conclude, it may be said that Unani system of medicine which owes its origin to Greece and entered into India at the close of twelfth century and more specifically in the thirteenth century after the establishment of the Sultanate rule in Delhi passed primarily through four phases. In the first phase (Sultanate period: 1200–1526) the Unani-tibb system took its root in India but when the the Delhi sultanate declined after Firuz Shah Tughluq and the new provincial kingdoms in Gujarat, Malwa, Jaunpur, and the Deccan kingdoms came into existence, the Unani system spread to these areas too. The second phase (Mughal period: 1526–1707) is considered as the golden period for the growth of Unani when it received all kinds of patronage and support from the Mughal rulers. After decline of the Mughal Empire, the Unani system got patronage from the nawabs in Awadh, Bengal, Hyderabad, Punjab and other areas but soon it had to face the challenge of the British apathy and challenge of the Western medicine. During this phase, i.e. the third phase, the system survived on account of the support from the people and the masses who had faith in Unani system of healing. It was during this phase that leading Unani practitioners looked inward to modernize the system. The fourth phase in the growth of Unani medicine began after India's independence in 1947 when the Unani-tibb along with Ayurveda and other indigenous systems of medicine again began to receive the patronage and support of the government both central and state levels. With the foundation of AYUSH under the Ministry of Health and Family Welfare in 1995, Unani along with Ayurveda and other indigenous systems of medicine entered into a new phase of growth and promotion on scientific lines by maintaining certain parameters of check and balance as well as expanding teaching and research in order to provide alternative health care systems to the masses at grassroot level. It was during this phase when the Unani along with other indigenous systems of medicine crossed the national boundaries and overseas doors began to open. It is significant that in recent years, a Degree course of Bachelor of Unani-Tibb Medicine (BUTM) is conducted by the University of the Western Cape Town in South Africa and graduates are registered as practitioners in Unani medicine. A degree course in Uighur medicine (Greeco-Arab medicine) at Xinjiang Uighur Medical College & Research Centre at West Beijing Road, Khotan City, Xinjiang, China is also popular course in medicine.

Appendix I

Gazette Notification of South African Government, 2007

6 No. 30286 GOVERNMENT GAZETTE, 14 SEPTEMBER 2007

Government Notices
Goewermentskennisgewings

DEPARTMENT OF HEALTH
DEPARTEMENT VAN GESONDHEID

No. 847 **14 September 2007**

ALLIED HEALTH PROFESSIONS ACT, 1982

ESTABLISHMENT OF THE PROFESSIONAL BOARD FOR AYURVEDA, CHINESE MEDICINE AND ACUPUNCTURE AND UNANI TIBB UNDER THE ALLIED HEALTH PROFESSIONS ACT, 1982 (ACT 63 OF 1982)

I, Dr M E Tshabalala-Msimang, Minister of Health, acting in terms of section 10A of the Allied Health Professions Act, 1982 (Act 63 of 1982), and in consultation with the Allied Health Professions Council of South Africa, hereby establish the Professional Board for Ayurveda, Chinese Medicine and Acupuncture and Unani Tibb.

DR ME TSHABALALA-MSIMANG
MINISTER OF HEALTH

Appendix II

Gazette Notification of South African Government, 2007

STAATSKOERANT, 14 SEPTEMBER 2007 No. 30286 7

No. 848 **14 September 2007**

ALLIED HEALTH PROFESSIONS ACT, 1982

INCLUSION OF THE PROFESSION OF UNANI TIBB UNDER THE PROVISIONS OF THE ALLIED HEALTH PROFESSIONS ACT, 1982 (ACT 63 OF 1982)

I, Dr M E Tshabalala-Msimang, Minister of Health, acting in terms of section 16 of the Allied Health Professions Act, 1982 (Act63 of 1982), and in consultation with the Allied Health Professions Council of South Africa, hereby declare the provisions of the said Act to be applicable to the profession of Unani Tibb, which profession has as its object the promotion of health, the treatment, prevention or relief of physical or mental defects, illness or deficiencies in humans.

DR ME TSHABALALA-MSIMANG
MINISTER OF HEALTH

Notes

1. S.I. Ahmad, *Introduction to Al-Umoor-Al-Tabi'yah*, Delhi: Saini Printers, 1980, pp. 1–3, 57–8.
2. Altaf Ahmed Azmi, *Basic Concepts of Unani Medicine: A Critical Study*, New Delhi: Jamia Hamdard, 1995, pp. 5–6.
3. Syed Zillur Rahman, 'Unani Medicine in India: Its Origin and Fundamental Concepts', in *History of Science, Philosophy and Culture in Indian Civilization, vol. IV, pt. 2, Medicine and Life Sciences in India*, ed. B.V. Subbarayappa, New Delhi: Centre for Studies in Civilizations, 2001, pp. 292–325.
4. Ziauddin Barani, *Tarikh-i Firuz Shahi*, Calcutta: Asiatic Society, 1862, p. 362.
5. M. Zubayr Siddiqui, *Studies in Arabic and Persian Medical Literature*, Calcutta: Calcutta University, 1959, pp. 1–40; Physician-Authors of Greeco-Arab Medicine in India, New Delhi: Institute of History of Medicine and Medical Research, 1970, pp. 1–17; Shabbir Ahmad Khan et al., eds., 'A Catalogue of Arabic and Persian Medical Manusripts', New Delhi: Institute of History of Medicine and Medical Research, pp. 5–22.
6. Two manuscripts of this work have so far come to light, one is available in the State Library (formerly called Asafia Library, Hyderabad, Andhra Pradesh) and the other in the Jamia Hamdard Library, New Delhi.
7. Tazimuddin Siddiqui, 'Unani Medicine in India during the Delhi Sultanate', *Indian Journal of History of Science*, vol. 15, no. 1, May 1980, pp. 18–24; Altaf Ahmed Azmi, 'Unani Medicine: Hakims and their Treatises', in *Medicine and Life Sciences in India*, pp. 326–31.
8. Sheikh Rizqullah Mushtaqi, *Waqi'at-i-Mushtaqi*, Eng. tr. I.H. Siddiqui, New Delhi, 1993, pp. 226–7.
9. Iqtidar Husain Siddiqui, 'Science of Medicine and Hospitals in India during the Delhi Sultanate Period', *Indian Historical Review*, vol. 39, no. 1, 2012, pp. 11–18.
10. Barani, op. cit., pp. 352–66.
11. Iqtidar Husain Siddiqui, op. cit.
12. Azmi, 'Unani Medicine', pp. 332–70; D.N. Marshall, *Mughals in India: A Bibliographical Survey*, Bombay, 1967, pp. 381–2.
13. Azmi, 'Unani Medicine', pp. 352–8.
14. Barbara D. Metcalf, 'Hakim Ajmal Khan, Rais of Delhi and Muslim Leader', in *Delhi Through the Ages: Essays in Urban History, Culture, and Society*, ed. Robert Erick Frykenberg, Delhi, 1985, pp. 299–315; S.Z. Rahman, 'Tazkira Khandan-i Azizi', Aligarh: Shifa-ul Mulk Memorial Committee, 1978, pp. 35–40; M.A. Razzack, 'Hakim Ajmal Khan: The Versatile Genius', New Delhi: Central Council for Research in Unani Medicine, 1987, pp. 9–14; M. Khalid Siddiqui, 'Paikere Fikro Amal: Hakim Abdul Hamid', New Delhi: Greto Enterprises, 2010, pp. 37–40.
15. Azmi, 'Unani Medicine', pp. 358–62.
16. Annual Report of the Central Council for Research in Unani Medicine, New Delhi: Ministry of Health and Family Welfare, Department of AYUSH, 2007.
17. *National Institute of Unani Medicine Bangalore: Memorandum of Association and Rules, Regulations and Bye-laws* (As amended up to April 2007), Ministry of Health and Family Welfare, Government of India, 1984, pp. 1–66.
18. WHO (World Health Organization), Legal Status of Traditional Medicine and Complementary/Alternative Medicine: A World Wide View, Geneva, WHO, 2001; Bangladesh Unani and Ayurveda Board. Present Status of Herbal Medicine in Bangladesh [On line]. Available from: www. Ics.trieste/media/134578/df2506/pdf, accessed on 24 October 2011; The Institute of Indigenous Medicine, Homepage, available from: http://iim.cmb.ac.lk/unani, accessed on 24 October 2011.

12

Unani Medicine in Indigenous Stain, with Reference to Some of its Notable Indian Resources

Ashhar Qadeer

Introduction

Presently in India, indigenous systems of medicine are governed by the Department of AYUSH under the Ministry of Health and Family Welfare. AYUSH stands for Ayurveda, Yoga and Naturopathy, Unani medicine, Siddha and Homoeopathy. Ayurveda (knowledge on longevity), Yoga and Siddha go back to the vedic scriptures of ancient India. Unani or the Greeco-Arab medical system was introduced in the subcontinent by the Muslims. Homoeopathy which was adopted and introduced by the German physician Samuel Hahnemann (1755–1843) has remained popular in India.

Unani originated at Unan or Greece and the renowned Greek philosopher and physician Hippocrates (460–377 BC) was its founder who planted it on the Greek soil. Then with the collaboration of Greek and Roman physicians, this system became deep rooted and by the medieval period its branches spread to the Middle East. In countries like Syria, Iraq and Persia it was developed to its zenith and was accepted internationally. Hence, it was also termed as the Greeco-Arab system of medicine.

Though, this system of healing is in touch with India since first century AD, it came into regular practice by the thirteenth and fourteenth centuries AD.[1] Unani system of medicine has a unique character of preserving its basic fundamentals with approval of new, advanced and progressive information. Wherever it is set up, it integrates with beneficial healing assets found at that place. There are no insensitive restrictions to intact distinctiveness. This superiority of Unani system of medicine converts its foreign character into national for every venue. The same happened to it in India and it has become indigenous.

This healing art was introduced and primarily practised in India by outsiders, mostly by the physicians of Turkish and Persian origin, who came to India with the establishment of the Muslim empires. In no time, they became familiar with the traditional medicines of India and enriched their system by amalgamation. Some of them gained knowledge of Sanskrit to understand Indian medicines in depth to use them for healing purposes.[2] Then, they produced medical notes, which proved to be pathbreaking for Unani medicine, to be practised here as an indigenous system. Even some Hindus came forward to become good Unani physicians. The scholar Abul Fazl, associated with the court of Akbar, in his famous book *Ain-i Akbari* gives the list of the court physicians. The names like Hakim Mahadeo, Hakim Bhim Nath, Hakim Narayan and Hakim Shivji have also been mentioned in the book. The practice of Unani medicine in India is continuing till date in the same manner.

Some of the notable Indian writings from the extension of *Tibb* (Unani medicine) to the knowledge of classical Indian medicines like Ayurveda, Yoga and Siddha are as follows:

1. *Kitab al-Saidna Fi al-Tibb* by Aburehan Mohammad Albairuni (d.1005).
2. *Majmu'a-i Shamsi* by Khwaja Shams al-Din Mustafi (d.730 H).
3. *Majmu'a-i Ḍiay'i* by Ḍiya Muhammad Mas'ud Rashid Zangi (d.1351).
4. *Rahat-ul Insan* by Hakim Ilyas b. Shehab (written in 778 H/AD 1377).
5. *Tibb-i Shehabi* by Shehab ibn Abdul al-Karim Nagori (close to 1388).
6. *Dastur al-Atibba* by Muhammad Qasim Farishta (d.1623).
7. *Madan al-Shifa Sikandar Shahi* by Bahwa bin Khawas Khan (d.918 H).
8. *Ganj-i Badaward* by Aman al-Allah Khan (d.1637).
9. *Dastur al-Hunud* by Aman al-Allah Khan (d.1637).
10. *Mujarrabat-i Akbari* by Hakim Muhammad Akbar Arzani (d.1722).
11. *Yadgar-i Radai* by Hakim Rada Ali bin Muhammad (close to 1828).
12. *Talifa-i Sharifi* by Hakim Muhammad Sharif Khan (d.1807).

Only five most important resources, for example nos. 3, 4, 5, 6 and 9 are being selected to highlight the theme here.

Ḍiyai

Majmu'a-i Ḍiyai[3] was written by Ḍiya Muhammad Mas'ud' Rashid Zangi Umar Ghaznawi alias 'Mubarakbad'. He was a court physician of Sultan Muhammad bin Tughlaq (AD 1325–51). He completed this book in Persian during his stay in Tilang (Devgiri or Daulatabad) around 737 H/AD 1336 and named its title after his name. However, the author admits that his book's title follows the trend of the book by his uncle, Khwaja Shams al-Din Mustafi, called *Majmu'a-i Shamsi*.

One of its complete manuscripts is available in Hakim Mohammad Said Library, Jamia Hamdard, New Delhi (MS No. 11963). The size is 16 × 26 cm., with 23 lines on each page and spreading over 250 leaves. The text is based on Arabic, Persian and also on some Ayurvedic medical works. As mentioned above, there is a reference to another book *Majmu'a-i Shamsi*, compiled earlier by Khwaja Shams al-Din Mustafi and is said to be Persian translation of an Ayurvedic book. This work has not been found in any library or collection in India.

Majmu'a-i Ḍiay'i shows that the writer was conversant with not only Persian and Arabic but also Sanskrit. The author has mentioned the sources of *Majmu'a-i Ḍiay'i* under which a number of books are enlisted. For the knowledge of Indian medicine, he had considered books like *Nag Arjun Sagar* of Nag Arjuna as a direct source and *Firdaus al-Hikma* of Ali bin Rabban Tabari and *Majmu'a-i Shamsi* of Khwaja Shams al-Din Mustafi as indirect sources.

This book has 46 chapters on different topics. Chapter 41 has been devoted to teach Indian physician about the extensive knowledge of the book. By this creation, considerable additions were made in *Tibb*, particularly in view of Indian climatic conditions, temperament and disposition of the people, and that Ayurveda was studied in depth to incorporate foreign medical knowledge.

In this book, *Tibb* is reviewed in the context of Indian climatic conditions, nature of the people, their living habits, particularly their diets and dietary sources. Drugs, simple, compound and of great efficacy found in India, were included in *Tibbi* Pharmacopeia. 1,150 simple drugs are listed there with their *Tibbi* and Hindi names. Some of the drugs were remained famous by their Hindi names. Even today, they are used by the *Tibbi* physicians with the same name like, *Halela, Balela, Amla, Alsi, Chaksu, Indra Jau, Kalaunji, Jawakhar, Bakain* and *Sanhka Holi.*

Some compound formulations like *Majun Suparipak, Maju Jograj Gugal,* and *Chewanprash* were included in *Tibbi* formulary and till date are in practice by the same names. Pharmacy unit processes, which were learnt from Indian physicians, are mentioned, which are being taught and followed till now. Some of them are: *Put, Jantar, Kharal,* etc.

Rahat-ul Insan

Another important book, composed during the reign of Firoz Shah, was introduced as *Rahat-ul Insan*.[4] The physician called Hakim Ilyas b. Shehab wrote it in 778 H/AD 1377 and dedicated it to Sultan Firoz Shah. The influence of Indian medicine (Ayurveda) is quite prominent in this book. The manuscript from which following information has been derived exists in Andhra Pradesh Government Oriental Manuscript Library and Research Institute Hyderabad, Andhra Pradesh.

It has three sections and 74 chapters as mentioned in the Preface by the author and he writes: 'It was written on 2nd *Muharram* 778 H at the insistence world-protecting master, Abu Muzaffar Firoz Shah. The Sultan, may his country and kingdom ever remain under the security and mercy of God, and was named *Rahat-ul Insan* comprising three sections and 74 chapters.'

The text shows that the influence of Indian medicine (Ayurveda) is remarkable in this book. Beside the Hindi names of the drugs, the author has also given Hindi names of the diseases. For example, in Unani medicine one of the fevers is called *Humma-i Saudavi*, caused by *Khilt-i Sauda.* The author writes: '*Tap-i Saudavi* is called *pat jar* in Hindi'. The prescription that has been given for *Tap-i Saudavi* is based too on the drugs of Hindi names as: '*Satawar*-3 *diram*, *Kulvi*-3 *diram*, *Bansa*-3 *diram*; pound each item and boil in 6 bowls of water until one bowl remains.'

Indeed, this book is a good example to observe the amalgamation of Unani medicine with Ayurveda to develop a comprehensive indigenous system of medicine.

Tibb-i Shehabi

Tibb-i Shehabi,[5] also known as *Shifa al-Amraz* was authored by an outstanding physician and scholar of his time called Shehab ibn Abdul al-Karim Nagori of Nagor in Gujarat close to 790 H./AD 1388.

It is written in verse in Persian language containing the knowledge based on previous medical references and personal observations of the author about the causes, symptoms and the treatment of the diseases. It also has the knowledge about the properties and actions of certain drugs and food. This work had been dedicated to the ruler of that time and is recognized as *Tibb-i Shehabi.*

The manuscripts are available in different Indian libraries. Hakim Mohammad Said Library of Jamia Hamdard, New Delhi also has a copy of it. It has 110 folios of size 16 × 11.5 cm. with 17–20 couplets on each page.

The text is composed on the basic fundamentals of Tibb and principles of treatment with an extension of Indian medical stain. There are a number of terms and vocabularies in relation with typical Indian customs. This is an apt example of rewriting of Tibb according to the practical need of a habitat.

In the last part of the text, the author admits that he borrowed heavily from the books of Indian writers. In the narration of basic principles, comparative description of Tibb and Indian medicine is provided in the book and many Indian terms like *Tatva, Panch Tatva, Dosha, Tridosha, Vata, Pita, Kafa, Rasa, Rakta, Mansa, Maidya, Manja, Dhata*, etc., have been mentioned.

The portion that deals with therapeutic has the description of the diseases by their Indian names like: *Khansi, Pindrog, Rengan, Phunsi, Phori, Pilia, Pitti*, and *Motia Bind.* These have been very much in use in *Tibbi* books by the subsequent authors.

At the end of the book, the physician has described the experiences of his life, which are particularly concerned with the nature and behaviour of Hindu and Muslim patients as follow:

> In this world, I found faithfulness in Hindus and I sought retribution on behalf of Muslims from God. The infidel had not given me wealth (treasure) in secret that the Muslim spoiled necessarily my wealth. When a Hindu suffers from any ailment, he goes

to a reliable physician; he does not disobey his orders regarding precautions, etc., and gets well after some time and accepts him as his master for all times to come. And if he dies during the treatment, they render greater service to the physician by his magnanimity [and say] that this man did his utmost to restore him to health but as God predestined it, medicine did not prove beneficial.

Now, when a Muslim gets afflicted by a disease and brings his urine to me for diagnose, by God, I treat him with full attention and give him tested medicines, and advise precautions. But, if I ask him to take honey, he drinks buttermilk, and if I ask him to take rice, he eats pottage. If he survives, his attendants say that was the grace of God, which saved him, and if he dies, they say that he has been killed by the physician. This is the position of the [followers of] Islam in this region and I do not know about other places.

The above experiences clearly indicate that at the time of Nagori, Unani medicine had not remained a foreign path and was well accepted by the Hindus who had full faith in Muslim physicians. There was no discrimination between Unani medicine and Ayurveda on the basis of region and religion.

Nagori did outstanding work to give Indian stain to Unani medicine. He also prepared a medical dictionary, and entitled it *Farhang-i Shehabi*. It has Hindi names of medicines along with Arabic and Persian names, e.g. *Baṣal* (Arabic) = *Piyaz* (Hindi), *Biladur* (Arabic) = *Bhilawan* (Hindi). This dictionary is incomplete and has only 12 folios, but it is a good evidence of efforts made by the physicians to amalgamate Unani medicine with Ayurveda to make an inclusive indigenous system of medicine.

Dastur al-Atibba

Dastur al-Atibba,[6] is the result of indepth research on medicine of the time by a renowned historian and physician Muhammad Qasim Farishta, who was born at Astrabad in northern Persia in 1552 and died in India in 1623. He migrated from Persia to India and reached Ahmadnagar during the reign of Hussain Nizam Shah (r.1553–65), and settled there.

Farishta had a command over medical knowledge. He learnt it from the masters like Hakim Sheikh Mohammad Misri, Hakim Cheter Bhoj and Hakim Sheikh Bin Nasrullah. In 1950, Farishta went to Bijapur and associated himself with the court of Ibrahim Adil Shah II (reigned 1580–1628). There, he wrote this book. To his name this work is also well known as *Ikhtiarat-i Qasmi*.

Copies of this manuscript are available in many Indian libraries like Hakim Mohammad Said Library, Jamia Hamdard, New Delhi; Khuda Bakhsh Oriental Public Library, Patna; Raza Library, Rampur, UP; Salarjung Museum, Hyderabad; Asiatic Society, West Bengal; and Maulama Azad Library, Aligarh Muslim University, Aligarh.

Hakim Mohammad Said Library, Jamia Hamdard has three copies. The copy (MS no. 160) is clearly readable. It has 161 folios, of size 19.5 × 10.5 cm. with 10 lines per page. This is the resource from which I have taken the following notes.

In his introduction to this book, what Farishta says is important as far as the interest of Unani physicians in classical Indian medicine is concerned. His narration is as follows:

> Writer of these pages, Muhammad Qasim, entitled as Hindu Shah, commonly known as Farishta, studied the noble science of medicine as deeply as possible and spent a part of his valuable life on it. After perusal of the books on the subject commonly consulted in Iran, Turkey and Arabia, his mind turned towards the study of the works of the Indian physicians. He found the theories as well as the practices of their medical sciences extremely well founded. He, therefore, thought it necessary to complete a book dealing with their medical principles, the applications of these principles and their method of principles of treatment of diseases, which at the outset, appeared to be strange. Since, there were many Muslim friends living in this country, who had no thorough knowledge of the ever-changing climate of this country, nor were they well aware of the system of treatment followed by the Indian physicians. He, therefore, mentioned the properties of drugs and victuals and their names which are difficult to pronounce. Besides, he also wanted to leave behind something by which he might be remembered.[7]

The text of *Dastur al-Atibba* contains a Preface, three sections and a Conclusion. The whole text is a beautiful amalgamation of Tibb and Ayurveda. Here, Unani medicine is completely stained in classical Indian medicine. The book not only contains the name of simple and compound drugs used in both the disciplines but also the author has included the experiences of Ayurvedic physicians, based on their investigation and prescriptions.

The Preface deals with the basic principles of Ayurveda. The knowledge derived from Indian medical books, like *Caraka Saṁhitā, Suśruta Saṁhitā,* is also mentioned. There are many terms associated with Ayurveda. The things mentioned include *Dhatus* (basic components of the body, *Tridosa*, there are humours, viz., *pitta, kafa, vayu*), *Tatva* (five preliminary elements), and six temperament (three simple and three compounds). Indian seasons are described under *Ritu.* Indian vegetables, cattle are enlisted as food resources. Seasonal variation and their affects on human heath with respect to Indian climate, foods and drinks are described. Indian regions are classified into three; according to the underground water level namely *Jangal Des* (with low level), *Anup Des* (high level) and *Sadharan Des* (average level). Thereafter, the affects of these levels on the soil, vegetables and life are also mentioned. As per the quality of dietary resources this classification is very important. Later on, Unani physicians always kept this classification in mind during the practice.

The first section describes about 700 herbs in alphabetical order; Ayurvedic physicians used most of these drugs at that time. The second section, which has been classified into 15 chapters, include the narration of compound drugs to treat different diseases. The Ayurvedic compounds like: *Ram Ban* and *Ghorachari* are described and have even been given *Tibbi* names like *Habb-i Ruh Parwar* and *Habbi Miskeen Nawaz* respectively. The third section is on 160 specific diseases and their treatment. Therapeutics are amalgamated from Tibb and Ayurvedic resources.

Dastur al-Hunud

Dastur al-Hunud[8] was written by Aman al-Allah Khan Amani (d.1637). His father Mahabat Khan is well known as Mughal army commander during the reign of Akbar. He had specialization in multiple disciplines, and he was also affectionate with medical knowledge and practice. He had keen interest in Ayurveda too and translated an important Indian medical work entitled *Madan Vinod*, composed by the King Madan Pal in 1375.

Its manuscripts are preserved in many libraries like Library of California University, New York; Khuda Bakhsh Oriental Public Library, Patna; and Salarjung Museum Library, Hyderabad. One of its manuscripts is available in Hakim Mohammad Said Library, Jamia Hamdard, New Delhi (MS no. 9864), which has been selected here to forward the information.

The size is 15.5 × 8.5 cm. with 16 lines on each page and spreading across 119 pages. The colophon does not show the date of translation. The Preface or Introductory remarks deal with scientific details and the essential causes. It covers 15 pages of the manuscript and is divided into 9 sections.

The text deals mostly with information on hygienic principles and Indian drugs. Some of its distinctions in Indian perspective are as follows:

There are nearly 700 drugs which have been explained. Majority of drugs is of Indian origin. Arabic and Persian names of those drugs are also mentioned. In case of Indian names, emphasis is given on pronunciation in most of the cases with the vowel points *Zabar, Zayr* and *Pesh*. At some places, Persian, Arabic and Greek translations for correct understanding have also been provided by the author. He writes in the beginning of the book: 'Most of the names of the drugs have been pronounced and their equivalents as found in our books in Persia and Greek languages have been translated into famous and popular words.'

Metals and minerals were not used in Tibb for medicinal purposes as ever used by Indian physicians. This book refers to their use and which is now in practice in Tibb also.

The first chapter discusses simple drugs and foods in an alphabetical order. The first alphabetical letter *Alif*, counter of 'A' comprises of 48 drugs; first one is *Aparjita*, the drug with an Indian name. Many other Indian named drugs like *Jetraj, Ilaichi, Tuj, Nagkesar, Jaiphal, Darhald, Lakh*, and *Heeng* are mentioned under their respective letters.

The second is on cooked foods, drinks, sweets and sweet pickles. Terms such as *Ahar*, and *Bojan* are mentioned. Some items like *Dal, Bhat, Khushkah, Dahi, Chatni, Phulka*, and *Achaar* clearly show the influence of Indian foods as advice for healing.

The information given in *Dastur al-Hunud* is ample evidence that the writer was familiar with the nature and properties of numerous Indian flora and other wealth, which can be used as drugs and nutritive agents. For example, a section where the flesh of the elephant has been described, the elephant is called by an Indian name *hathi* and the Arabic word *fil* for the same has not been used.

It is also interesting to note that the author has not mentioned the famous word *sharab* for wine under the letter *sheen* but has mentioned under *meem* with the Indian name *madhu*. This indicates that the author has cited Indian names of the healing assets prevalent during his time.

Later on, a renowned Unani physician of nineteenth century Hakim Muhammad Sharif Khan was also convinced with the information of *Dastur al-Hunud*. He himself wrote a book entitled *Talifa-i Sharifi*, which contains the description of about 1,053 Indian drugs and also has the reference of that book.

Tibb in Indigenous Stain

Following are some examples taken from notable texts to show the Indian influence on *tibb*:

Simple Drugs Cited in *Tibbi* Pharmacopeia by Indian Name:

Misk, Saunth, Rasaut, Halela, Balela, Amla, Mulaithi, Khaksi, Lajward, Kath, Gandhak, Gurhal, Geru, Amaltaas, Asgandh, Aalu Balu, Karanjwah, Tamar Hindi, Gugal, Kakra Singhi, Shahtra, Chiraita, Mundi, Makoh, Kasni, Balchhar or *Jatamansi, Kunjad, Ilaichi, Arad, Arosa, Supari, Kuchla, Ambar, Kaknaj, Majeeth, Khand, Gandna, Akash Bail, Tutia, Moong, Pan, Arand, Jhau, Kasaundi, Kachnal, Kanair, Shingarf, Kauri, Makhana, Tejpat, Gokhru, Kutki, Imli, Indrejau Sheerin, Sankha Holi, Ajwain, Zeera, Neshkar, Atees, Silajeet, Piplamol, Kalaunji, Haldi*, etc.

Compound Drugs Cited in *Tibbi* Pharmacopeia by Indian Name:

Itriphal, Dawaulmisk, Majun Suhag Saunth, Majun Gokhru, Majun Kikar, Majun Muchras, Majun Ispand, Majun Dhaturah, Jawarish Kafuri, Jawarish Behingrah, Jawarish Bikirmaditiya, Qurs-i Pahara, Qurs-i Saad Hindi, Habb-i Rasaut, Habb-i Lajward, Habb-i Seemaab, Habb-i Shanjirf, Habb-i Ramban, Habb-i Siljit, Habb-i Biladur, Habb-i Tutia-i Hindi, Habb-i Gandhak, Marham-i Gandhak, Marham-i Shanjirf, Zimad Bachhnak, Zimad Mainphal, Churan Waji, Safoof Halailah, Sharbat-i Gurhal, Habb-i Geru, Habb-i Kath, Habb-i Asgandh, Sharbat-i Alu Balu, Habb-i Karanjwah, Zulal-i Tamar Hindi, Safoof-i Kakrasinghi, Majun Jograj Gugal, Arq-i Shahtra, Arq-i Makoh, Arq-i Kasni, Arq-i Ajwain, Arq-i Zeera, Arq-i Mundi, Roghan-i Balchhar, Roghan-i Kunjad, Roghan-i Halilah, Roghan-i Bachhnak, Roghan-i Bahengrah, Safoof-i Ilaichi, Arad-i Khurma, Sharbat-i Arosa, Panch Khar, Panch Laun, Panchmool, Dasmool, Malti Basant, Majun Supari Pak, Zurur-i Kath, Roghani Kuchla, Arq-i Ambar, Habb-i Kakanaj, Majur Suparipak, Lauq-i Aab Neshkar, Majun Petha Pak, Majun Muchras, Majun Nakchhikni, Marmam-i Aatshak, Tiryaq-i Pechish, Chaywanprash, Matbukh Kachnal, Matbukh Muqil, etc.

Drug Unit Process Cited in *Tibbi* Pharmacy by Indian Name:

Jalmundra, Kaprauti, Bajar Put, Saam Put, Bhand Put, Balu Put, Bhoder Put, Dhunab, Bhulbhulana, Pharaira, etc.

Drug's Shapes Cited in *Tibbi* Formulary by Indian Name:

Goli, Chatni, Churan, Surma, Kajal, Ubtan, Laip, Sat, Ras, Rasain, Kara, Sharbat, etc.

Drug Processing Equipments Used in *Tibbi* Pharmacy by Indian Name:

Chhalni, Kharal, Dabi, Patal Jantar, Jal Jantar, Garbh Jantar, Balu Jantar, Nari Jantar, Nal Bhapka, etc.

Diseases Mentioned in *Tibbi* Medicine by Indian Name:

Khansi, Kali Khansi, Rengan, Phunsi, Pilia, Pitti, Pind Rog, Motia Bind, Mirgi, Pechish, Bawasir, Lakuwah, etc.

Kushtajat or Calx (Calaxes): Particular Formulations Used in Unani Medicine:

Kushtah is a particular formulation used in Unani medicine. Its unit processes are similar to the 'Bhasam' used in Ayurveda. It is has been disclosed in Unani literature that the course of making *Kushtah* follows the procedure of *Bhasam* which has the types of matter termed as *Ras* and *Rasayāna*. There are many *Kushtajat* being used by Unani physicians based on Indian drugs like: *Kushtah Gaudanti, Kushtah Abrak, Kushtah Sisa, Kushtah Hartal, Kushtah Jast, Kushtah Sankhya, Kushtah Shanjirf, Kushtah Raskapoor, Kushtah Darchikna*, and *Kushtah Parah*.

Thus, Unani medicine assimilated with the indigenous system and became indigenous, but kept its basic identity elements and principles alive in the Indian subcontinents.

Conclusion

Unani medicine gradually extended and developed in different parts of the world after its birth in Unan or Greece.

In India, it came through Central Asia, mostly introduced by the Muslims. After its introduction, the experts had taken the charge to mould it according to the nature and need of a new habitat. They developed the texts composed of the matter from the literature of the *Tibb* and pre-existing Indian medicines, some of which have been briefly mentioned earlier.

As a result, Unani medicine or *Tibb* has been stained deeply as per the Indian temperament and character. It is now no more foreign and has been identified as one of the indigenous systems of medicine on a national and international level.

Notes

1. R.L. Verma, 'The Growth of Greco Arabian Medicine in Medieval India', *Ind. J. Hist. Sci.*, vol. 5, no. 2, 1970, pp. 348–76.
2. Ibid.; M.Z. Siddiqui, *The Unani Tibb (Greek Medicine) in India, A Concise History of Science in India*, New Delhi, p. 270.
3. A. Farooqui, *Majmu'a-i Ḍiya'i: Ehd-i Tughlaq ka ek Nadir Tibbi Makhtootah, Tibb-i Islami Barri Sagheer Mein*, Khuda Bakhsh Public Oriental Library, Patna, 1983, p. 226; Tazimuddin Siddiqui, 'Unani Medicine in India during the Delhi Sultanat', *Studies in History of Medicine*, vol. 4, no. 3, New Delhi, 1978, pp. 183–9.
4. M.A. Azmi, *History of Unani Medicine in India*, Centre for History of Medicine and Science, New Delhi 2004, pp. 12–13.
5. A. Farooqui, 'Tibbi Shehabi: A Rare Medical Manuscript', *Studies in History of Medicine*, New Delhi, 1985.
6. M.A. Azmi, op. cit., pp. 34–5.
7. A. Hassain and A. Qadeer, 'Ikhtiyarati Qasmi: A Sixteenth Century Medical Manuscript by Mohammad Qasim Farishta', *Hamdard Medicus*, April–June 2006, vol. XLIX, Pakistan, pp. 53–5.
8. A. Baari, *Dastur al-Hunud: A Persian Medical Manuscript, Salient Features of History of Medicine*, New Delhi: Al-Qazi Publishers, 2007, pp. 97–105.

13

Medical System in Ancient India

History, Myth or Mist!: A Contemporary Relevance

Parthasarathi Giri

'At all defining moments in history, either the man defines the moment or the moment defines the man.'[1] With passage of time a group of 'The man' tried to make the balance between *obtained skill* and application of the *acquired knowledge* on a sick person—exclusively asking *relief from pain.* The mankind gradually gained *knowledge* and then applied the *power* to get the desired result by developing the changing *attitude* towards the scientific facts. The 'application of medicine' slowly took its change from *folklore* to a sequence of science. The art of practice of modern medicine gradually became 'evidence based' and not based on traditional belief or *folklore.*

The mankind is indebted to the major field of ancient medicine, the Ayurveda, Siddha and Unani to gather and refresh our learning curve in categorizing and treating a 'man as a whole with its surroundings' and not concentrating on the segment of a diseased person, i.e. a modern concept of categorizing the work in a sequential and priority basis known as *triage.* This is also related to the management sequence of patients in the ancient system of medicine.

The art of modern medicine is based on the 'quality of life improvement' where *cure* is not possible and appreciation of *care* is all that improves the quality of life—the equivalent concept of 'healing touch' in medicine has been well described by Acharya Sushruta in *c.*600 BC. The Unani system of medicine owes, as its name suggests, its origin to Greece. The Greek philosopher-physician Hippocrates (460–377 BC) freed medicine from the realm of superstition and magic, and gave it the status of Science. In India, the Unani system was introduced by the Arabs. Siddha is another system of ancient medicine lost in time. According to this system, the human body is the replica of the universe and so are the food and drugs irrespective of their origin. Siddha system was developed in the south while Ayurveda in the northern part of India.

Ayurveda: A Myth or Mystery!

Ancient Indian wisdom of healing system goes back to at least 6000 BC if not more. Hindu mythology denotes that Lord Brahma, the creator of the Universe was the first teacher in Ayurvedic texts. He later bridged it into eight parts of which *kayachiktsaya* or medicine and *shalyatantra* or surgery appeared as the main subjects. Lord Brahma taught the knowledge of healing to celestial physician Prajapati Daksha who, in turn, transmitted the acquired knowledge to the divine twin sons of the Sun God called Ashwini Kumars who are regarded as the heavenly healers. The Ashwinis imparted the science to Indra. Up to this time, the knowledge of Ayurveda was known only to celestial personalities. It is believed that it was Lord Indra who passed on this knowledge of Ayurveda, the 'science of life', to sages and rishis (mortals), the first pupil being Bharadwaja. Bharadwaja, in turn, taught this subject to others including Atreya. Atreya, it is believed, lived in the period 700–600 BC and became a renowned teacher at Taxila.

Another mythological belief runs that Lord Vishnu was an eminent heavenly physician. Several sages approached the Lord to appear as a saviour of mankind from the impending disasters and distress. In response to their prayers, Lord Vishnu ordered the churning of the ocean of milk with the consent of *Vasukis* and *Asuras*. Dhanvantari came out of the ocean with a pot of *amrita.* It is also believed that Lord Indra favoured and blessed Dhanvantari with the knowledge of Ayurvedic medicine. Dhanvantari later became a renowned teacher in the art of surgery and started teaching his disciples at Kashi or Varanasi. He was regarded as the 'patron saint of surgery' and elevated to divinity of classical medical wisdom. It is supposed that he lived sometime around sixth century BC.

Bramha > Prajapati Daksha > Aswani Kumars > Indra

Bharadwaja > Atreya > Agnivesha

Dhanvantari
Sushruta

The Vedic rishi physicians and surgeons who came to be known as *vaidyas* were deeply devoted to the art of practising the divine knowledge and training through direct cognition during meditation. They realized the health as an integral part of spiritual life. The period of Vedic medicine lasted until about 800 BC. But it is also a fact that the Vedas are rich in magical practice and charms for the treatment of diseases and for the expulsion of the demons and deities who were believed to cause diseases.[2]

Basic Philosophy of Three Major Ancient Medical Systems

Basic Concepts of Ayurveda

There are four key concepts in Ayurveda or the science of life. They are: *Panchamahabhutas, Tridosha, Dhatus* and *Malas.* According to the theory of *Panchamahabhutas* the entire universe is made of five *Mahabhutas,* or the great elements which are not material in usual sense of the term. They are various types of energy identified as:

1. *Akasa* or space,
2. *Vayu* or air,
3. *Tejas* or luminous light,
4. *Ap* or water, and
5. *Prithvi* or the earth.

Vyādhi or disease in Ayurveda is due to an imbalance of three fundamental elements of the body. They are *vata, pitta* and *kapha. Vata* or *vayu* is an important ingredient of human body and mainly associated with *Akasa.* Due to *vata* along with *tejas, ap* and *prithvi* our universe is running with ease. *Vata* interacts with each other in the environment. Accordingly, *vata* transmits sense to the mind. The sensory organs of touch and sound are dependent partially on *vata.* The *dhatus* or tissue material and *malas* or waste matters are transported by *vata.* The combination of these energies stimulates *agni* and produces joy. This whole procedure was believed to interact to form the embryo in the womb. Embryo represents the evidence of life. On the other hand, *pitta* is also the primary constituent of a living body whose structure is close to *tejas,* the luminous light. Its function is to balance and transform the vision, digestion, production of heat, hunger, thirst, softness and suppleness of body, luster, cheerfulness and intelligence. *Kapha* is the third primary constituent of the body. It has water and earth as the major elements. The function of *kapha* is to conserve and stabilize the metabolic state. It organizes tissues into their microscopic and macroscopic form.[3] The lack of harmony in *vata, pitta* and *kapha* causes disease including *karkat* or cancer.

Vyadhi or disease in Ayurveda is divided into three broad classification as:

1. *Adhyatmika*: physical and psychic type and constitutional symptoms
2. *Adhibhautika*: caused by environment
3. *Aadhidaivika*: caused by gods or spirits

The treatment of various kinds of *doshas* or diseases has been practically classified[7] in seven different ways which are:

Aadi-bala pravritta	Genetically predisposed
Janma-bala	Congenital
Dosha-bala	Caused by imbalances in *vata, pitta* and *kapha*
Sanghata-bala	Traumatic
Kaala-bala	Seasonal or time linked
Daiva-bala	Gods or demons
Svabhaava-bala	Natural changes

There are few examples to understand the state of diseases as explained in ancient medicine in comparison to the text of present evidence-based modern medicine. Fever is explained as a *dosha* and it is caused due to disturbance in the primary constituents like *vata, kapha,* and *pitta* either as a single unit or in combination. While overeating of incompatible foods invites a *dosha* or disturbance in the gastrointestinal tract and expel the internal gastric *fire* which is responsible for indigestion. Treatment is described as to set the *fire* element in its right place. Obesity is mainly due to the absence of physical activity. Other causes may be due to sleeping during the day. Increased *kapha* on account of increased intake of foods finally results in the accumulation of fat. This develops a block in the channels of nutrition. This block causes an increase in hunger as a result the body does not get nutrition. In diarrhoea a large amount of water and minerals is lost. Treatment is carried out by restoring balance of water and mineral elements in body. Overeating of foods that are too salty, sour, alkaline, fatty, improperly cooked, meat of the animals or birds of marshy and desert regions soaked in water, excessive drinking of sugarcane juice, exposure to cold winds, sleeping in the daytime and not in the night, travelling long distances at stretch may cause gout in susceptible persons. Peptic ulcer and colic pains are caused due to increase of *vata* on account of excessive intake of astringent and dry hot bitter foods, long and durable grief, starvation, fasting and keeping awake at night. *Vata* in turn increases gastric fire which sometimes leads to develop peptic ulcer and induces colic in abdomen. The Ayurvedic doctors prefer that the balance of the body is restored.[4]

Fundamentals of Unani Medicine

Every person is supposed to have a unique humoural constitution which represents his healthy state of body and mind. To maintain the correct humoural balance there is a power of self-preservation or adjustment that is called *quwwat-i mudabbira* or *medicatrix naturae* or healing power of nature. A great reliance is placed in Unani on this aspect of *power.* The humoural hypothesis is explained as the basic form of body constituents that is *dam* or blood, *balgham* or phlegm, *safra* or yellow bile and *sauda* or black bile. The humours themselves are assigned as temperament or *mizaj* like:

1. Blood is hot and moist,
2. Phlegm is cold and moist,
3. Yellow bile is hot and dry, and
4. Black bile is cold and dry.

The temperament or *mizaj* of a person in Unani is expressed as sanguine, phlegmatic, bilious and melancholic. These are according to the presence and dominance of four humours like blood, phlegm, yellow bile and black bile in the body of a person. The correct selection of diet and its digestion are considered to be necessary pathways to maintain the humoural balance or a state of equilibrium.[5]

Diagnosis

Another distinctive feature of the Unani system of medicine is its emphasis on diagnosis of a disease by:

1. *Nabz* or pulse, a rhythmic expansion of arteries which is felt by fingers.
2. Examination of *baul* or urine and *baraz* or stool, etc.

Prevention of Disease

Unani system of medicine recognizes the influence of surroundings and ecological conditions on the state of health of human beings. The system aims at restoring the equilibrium of various elements and faculties of the human body. There are six essential prerequisites for the prevention of diseases and keeping water, food and air free from pollution. These essentials are known as *Asbab-i sittah zaruriya*,[6] and include:

1. Air,
2. Food and drinks,
3. Bodily movement and rest,
4. Psychic activity and repose,
5. Sleep and wakefulness, and
6. Excretion and retention.

Unani medicine has enriched by imbibing what was best in the contemporary system of traditional medicine in Egypt, Syria, Iraq, Persia, India, China and other Middle East and Far East countries. The theoretical framework of Unani medicine is based on the teachings of Hippocrates. After Hippocrates, a number of other Greek scholars enriched the system considerably. Galen (AD 131–210) stands out as the one who stabilized its foundation. Later, Arab physicians like Rhazes (AD 865–925) and Avicenna (AD 980–1037) constructed an imposing edifice. In India, the Delhi Sultans, the Khiljis, the Tughlaqs and the Mughal Emperors provided state patronage to the scholars. The sultans enrolled some of them as state employees and court physicians. The system became popular to the common people and spread all over the country.[7]

Basic Philosophy and Theory behind the Siddha System

Sidhha (lit. 'established truth'), a traditional Indian medical system of Dravidian origin with its root in Tamil literature, believes that human body, a microcosm, is the replica of universe, a macrocosm. Food and drugs, irrespective of their origin, are also interpreted and treated in the same way. Ayurveda and Siddha believe in the hypothesis that 'anything and everything under the universe is its replica'.

Siddha system of medicine treats not only the body but also the mind and soul. According to Siddha, human body is composed of five basic primordial elements, namely earth, water, fire, air and space. Human body is a conglomeration of three *doshas* or humours, i.e. *vatham* (air), *pitham* (fire) and *kapham* (earth and water) as well as seven physical components which are:

1. *Saram* (plasma) responsible for growth, development and nourishment;
2. *Cheneer* (blood) responsible for nourishing muscles, imparting colour and improving intellect;
3. *Ooun* (muscle) responsible for shape of the body;
4. *Kollzuppu* (fatty tissue) responsible for oil balance and lubricating joints;
5. *Enbu* (bone) responsible for body structure, posture and movement;
6. *Moolai* (nerve) responsible for strength; and
7. *Sukila* (semen) responsible for reproduction.

Equilibrium in humours or *doshas* ensures good health while disturbance in any form in the universal elements develops diseases. In normal or healthy condition, the ratio of these three humours (*vatham, pitham* and *kapham*) is 4 : 2 : 1 respectively.

Food is considered to be the basic building material for human body, which gets processed into humours, tissues and wastes. Diet and lifestyle play a major role not only in health but also in curing diseases. It is said that our body, mind and universal elements are interdependent. Siddha also deals with the concept of salvation in life. Achievement by salvation in life is considered to be the best way to gain stability, possibly by combining the mode of meditation and medicine.[8]

Every taste in Siddha system has relation with the three *doshas*. Herbs with a particular taste should be favoured to balance the *doshas* and restore health. Three *doshas*, i.e. *vatham, pitham* and *kapham* are related to *arusuvaigal* or six tastes which are based on the theory of *panchabhuta* or five elements which are as follows:

1. Sweet relates to *vatham* (water + earth),
2. Pungent relates to *pitham* (fire + air),
3. Sour relates to *kapham* (fire + earth),
4. Bitter relates to air + space,
5. Astringent relates to earth + air, and
6. Salt relates to fire + water.[9]

Ayurveda, Unani and more particularly Siddha system of medicine define and emphasize priority in the management of pregnant women and children over the adult male. Priority in the management policy is strongly advocated in Siddha; for a girl child at every stage of her life beginning from birth to menarche, from menarche to motherhood and breastfeeding, then menopause to the geriatric morbidity. This is similar to the simulating modern French model of *triage* system which is a system of management of patients according to its priority.[10]

There is no doubt that Siddha medicine is derived from alchemy. The use of metals and minerals are more predominant in Siddha in comparison to other Indian traditional medicine systems. According to the Siddha system, metals and their alloy affect the health and in disease as one knows that human body needs various kinds of minerals for maintaining health and their lack or abundance causes disease. Based on the theory of *Panchabutas* (metals of gold, lead, copper, iron and zinc) the Siddha medicines are prepared with these metals and minerals. Gold and lead are used for the maintenance of the body. Iron, the only metal attracted by the electric power of the magnet, and zinc, used for generating electricity, are employed in the medicines which are administered for the extension of life and copper is used for the preservation of heat in the body. But the use of metals and their alloy in making drugs is highly selective and applied on the individuals after multi-factorial assessment; they include history, age, sex, nutrition, state of mind, and many others.

Three broad categories of drugs are fundamentally used in Siddha. They are *thavaram* or the drugs of herbal product, *thathu* or the drugs of inorganic substances and *jangamam* or the drugs of animal products. The *thathu* drugs are further classified as *uppu* (water soluble inorganic substances or drugs that give out vapour when put into fire), *pashanam* (drugs not dissolved in water but emit vapour when fired), *uparasam* (similar to *pashanam* but differ in action), *loham* (not dissolved in water but melt when fired), *rasam* (drugs which are soft) and *ghandhagam* (drugs which are insoluble in water, like sulphur).[11]

Minerals

'Uppu' or Hydrophilic
mostly alkali and salts (water soluble)
Hydrophobic

natural artificial

Hydrophobic materials are again divided into natural and artificial. These materials are mostly capable of emitting vapour when put on fire. They also solidify on cooling. These items are gold, silver, copper and iron. Sublimation on heating mercury yields a different non-toxic form of red oxide that helps serving medicinal effects in various alchemical and molecular level of the disease. Siddhas are aware of several alchemical operations like calcinations, exaltation, sublimation and distillation. These methods of poly pharmacy were very much applied in Siddha system of medicine.[12]

Ayurveda, Unani and Siddha: A Comparison

The system of ancient medicine in India has basically followed the common path of management of disease taking 'man and environment' as a single unit. All the three systems (Ayurveda, Unani and Siddha) share a common point of 'homeostasis in the fluid balance to maintain a state of equilibrium', a modern concept of pH that dictates modern regulatory in fluid balance.

In Unani system of medicine various types of treatment are employed, such as: *Ilaj bil-tadbeer* or regimental therapy, *Ilaj bil-ghiza* or dietotherapy, *Ilaj bil-dawa* or pharmacotherapy and *Ilaj bil-yad* or surgery. The regimental therapy includes venesection, cupping, diaphoresis, diuresis, Turkish bath, massage, cauterization, purging and emesis, exercise and leeching, etc. Dietotherapy aims at treating certain ailments by administrating specific diets or by regulating the quantity and quality of food.[13] Pharmacotherapy deals with the use of naturally occurring drugs, mostly herbal, though drugs of animal and mineral origin are also used. Surgery has also been in use in this system for quite long. The ancient physicians of Unani medicine were pioneers in this field and had developed their own instruments and techniques. Single drug or their combinations in raw form are preferred over compound formulations. Compound formulations are also used in the treatment of various complex and chronic disorders. Modern pharmacopeia does not support the combination of drugs. The medicines are administered with the temperament of the patient, thus accelerating the process of recovery and also eliminating the risk of drug reaction.

There is a close similarity between Siddha and Ayurveda, with specialization in iatro-chemistry. According to this system, the human body is the replica of the universe and so are the food and drugs irrespective of their origin. The equilibrium of humours is considered as health and its disturbance or imbalance leads to the development of a disease.

Thus, there are medicines in the Siddha system supposed to have the effect of arresting the degeneration of the cells in body. Alchemy is an important aspect of this form of medicine. However, the success of this aspect of the system is not established although there are some experts of the system who even today claim to transmute metals.

However, alchemy was not the primary work of Siddha. Siddhas essentially wanted to evolve drugs which would arrest the decay of the body. They believed that this could be achieved when drugs were prepared from non-decaying material like metals and minerals. The advantage of this was that they could be prepared and preserved at all times and seasons, whereas the vegetable-based drugs could be collected and prepared only during their respective seasons. Under such unpredictable environment they thought that it was not safe to depend on vegetable-based drugs only.

Mercury and sulphur play a major role in the therapeutics of this medical science and often, they are used in combination. The addition of sulphur is expected to control the fluidity of mercury. Siddha medicine has an interesting way of categorizing the drugs. On the basis of mutual interaction, they are called enemies or friends. The drugs which are compatible with each other are called friends and those which do not are enemies. The Siddha practitioner considers these aspects while administering them. The diagnosis is based on findings from eight aspects called *ashtasthana pareeksha*, viz., *nadi* (pulse), *kan* (eyes), *swara* (voice), *sparisam* (touch), *varna* (colour), *na* (tongue), *mala* (faeces) and *neer* (urine).[14]

Siddhas developed a longevity discipline called *kayakalpa* (or 'making the body competent for long life'), something akin to gerontology of the modern medicine. Gold and mercury figure prominently for rejuvenation. More than the medicine, it is the discipline of life that the Siddha system advocates for longevity. Control in the breathing and diet is the basic method as suggested in this system.[15] Meditation and Yoga are also significant aspects of the Siddha system. Ayurveda and Unani also maintain such practices.

Relation between Ancient and Modern Medicine

If one traces the progress of the Indian medical system since the pre-Vedic period (*c.*6000–1500 BC) it would become evident that the system of medicine mostly deals with the *fear psychosis.* Diseases during the pre-Vedic period were attributed to supernatural powers and magic, etc. Hence, the treatment consisted of prayers to appease the supernatural powers, and religious rites, talismans, amulets, etc., to counter evil magic. People offered their most lovely items to the concerned god or demon to save their lives and had to fight against the evil that created panic and distress in their critical life cycle. This period is not a clearly defined span so far as the ancient medical practice was concerned.

Changes in medicine practice became more rational and sequential in the later part or the post-Vedic period (800 BC–AD 200). The people in this latter part of Vedic period started learning about the ways of life with reduced stress. This was the period of learning and evaluating the 'cause and effect' relation of disease and may well be denoted for initiation and evaluation of scientific base behind the disease. A systemic review of the ancient medicine system would lead one to form the idea that the science was applied in the form which was not essentially and wholly irrational in treating a man suffering from pain and distress. It was the pain, the highest form of disease sensation that helped man to seek advice from the physician and survive. It is a fact that modern modalities of correlation and sequential thinking were the primary deficit in the process of practice of medicine in those days; observation-based experience was the prime learning mode for the ancient medical practitioners.

Later, medicine assumed more rational approach under the great gurus Atreya, Dhanvantari, Charak and Sushruta most specifically the last two. Nagarjuna (100 BC–AD 100) who was a practitioner of Ayurveda and became famous for many of his unique conceptualizations, such as his descriptions of the circulatory system and blood tissue (uniquely described as *rakta dhātu*) and his pioneering work on the therapeutic value of specially treated minerals known as *bhasmas*. Nagarjuna is also known as the 'father of Rasashastra' (or iatro-chemistry = chemistry + medicine).[16]

There is adequate evidence that anatomical study of the human body was carried out with proficiency to gain precise knowledge of human body. Detailed knowledge of anatomy, physiology, etiology, embryology, digestion, metabolism, genetics and immunity is also found in many texts. Over 121 surgical instruments have been described by Acharya Sushruta whose famous work of surgery, *Suśruta Saṁhitā* which was translated into Arabic in AD eighth century by Rhazes and was called *Kitab-i Susrud* has described about the observation of internal part of human anatomy for medical surgery and treatment.[17] To quote the appropriate translation, 'any one, who wishes to acquire a thorough knowledge of anatomy, must prepare a dead body and carefully observe and examine all its parts'. The method of study was to submerge the body in water and allow it to decompose before an examination was carried out at intervals to study structures, layer by layer, as they got well exposed following decomposition.[18] The dead animals were also the subject of study in the same manner.

Some of the practices, especially in context of surgery, developed during the ancient period in India which appeared to have close proximity with our modern methods in surgery. It is believed that the ingenious methods were employed for suturing the severed ends of intestine. The cut ends of the intestine were apposed to each other and big black ants, collected specifically for this purpose, were made to bite the apposed ends and their heads were severed when their pincers had closed. Thus, the pincers remained in situ due to rigor mortis retaining the cut ends of the intestine in apposition for sometime. The heads and the pincers of the ants being organic matter got digested in due course of time resulting in healing of the wound. This is close to the use of *staples* in the present day open and laparoscopic surgery. Rhinoplasty reconstruction of sliced nose, like grafting of skin in modern surgery was also performed for restoration of severed or cut noses as punishment for certain offences such as adultery. Sushruta carried out plastic surgery, giving his patients a new nose or a new ear by the process of skin grafting. N.K. Pattenshetty contemplates that 'knowledge of surgery in India must have been known many centuries before the Christ'.[19] While modern techniques of plastic surgery began after the First

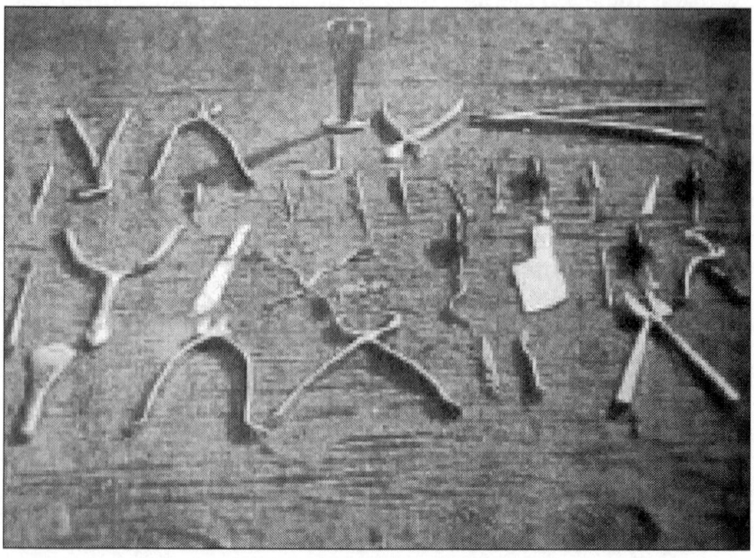

Plate 13.1: Surgical Instruments Described in *Suśruta Saṁhitā*

World War when Sir Harold Gallilies operated for facial injuries at the Royal College of Surgeon in England.[20]

Surgery also advanced through wars and battle wounds. It is said that Visapala, a woman related to Raja Chola, accompanied him into the battlefield and lost a leg. A surgeon fitted her with an artificial leg. The first evidence of a brain surgery is supposed to have taken place during the Harappa period as is claimed on the basis of finding a human skull with multiple trepanations. Trepanation was the oldest 'craniotomic surgical procedure practised by mankind since the Stone Age by way of drilling or cutting through the skull vault of a living or recently deceased person'.[21] Raja Bhoja (AD 1010–53) was managed by skull trephine by removing a portion of the brain. It is said that Raja Bhoja was afflicted by a tumour in his brain which used to cause him intense headache. Two learned Brahmin brothers from the school of Ujjain, who were pre-eminent surgeons of the era, performed a surgery on his brain and relieved him of his tumour. The description of the surgery that survives suggests that they artificially induced a coma with a special preparation known as the *sammohini* and then opened his skull to remove the tumour. He was then brought back to consciousness with another drug. Use of *sammohini*, herbal medicine, clearly indicates that stage of anesthesia was well known in ancient India. Later, people also used opium poppy, coca leaves, mandrake root, alcohol, and even phlebotomy (to let out venous blood to the point of unconsciousness) to allow surgeons to operate without pain sensation. Till the nineteenth century, this branch of surgery had made little advance anywhere in the West.[22]

The ancient surgeon Sushruta classifies the accidental wounds into six kinds. This classification is still followed except for gunshot or blast wounds. This classification is:

1. Wound causing severance of a part or a whole limb (*chinna*).
2. Wound into a hollow viscus puncturing it (*bhinna*).
3. Puncturing wound of any structure other than a hollow viscus (*viddha*).
4. Uneven or lacerated wound (*ksata*).
5. Crushed wound (*Picchita*).
6. Superficial abrasion (*ghrsta*).[23]

Food is now proved to be an essential ingredient for modulation of many diseases. Nutritional elements must be fragmented to a micro level for assimilation. If one could relate the facts, it appears that the *food as a medicine* was a distinct hypothesis of Ayurveda, Unani and Siddha. Pathophysiology categorizes and classifies them into:

1. Enteral nutrition and parenteral nutrition.
2. Immunocompetent food and antioxidants.
3. Food rich in fibres.
4. Probiotics are live microflora when administered in optimum concentration confer a health benefit on host.

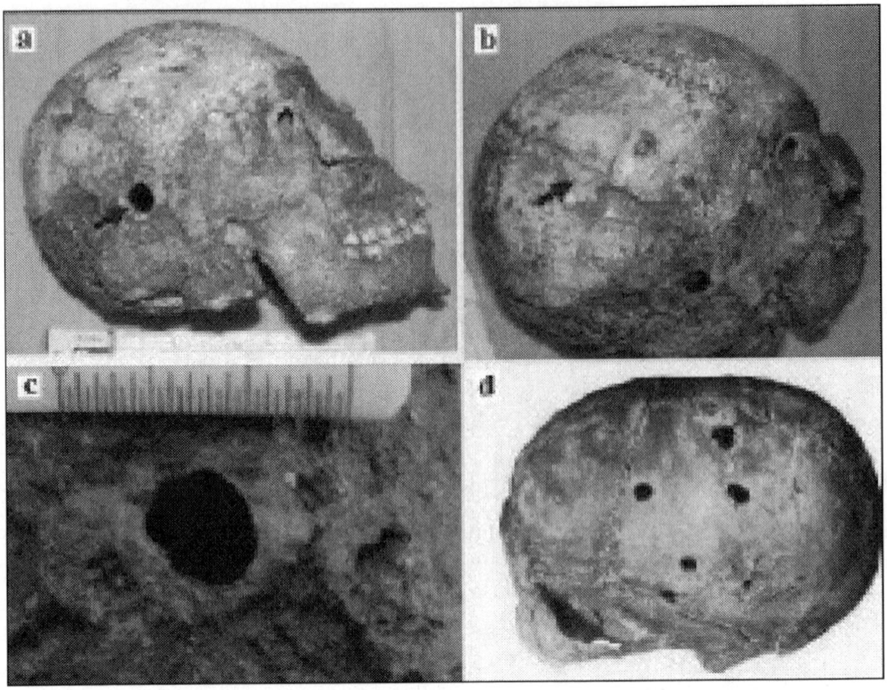

Plate 13.2: The Trepanated Harappan Male Skull
The Palaeoanthropology Repository (H-796/B)
Anthropological Survey of India, Kolkata

Details of Plate 13.2:

(*a*) the left lateral view showing the trepanated hole;
(*b*) the postero-lateral view showing the horizontal linear traumatic fracture on the occipital bone;
(*c*) an enlarged view of the trepanated site showing the rim of callous formed due to healing; and
(*d*) the trepanated Burzahom female skull showing signs of multiple trepanations.[24]

5. Prebiotics are non-digestible food ingredients that has the power of selective stimulation for controlling effects on gut flora.

The modern modalities explained that 'A 70 kg man has 60 per cent total body water of which one-third is extra cellular and two-third being intra cellular'. So to say, a man or an animal is predominantly made up of water and about 60 per cent of a mammalian body is made up of water. So tissues (*malas*) need water to transport nutrition for oxidation. Air (*vayu*) and water (*ap*) = energy (*teja*). CO_2 + water. O_2 is utilized by the tissues as energy.

It is also notable that the soldiers and war team in ancient India was accompanied by some physicians and there was priority in the management of warriors who suffered wounds and trauma. The physicians followed the priority depending on the types of wound, age, sex, and severity. Pregnant women, wounded soldiers and children were treated with priority over adult women and men. This system of priority management in treatment appears very close to the procedure of the *triage* system in the modern disaster management.

An important aspect of management of a diseased person in Unani and Siddha systems is to keep a close observation of urine of the patient. This is considered a definite guide in the management of a critically ill person in the modern line of treatment too.

Conclusion

Myth or folklore cannot exist until there is strong evidence-based science behind it. It is the time when one should re-evaluate the ancient art in the light of the modern scientific facts. Extensive research is essential to justify the facts beyond myth. Charles Darwin expressed in the *Origin of Species* the idea of primary thinking related to the fact that living being on earth is interrelated. He wrote, '. . . all animals and all plants throughout all time and space should be related to each other in group and subordinate to group, in the manner which we everywhere behold. . .'.[25] This is the basic in the hypothesis of Siddha system—'anything and everything under this universe is its replica'. Yesterday's myth appears to be the science today.

The advancement in surgery was less developed in the West till nineteenth century. But it was well developed in the East. 'Its origin can be traced back to ancient Egypt, with wound care depicted in hieroglyphs on papyrus to India in the sixth century BC, where Sushruta described using the forehead flap to reconstruct a nose, and to Al-Zahrawi, the tenth century Islamic surgical scholar from Cordoba.'[26] Similarly, anchoring the cut margins by apposing with the pincers of ant-heads is close to the use of modern staples for various types of anastomosis in present-day surgery. A.L. Basham has rightly observed, '. . . the compendia of Caraka (AD first–second centuries) and Susruta (*c.* AD fourth century) are the products of a fully evolved system which resembled those of Hippocrates and Galen in some respects, and in others had developed beyond them.'[27]

During the period of myth the fact was evident but not documented for want of modalities. Charaka, Sushruta, Jeebak, Nagarjuna and others followed the hypothesis of *vata*, *pitta* and *kapha*. The Unani system was the hypothetical approach with the humour, *dam* and the bile for balancing the body to attain homeostasis. These terms are very close to the present theory of 'fluid balance'.

Despite the advancement and progress to certain degree on scientific line the ancient art of healing declined or passed through a period of regress. There are reasons behind the decline of the golden state or art of ancient medicine. Some of the facts or evidences responsible for the decline may be:

1. Non-availability of written scripts over a period of several centuries.
2. Court physicians believed to keep the secrets within the selected groups. A few practitioners believed in keeping the records in writings.

3. During the period of British rule in India, Western medicine took the flight of development by scientifically transferring the knowledge of ancient medicine in India, China, Tibet, Middle East and many others.
4. Indian medical system and the native practitioners did not get the patronage by the British rulers.
5. Lack of confidence of country people on the traditional medicine to control emergency medical needs and epidemics like smallpox, malaria, kala-azar and fever of different origins. They were controlled by the evident Western medicine though the basic ingredients were very much known to our ancient system of medicine.
6. Series of attacks on India from outside broke the learning curve of knowledge in ancient India like the one that ceased in Nalanda.
7. A great lacuna in research is still very much evident even after India became independent from the British rule.

Denial of the label of 'science' creates an obvious bias—Ayurveda is seen as 'lesser' than the Western medical system.[28] Clearly, this is not an empowering process for indigenous medicines.

Some practices of Ayurveda are still followed, in terms of seasonal regiments, diet and the use of local medicinal plants. A villager suffering from diarrhoea may already know to use crushed pomegranate rind for his condition. But, an expert in a city hospital or the internet would advice for the use of an anti-diarrhoeal drug. There is no way for the villager can determine what the iatrogenic effects of the anti-diarrhoeal are![29] Clearly, this is not an empowering process. The greater coherence between folk health traditions and Ayurveda needs to be leveraged to strengthen local knowledge and understand the national heritage of the art of healing through the lens of modern science of medicine.

Notes

1. Ron Shelton, 'From the Film "Tin Cup" quoted in Mamoon Rashid, 'Disaster Surgery', *Bailey and Love's Short Practice of Surgery*, ed. S. Norman Williams, John Christopher, Bulstrode Kent and P. Ronan O'Connell, 25th edn., Florida: CRC Press, 2008, p. 410.
2. Vaidya Bhagwan Dash and Acharya M. Manfred Jounious, *A Handbook of Ayurveda*, New Delhi: Concept Publishing Company, 1983, pp. 6–7; Kenneth Zysk, 'Mythology and the Brahmanization of Indian Medicine: Transforming Heterodoxy into Orthodoxy', Internet Exhibitions Moesgaard www.hindu.dk, pp. 1–11.
3. Dash and Jounious, op. cit., pp. 15–18.
4. Priya Vrat Sharma, *History of Medicine in India: From Antiquity to AD 1000*, New Delhi: Indian National Science Academy, 1992, pp. 325–53.
5. Rahat Usmani, 'Role of the Internet in the Access and Dissemination of Information in the Unani System of Medicine', in *Information Management in the New Millennium*, ed. Ramesh Kundra, Usha Mujoo Munshi, New Delhi: Allied Publishers Pvt. Ltd., 2002, p. 660.

6. A.A. Azmi, *Basic Concepts of Unani Medicine: A Critical Study*, New Delhi: Jamia Hamdard, 1995, pp. 5–6; Syed Zillur Rahman, 'Unani Medicine in India: Its Origin and Fundamental Concepts', in *History of Science, Philosophy and Culture in Indian Civilization, Medicine and Life Sciences in India*, ed. B.V. Subbarayappa, vol. IV, pt. 2, New Delhi: Centre for Studies in Civilizations, 2001, pp. 292–325.
7. T. Siddiqui, 'Unani Medicine in India during the Delhi Sultanate', *Indian Journal of History of Science*, vol. 15, no. 1, 1980, pp. 18–24; idem, 'Unani Medicine in India: AD 1524 to 1605', *Indian Journal of History of Science*, vol. 16, no. 1, 1981, pp. 22–5.
8. B.V. Subbarayappa, 'Sidhha Medicine: An Overview', *Lancet*, vol. 350, issue 1994, 1997, pp. 1841–4; S.S. Shukla, and S. Saraf, 'Fundamental Aspect and Basic Concept of Siddha Medicines', *Systematic Reviews in Pharmacy*, vol. 2, issue 1, 2011, pp. 48–54.
9. Dr S.K. Sasi and Dr S. Chitra, 'A Validation of Siddha: Basic Principles Using a Scientific Parameter', *International Journal of Pharmacy and Pharmaceutical Sciences*, vol. 4, suppl. 2, 2012, pp. 7–8.
10. Iain Robertson-Steel, 'Evolution of Triage Systems', *Emergency Medicine Journal*, vol. 23, issue 2, 2006, pp. 154–5.
11. Shukla and Saraf, op. cit.
12. Ibid.
13. Azmi, op. cit.; Rahman, op. cit.
14. B. Ravishankar and V.J. Shukla, 'Indian Systems of Medicine: A Brief Profile', *African Journal of Traditional, Complementary and Alternative Medicine* (*AJTCAM*), vol. 4, suppl. 3, 2007, p. 331; Dr R. Kumar, *Medical Tourism in India: Management and Promotion*, New Delhi: Deep & Deep Publications, 2008, p. 201.
15. V.A. Shanmuga, 'Sidhha's Science of Longevity and Kalpa Medicines of India', Madras: Sakti Nilayam, 1963, pp. 202–13; K.H. Krishnamurthy and G. Chandra Mouli, 'Siddha System of Medicine: A Historical Appraisal', *Indian Journal of History of Science*, vol. 19, no. 1, 1984, p. 51.
16. S.S. Savrikar and B. Ravishankar, 'Introduction to *Rasashastra* the Iatro-chemistry of Ayurveda', *AJTCAM*, vol. 8, suppl. 3, 2011, pp. 66–82.
17. K. Natarajan, 'Surgical Instruments and Endoscopes of Susruta: The Sage Surgeon of Ancient India', *Indian Journal of Surgery*, vol. 70, issue 5, 2008, pp. 219–23.
18. S. Saraf and R.S. Parihar, 'Sushruta: The First Plastic Surgeon in 600 BC', *The Internet Journal of Plastic Surgery*, 2007, vol. 4, no. 2, DOI: 10.5580/1456.
19. N.K. Pattenshetty, 'Surgery in Ancient India: Its Evolution and Progress', op. cit., ed. B.V. Subbarayappa, New Delhi: PHISPC, 2001, pp. 157–91.
20. Tim Goodacre, 'Plastic and Reconstructive Surgery', in *Bailey and Love's Short Practice of Surgery*, p. 394; Surajit Bhattacharya, 'Sushrutha: Our Proud Heritage', *Indian Journal of Plastic Surgery*, vol. 42, no. 2, 2009, pp. 223–5.
21. A.R. Sankhyan and G.R. Schug, 'First Evidence of Brain Surgery in Bronze Age Harappa', *Current Science*, vol. 100, no. 11, 2011, pp. 1621–2.
22. In 1843, Easdale reported surgical operation under mesmeric anaesthesia in Hoogly Hospital in West Bengal. Ether anaesthesia was used in India only six months after its official demonstration on 16 October 1846, Massachusetts General Hospital, USA. Subodh Kapoor, ed., *The Indian Encyclopaedia*, vol. 3, New Delhi: Genesis Publishing Pvt. Ltd., 2002, p. 833.
23. D.P. Agarwal, 'Military Surgery in Ancient India', www.indianscience.org; Sharma, op. cit.
24. Sankhyan and Schug, op. cit.
25. Charles Darwin, *Origin of Species: 150th Anniversary Edition*, Florida: Bridge Logos Foundation, 2009, p. 122.
26. Goodacre, op. cit., p. 394.

27. A.L. Basham, 'The Wonder that was India', 3rd revd. edn., London: Picador, 2004, pp. 500–1.
28. Arvind Ranganathan, 'Using ICT to Place Indigenous Knowledge Systems at the Heart of Education for Sustainable Development', 2004, p. 8, http://www.globalknowledge.org/ict4d/index.cfm?menuid=56&parentid=52>
29. Ibid., p. 4.

14

Indian Herbs and Plants for Treatment of Liver Disorder/Hepatitis B

Mohit Saha

INDIAN CIVILIZATION HAS been well known for its rich heritage of varieties of herbal plants. The *Rig Veda* (*c.*1700–1100 BC), the earliest Vedic literature has recorded around 67 medicinal plants, the *Yajur Veda* (*c.*1400–1000 BC) 81 and the *Atharva Veda* (*c.*900 BC) has described 290 medical plants. The two earliest treatises on medicine and surgery, viz., *Carak Saṁhitā* (*c.*300–200 BC) and *Suśruta Saṁhitā* (*c.*200 BC) have mentioned properties and uses of 1,100 and 1,270 species of plants and herbs respectively. In this way, drugs of herbal origin have traditionally been used in India since very inception of the Indian civilization. Apart from Ayurveda, the oldest system of indigenous medical system Unani is the later developed healing system which together use over 700 species of herbs for medicine; modern medicine and even allopathic also use a good large number of herbs in preparing drugs generally derived from different parts of plants like leaves, stem, bark, root, flower, seed, etc.

Bhui Amla (Phyllanthus Niruri), *Kutaki* (Picorrhiza Kurroa), *Haritaki* (Terminalia Chebula), Indian Rhubarb/*Revand Chini* (Rheum Sps.), *Amla* (Emblica Officianalis), *Tulsi* (Ocimum Tenuiflorum), *Kalmegh* (Andrographis Paniculata), *Makoi* (Solanum Nigrum), *Kasni* (Cichorium Intybus), *Neem* (Azadirachta Indica), *Daruharidra* (Berberis Aristata), *Yashti Madhu* (Glycyrrhiza Glabra), *Sharpunkha Mool* (Tephrosia Purpurea), *Giloy/Guduchi* (Tinospora Cordifolia), *Bhringraj* (Eclipta Alba) and *Punernava* (Boerhaavia Diffusa) are some of the significant herbs and plants which have been traditionally used by the indigenous medical practitioners. Some information, particularly the use of herbal medicine to cure jaundice and Hepatitis B, is provided by Aimil Pharmaceutical (India) Ltd. on its website.[1]

Jaundice was already known to the people from very ancient time. But Hepatitis B that is an infectious inflammatory illness of the liver caused by the

Hepatitis B virus (HBV) that affects hominoidea, including humans, was first discovered in 1885 by Lurman, a German researcher who found prolonged jaundice in several shipyard workers. However, the credit for discovery of the virus goes to Baruch Blumberg, an American doctor, who along with his team developed in 1965 the blood test in some Australian aborigines, that is used to detect the virus for which the virus came to be known as Australia antigen (Au antigen). In 1969, Blumberg invented the first Hepatitis B vaccine for which he was awarded the Noble Prize in Medicine in 1976. D.S. Dane, a British Pathologist, discovered complete HBV particle in 1970 that is also known as Dane particle. This was followed by discovery of HBeAg by L. Magnius in 1972.

The acute illness with the virus causes liver inflammation, vomiting along with jaundice and sometimes death. Chronic Hepatitis B may eventually cause cirrhosis and liver cancer. The infection with Hepatitis B virus begins with general ill-health, loss of appetite, nausea, vomiting, body aches, mild fever, and dark urine, and then progresses to development of jaundice. It has been noted that itchy skin has been an indication as a possible symptom of all Hepatitis B virus that primarily interferes with the functions of the liver by replicating in liver cells, known as hepatocytes. The tests, called assays, for detection of Hepatitis B virus infection involve serum or blood tests that detect either viral antigens (proteins produced by the virus) or antibodies produced by the host. The Hepatitis B surface antigen (HBsAg) is most frequently used to screen for the presence of this infection. Individuals who remain HBsAg positive for at least six months are considered to be Hepatitis B carriers.

Although none of the available drugs can clear the infection, they can stop the virus from replicating, thus minimizing liver damage. Currently, there are seven medications licensed for treatment of Hepatitis B infection in the United States. These include antiviral drugs lamivudine (Epivir), adefovir (Hepsera), tenofovir (Viread), telbivudine (Tyzeka) and entecavir (Baraclude), and the two immune system modulators interferon alpha-2a and PEGylated interferon alpha-2a (Pegasys).

Apart from the use of some drugs and vaccine, herbal medicines are well known for this treatment in India. Some popular herbs and plants of India traditionally used for the cure of jaundice and Hepatitis B are discussed hereunder.

Bhui Amla **(Phyllanthus Niruri) as a Drug for Liver**

As a Potent Anti Viral

Bhui Amla or Phyllanthus Niruri also known as Chanca piedra is a small herbal plant growing up to 30 to 40 cm. in height. Indian and Brazilian research groups were the first to conduct studies in mid-1960s on this plant since it was indigenous to these countries. The plant has also been known in the Amazonian basin as well as China. It is used for the treatment of viral

Hepatitis. The plant got worldwide attention in the late 1980s due to its antiviral activity against Hepatitis B. A study conducted in India in 1982 established that *Bhui Amla* eliminated Hepatitis B in mammals within 3–6 weeks (Sousa et al., 1991: 377–8).

Use of *Bhui Amla* or Phyllanthus Niruri on chronic carriers of Hepatitis B virus has been very effective.[2] Fifty-nine per cent of the treated patients with *Bhui Amla* lost HBsAg after the treatment as compared to only 4 per cent controls. In no case the surface antigen returned upto nine months clinical observations revealed no toxic effects. While in carrier patients, positive for HBsAg but negative for HBeAg, 93 per cent cleared the carrier stage. In HBsAg and HBeAg positive carriers but negative for anti HBcigM, 44 per cent patients were cleared. Of the patients positive for all the three markers, 13 per cent were cleared. In treated carriers positive for HBsAg, anti HBcigM but negative for HBeAg, 67 per cent lost the carrier stage. The mode of mechanism suggested is by inhibiting the reaction between HBsAg (surface antigen of HBV) and the antibody (anti-HBsAg) and by inhibiting the endogenous DNA polymerase of HBV.

As Antihepatotoxic

It is notable that *Bhui Amla* or Phyllanthus Niruri helps in quick elimination of toxicants from body fluids. *Bhui Amla* (Phyllanthus Niruri) exerts hepatoprotective effects against drugs like paracetamol, chemicals, and countrymade liquor probably due to counteracting the inhibition of cytochrome P450 and decreasing glutathione depletion. This causes quick elimination of toxicants from body fluids.[3]

Bhui Amla Reduces Fat from Liver

Further, *Bhui Amla* along with *Giloe/Guduchi* or Tinospora Codifolia possess the potentiality to reduce extra fat from liver. Intoxication with carbon tetrachloride causes liver damage by increasing liver weight due to accumulation of fat. It results in elevated levels of SGPT, SGOT, Bilirubin and increased pentobarbitone induced sleep time in experimental subjects. Treatment with *Bhui Amla* and *Giloe/Guduchi* (Tinospora Codifolia) exhibited statistically significant anti-hepatoxic activity in terms of reduction on liver weight, SGPT, SGOT, Bilirubin and pentobarbitone induced sleep time.[4]

***Kutaki* or Picorrhiza Kurroa Works as Anti-HBsAg and Anti-HBeAg**

Kutaki, scientifically known as Picorrhiza Kurroa, has been traditionally used to treat various liver disorders in the Ayurvedic system of medicine. Found in higher Himalayan ranges, the dried rhizomes of the plant constitute the drug recognized for *Yatrik-uttejak* or liver-stimulator mainly used for treating various liver disorders including viral jaundice.

Kutaki (Picorrhiza Kurroa) with picroliv functions as a promising anti-HBsAg and Anti-HBeAg like activity as was noted in acute and chronic liver disease and healthy HBsAg carriers. Picroliv also inhibited purified HBV antigens (HBeAg and HBsAg) prepared from healthy HBsAg carriers.[5]

Kutaki (Picorrhiza Kurroa) as Hepatoprotective Modifier

Glucosidic fraction from *Kutaki* prevent the induced histopathological changes characterized by diffused hepatocytes alteration in the form of ballooning, granular cytoplasm, indistinct cell outlines, nuclear changes, focal necrosis and vascular damage.[6]

It is notable that Hepatoprotective effects reduces formation of toxic metabolites also in human body. Picroliv, the irridoid glucoside mixture from *Kutaki*, shows anti-hepatoxic action which seems likely due to an alteration in the biotransformation of the toxic substance like ATT drugs, paracetamol and alchohol, etc., resulting in decreased formation of reactive metabolites. Under a dose comparable study, it showed better hepatoprotection than silymarin.[7]

Haritaki or Terminalia Chebula and *Revand Chini* or Rheum Sps. as Potential Anti-Viral

Terminalia Chebula known as *Haritaki* in Sanskrit and *A-ru-ra* in Tibetan is about 98 ft. tall plant with nut like fruit. It is found in India, Nepal, Sri Lanka, China and some other countries. In Bengali, it is called *horitoky* while in Hindi and Urdu it is called *Harad*. In general use it stimulates the liver and is used in liver enlargement. It protects liver further by expelling the waste excretory products from the intestines.

The fruit of *Haritaki* and powdered roots of *Revand Chini* or Rhubarb, demonstrated anti-viral activity in ducks with Hepatitis B virus. During a period of four week, treatment measuring serum DHBV DNA (Duck

Dried Stems of *Revand Chini*/Rhubarb

Fruit of *Haritaki* or Terminalia Chebula

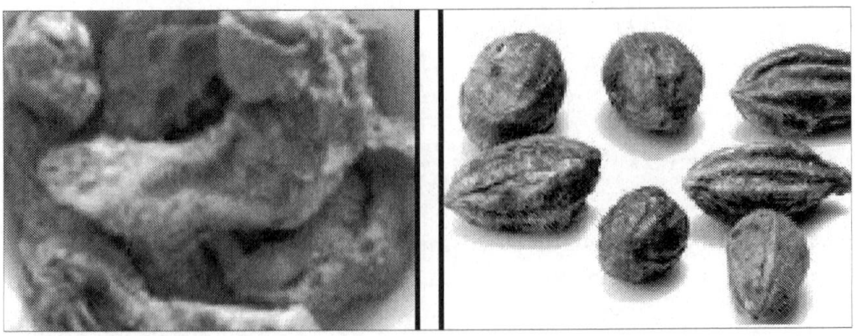

Plate 14.1

Hepatitis B virus DNA) levels and DHBV DNA polymerase activity as anti-viral indicators. During a four week treatment, decrease in serum DHBV DNA levels was clearly parallel by inhibition of DHBV DNA polymerase. Rhubarb contains the tannins and anthroquinone derivatives as the pharmacologically active components. More than 50 kins of tannins have been isolated from Rhubarb amongst which i-epicatechin, procynandine, rhatanin dominates in effects, delaying progression to severity. Indian Rhubarb, i.e. *Revand Chini* is an enriched source of emodin and chrysophanic acid satisfying United States pharmacopoeial standards, containing not less than 30 per cent, and have been recommended to replace Chinese drug.[8]

Free Radical Scavenging Anti-Oxidant Activity with Rhubarb

Stilbenes and Naphthalene glycosides from Rhubarb showed free radical scavenging activity for DPPH and oxygen free radical. In addition, most stilbenes inhibited lipid peroxidation of erythrocyte membrane by tert-butyl hydroperoxide and xanthine oxidase.[9]

Faster Clinical and Biochemical Recovery in Viral Hepatitis by *Kutaki* (Picorrhiza Kurroa): In a double blind controlled trial on 42 cases of acute viral Hepatitis, it was observed that clinical recovery of jaundice by using *Kutaki* reduction of hepatomegaly and biochemical recovery was much earlier and better in treated cases with $p < 0.01$ as compared to control reversion of enzymes SGPT, SGOT, and Serum alkaline phosphates were quick and values returned to normal level in sixth week of follow up. Result suggests that the drug made of *Kutaki* (Picorrhiza Kurroa) contains choleretic and cytoprotective action on hepatocytes against viral toxins, thus, helping in regeneration of hepatocytes.[10]

Glycyrrhizin as Biological Response Modifier: Glycyrrhizin that is a major component of *Yasthi Madhu*, the root Glycyrrhiza Glabra, has also been used for the treatment of Hepatitis B. It improves liver functions with complete recovery from Hepatitis. It is a supplement of interferon for the treatment of patients with chronic Hepatitis B and has also been used to treat non-responders to interferon therapy. The interaction between hepatocytes and lymphocytes may be altered in such a way due to glycyrrhizin that there is no rebound of transaminases after interferon therapy. Enhancement of interferon production in glycyrrhizin treated human peripheral lymphocytes in response to concanavalin A and to surface antigen of Hepatitis B virus, indicates the function of glycyrrhizin as a biological response modifier. RNA and protein synthesis of treated lymphocytes was increased compared to control cells.[11]

Clinical Study in Acute Viral Hepatitis and Hepatoprotective Effects: The clinical study in patients suffering from viral Hepatitis revealed that the mean reduction in the serum Bilirubin, SGPT, SGOT, and Alkaline phosphatase were significantly higher with $p < 0.001$ in the trial group as compared to control in the case of actual viral Hepatitis. There was progressive improvement in biochemical values and symptoms from the first follow up onwards in trial group while in control group, at the time of first follow up, the mean values were even higher than the basal.[12]

Sharpunkha-mool **(Tephrosia Purpurea)** also known as *ban-nil* or wild indigo, 0.5–1.0 m. high with 8–15 cm. long and 0.5–1.0 cm. thick cylindrical root and purple flower is known as a significant medicine in liver damage by intoxication. *Sharpunkha-mool* in case of intoxication subjects, has significant protection against increase serum bilirubin, SGPT, SGOT, and checked the central or submissive necrosis in hepatocytes. *Sharpunkha-mool* thus displays its restorative role in liver biochemical due to membrane stabilizing effects on hepatic cells.[13]

Hepatoprotective Effects Inhibits Toxic Metabolite Generation and Restores Hepatic Acid Phosphatase Enzymes: Leaf extract of *Bhringraj* (Eclipta Alba), a plant with white flowers is considered a powerful liver tonic. The hepatoprotective effects of *Bhringraj* have been studied at subcellular levels in experimental subjects. The study showed that hepatoprotective activity of Eclipta Alba is by counteracting the inhibition of hepatic microsomal drug metabolizing enzymes. The effects of Eclipta Alba on hepatic microsomal drug metabolizing enzymes indicate that pretreatment with Eclipta Alba counteracts the CCL4 induced inhibition of amidopyrine-N-demethylase activity, thus, showing its hepatoprotective effect by regulating the levels of drug metabolizing enzymes.[14]

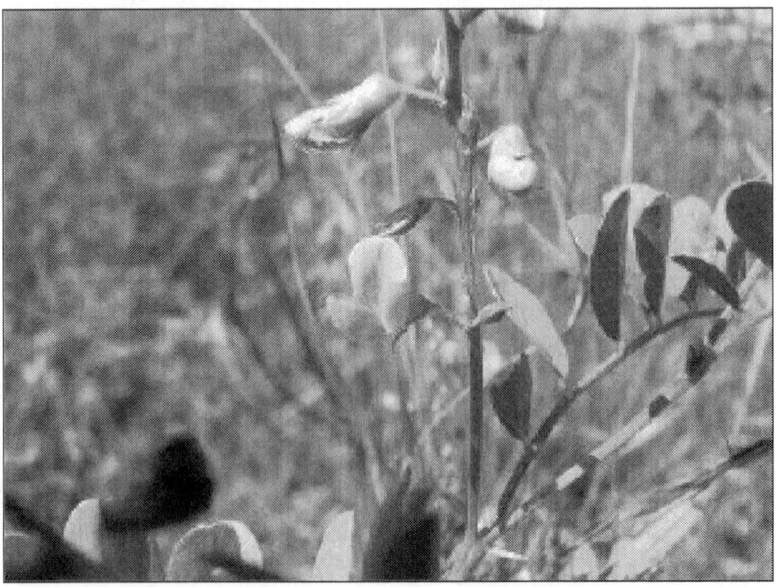

Plate 14.2: *Sharpunkha* or Tephrosia Purpurea

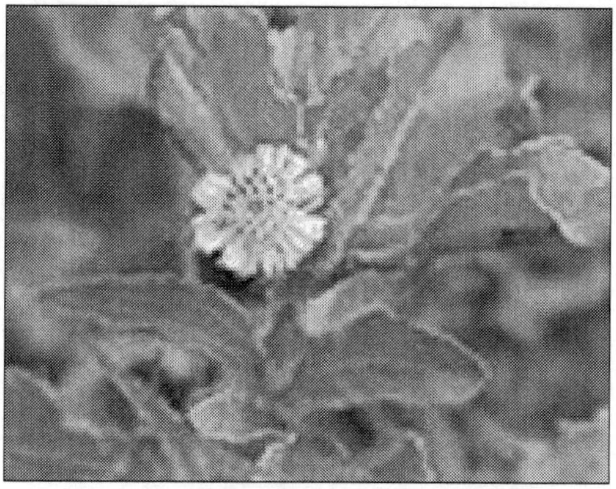

Plate 14.3: *Bhringraj* or Eclipta Alba

Anti-oxidant properties of Eclipta Alba ameliorated benzoyl peroxide induced lipid peroxidation, increased generation of hydrogen peroxide and depleted glutathione levels. In addition, it reversed benzyl peroxide mediated inhibition of antioxidant enzymes such as catalase, glucose 6-phosphate dehydrogenase, glutathione reductase and glutathione-S-transferase suggesting thereby, the amelioration of benzyol peroxide mediated toxicity to be because of anti-oxidant properties.[15] For this purpose, its juice may be taken mixed with black pepper and *mishri* or candy.

Giloy or *Amrita* as Preventer of Fibrotic Changes and Modulating Kupffer Cell Activity

Giloy (Tinospora Cordifolia), a climbing shrub with broad leaves known as *Amrita* in Ayurveda, has shown effect to prevent fibrosis tissue deposition in post-insult period. It has been proved that suppression of kupffer cells deprives the hepatocytes from cyto protective effects.

In experimental subjects, repeatedly injected horse serum antibodies, developed against the heterologous serum, combined with antigen ensuing an inflammatory process, suppressing kupffer cell activity, lead to fibrosis. On discontinuation of horse serum, perpetuation of fibrotic process was observed in damaged liver. Therapy with *Giloy* has been shown to prevent fibrous tissue deposition in post insult period. This appears to be due to its macrophage activating property, which opposed any suppressant influences on kupffer cells. It has been proved that suppression of kupffer cells deprives the hepatocytes from cytoprotective effect.[16]

Kalmegh (Andrographis Paniculata) Significantly Reduces Enzymatic Leakage of SGPT and Alkaline Phosphatase and Acting as Anti-Oxidant

Kalmegh (Andrographis Paniculata) or *Kalmegha* also known as *Bhui-neem* or *neem* of the ground for its bitter taste, significantly reduces leakage of SGPT

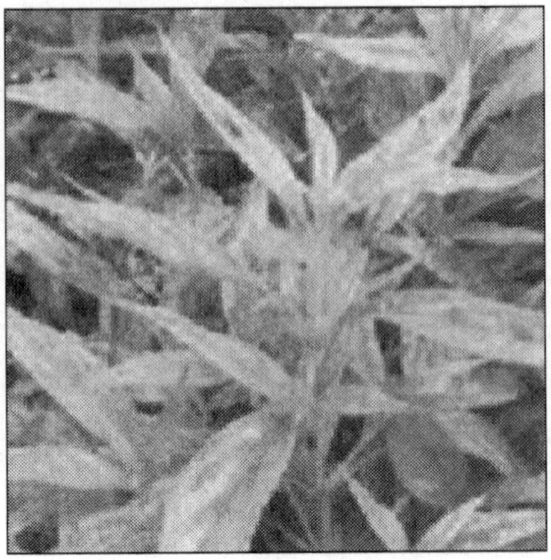

Plate 14.4: *Kalmegh* (Andrographis Paniculata)

and Alkaline phosphatase and inhibits glutathione depletion by exerting strong antioxidant effect. A significant increase in the level of cytocrome P450, cytochrome P450 reductase, cytochrome B5 reductase, glutathione S transferase, DT diaphorase, superoxide dismutase, catalase, glutathione peroxidase and glutathione reductase and significant decrease in activity of lactase dehydrogenate were observer in the liver, indicating antioxidant activity of the drug and chemopreventive potential against chemotoxicity including carcinogenicity.[17]

Makoi and *Kasni* Protect DNA against Oxidative Damage

Makoi (Solanum Nigrum), a plant of 12–48″ and 6–8 mm. berry of black and red colour has been traditionally used as medicine in India and abroad. Boiled extracts of leaves and berries are used to alleviate liver-related ailments, including jaundice. On the other hand, Chicory which is commonly known as *Kasni*, a perennial herb widely grown and cultivated in India is widely known for its medicinal benefits.

The extracts of *Makoi* (Solanum Nigrum) and *Kasni* (Cichorium Intybus) in the reaction mixture containing calf thumus DNA and free radical generating system, protect DNA against oxidative damage to its deoxyribos sugar moiety.

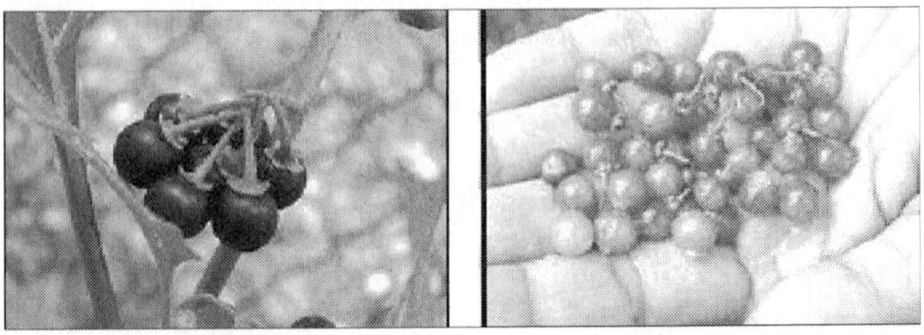

Plate 14.5: Black *Makoi* and Red *Makoi*

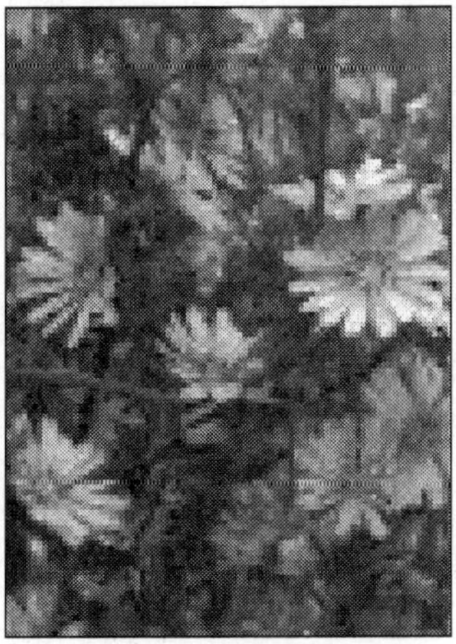

Plate 14.6: *Kasni* (Cichorium Intybus)

The effect was dependent on the concentration of the plant extracts. These studies suggest that the hepatoprotective effect of these crude plant extracts may be due to their ability to suppress the oxidative degradation of DNA in these debris.[18]

Makoi as Immuno Modulators

Makoi also reduces mortality, improving Phagocytosis and intra-cellular bactericidal capability of Neutrophils. It has been found that pretreatment of experimental subjects with certain plant drugs protects them against E. coli, Staphylococcus aureus and mixed bacterial species. It has also been found to increase the phagocytic and killing activity of peritoneal macrophages. *Giloy* (Tinospora Cordifolia) and gentamicin reduced mortality in mice injected Ix10(8) E. coli intra-peritoneally from 100 per cent in controls to 17.8 per cent and 11.1 per cent respectively. Tinospora Cordifolia treated group showed significantly improved bacterial clearance as well as phagocytic and intracellular bacterial capacities of neutrophils. In the Gentamicin treated mice, although clearance was rapid but polymorph phagocytosis was depressed. Tinospora Cordifolia did not possess in-vitro bactericidal activity.[19]

Makoi Works also as Anti-Ulcerogenic

Makoi has been found to exert anti-ulcerogenic effect due to decrease of acid and pepsin output and enhances gastric mucosal strength suggesting Gastric mucosal protection activity.[20]

Tulsi (Ocimum Tenuiflorum) Protects Hepatocytes against Radiation Injury, Modulates Glutathione and Antioxidant Enzymes

Tulsi (Ocimum Tenuiflorum), an aromatic plant of 30–60 cm. with hairy stems and simple green strongly scented leaves with antioxidant properties has been traditionally used in Ayurveda for healing various diseases and is worshipped in India as a sacred plant. Due to its antioxidant properties it has the capacity to repair cells damaged by exposure to radiation.

Radiation interacts with biomolecules and produces toxic free radicals leading to DNA and membrane damage. Pretreatment with *tulsi* checks the radiation induced depletion (approx. 30–60 per cent of control) of glutathione (GSH) and antioxidant enzymes, viz., glutathione transferase, reductase, peroxidase and superoxidase dismutase and maintain their levels within or above the control range. Due to their initial significantly higher availability, they also reduce the lipid peroxidation, thereby significantly protecting DNA and membrane from free radical damage. Pretreatment with *tulsi* increases the ability to cope up with free radicals produced by radiation making them more radio resistant with faster recovery in liver cells.[21]

Tulsi Functions as Anti-Inflammatory Agent

Tulsi also shows anti-inflammatory activity against all the four phlogistic (viz., carageenin, serotonin, histamine and PGE) induced inflammation. It blocks both the pathways, i.e. cyclogenase and lipooxygenase of arachidonic acid metabolism. It may be inferred that Ocimum sanctum may be a useful anti-inflammatory agent.[22]

Anti-Inflammatory Herbs that Alter Cell Surface Biology and Modulates Immuno Suppression

Punernava (Boerhaavia Diffusa), a plant which spreads like spider, *Daruharidra* (Berberis Aristata), a Himalyan plant which grows up to two metres and *Kutaki* (Picorrhiza Kurroa) are anti-inflammatory herbs that exert anti-inflammatory action by Beta androgenic blockade suggesting alterations in the cell surface biology involving protein mediation. On the other hand, the components *Giloy*, *Kutaki* and the root of *Rasaunt* (or Barberries) have been found to modulate immuno suppression in dose dependent inhibitory effects, significantly exerting anti-inflammatory activity on acute, subacute and chronic type of inflammation produced by immunological and non-immunological methods, thus relieving inflammation of associated smooth muscles.[23]

Herbs Checking Inflammatory Mediators: The Free Radicals

Daruharidra and *Amla* exert protection against free radicals which induce lipid peroxidation, thus checking the inflammatory disease associated with membrane damage and tissue injury. The IC 50 for *Daruharidra* and *Amla* have been found to be 13 and 30 g/ml in bovine brain phospholipids lysosomes as model membranes.[24]

Cortisone Degradation Inhibiting Effect

Glycyrrhizin from *Yashti Madhu* (Glycyrrhiza Glabra) effectively decreased one of the most important classes of inflammatory mediators, i.e. reactive oxygen species (ROS) of three kinds which are generated by human neutrophils and not those generated in cell free system. The anti-inflammatory effect seems to be due to, in addition to a cortisone degradation inhibiting effect in the liver, its inhibitory effect on generation of ROS by neutrophils. It did not affect neutrophil chemotaxis or phagocytosis either.[25]

Neem Inhibits Chemiluminescence Generation

Neem or Azadirachta Indica, an evergreen tropical tree of 15–20 m. tall with medium to dark green leaves of 3–8 cm. has been traditionally used for its medicinal properties as panacea for several diseases. It also works as anti-inflammatory agent in certain diseases including liver enlargement as it is anti-inflammatory, anti-alergic, insecticidal, nematicidal, spermatocidal, anti-dermatic, anti-viral, anti-fungal, anti-AIDS, anti-cancer, antimalarial, anti-pyretic, anti-arthritic, hypoglycaemic, anti-gastric ulcer and immunomodulatory.

Inhibition of chemiluminescence generation (by activated human polymorphonuclear leuckocytes which is a measure of oxidative burst) activity of phenolic compounds from *Neem* may account for a major part of the anti-inflammatory activities and its therapeutic benefits.[26]

Conclusion

Over hundred Indian medicinal plants, some of which described above, are being used for jaundice and liver diseases under indigenous medical systems particularly Ayurveda and Unani. But only three terrestrial plants, i.e. *Yashti Madhu*

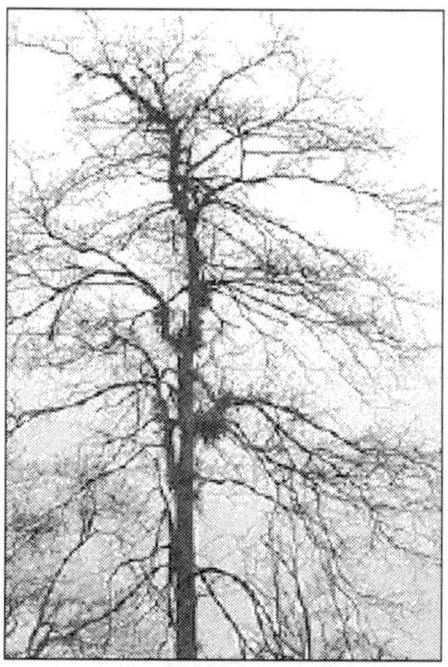

Plate 14.7: Leafless Tree of Terminalia Chebula

(Glycyrrhiza Glabra), *Kutaki* (Picorrhiza Kurroa) and *Bhui Amla* (Phyllanthus Niruri) have been scientifically elucidated while adhering to the internationally acceptable scientific protocols. A fourth plant Sylibum Marianum or milk thistle generally used in Europe also falls in this category and the medicines produced by using these plants are used for Hepatitis B and C viruses. For the first time in the Indian systems of medicine, a chemo-biological fingerprinting methodology for standardization of *Bhui Amla* (Phyllanthus Niruri) preparation has been patented.

Ayurveda is the most commonly practised form of CAM (Complementary and Alternative Medicine) in India fulfilling the medical needs of 80 per cent of the population. The National Centre for Complementary and Alternative Medicine (NCCAM) defines CAM practices as those not presently considered an integral part of conventional medicine. However, utilization of CAM is a universal phenomenon both in developing countries as well as developed countries like USA.

Since many alternative medicinal substances are legally considered dietary supplements, they do not come within the preview of FDA (Food and Drug Administration). However, these are governed under Current Good Manufacturing practice in Manufacturing, Packaging or Holding Human Food (CGMP) regulations. Moreover, according to Dietary Supplement and Health Education Act (DSHEA) passed by United States Congress in 1994, proof of safety or efficacy is not a prerequisite for the marketing of dietary supplements. A draft law reminiscent of the DSHEA is in development in India to regulate manufacturing, importing and marketing of health foods/dietary supplements and other nutraceuticals. The Indian Food Safety and Standards Bill, 2005, which became a law, promising a significant impact on the Indian dietary supplement industry and encouraging manufacturers to do new product development, emphasizes on developing reliable testing protocols, carrying out clinical studies and establishing structure-function claims based on these studies.

This would encourage cross-pathy practices among both qualified allopathic and Ayurvedic practitioners. It is notable that Clause 1.1.3 of Medical Council of India (MCI) prohibits the allopathic practitioners to prescribe drugs from Ayurvedic System of Medicine and Ayurvedic practitioners from allopathic system of medicine. Yet the benefit of the patient lies in the optimal balance and evidence-based use of the two systems and this need to be encouraged especially in developing countries like India with inadequate doctor patient ratio.

Notes

1. www.aimilpharmaceuticals.com.
2. S.P. Thyagarajan, T. Thirunalasundari, S. Subramanian, P.S. Venkateswaran and B.S. Blumberg, 'Effect of Phyllanthus Amarus on Chronic Carriers of Hepatitis Virus', *The Lancet*, vol. 332, issue 8614, 1988, pp. 764–6.
3. R.K. Gulati, S. Agarwal and S.S. Agarwal, 'Hepatoprotective Studies on *Phyllanthus emblica*

L. and quertetin', *Indian Journal of Experimental Biology* (*IJEB*), vol. 33, issue 4, 1995, pp. 261–8.

4. B.P. Reddy, V.N. Murthy, V. Venkateshwarlu, C.K. Kokate and D. Rambhau, 'Antihepatotoxic Activity of Phyllanthus Niruri, Tinospora Cordifolia and Ricinus Communnis', *Indian Drugs*, vol. 30, no. 7, 1993, pp. 338–41.
5. B.N. Dhawan, D.K. Kulshreshtha, G.K. Patnaik, Raj Mehrotra and Shashi Rawat, 'In Vitro Studies on the Effect of Certain Natural Products against Hepatitis B. Virus', *Indian Journal of Medical Research* (*IJMR*), vol. 92, 1990, pp. 133–8.
6. Y. Dwivedi, R. Rastogi, S.K. Sharma et al., 'Picroliv Protects against Monocrotaline—Induced Hepatic Damage in Rats', *Pharmacological Research*, vol. 23, no. 4, 1991, pp. 399–407.
7. R.A. Ansari, S.C. Tripathi, G.K. Patnaik and B.N. Dhawan, 'Antihepatotoxic Properties of Picroliv: An Active Fraction from Rhizomes of Picrorhiza Kurrooa', *Journal of Ethnopharmacology*, vol. 34, issue 1, 1991, pp. 61–8.
8. T.H. Chung, J.C. Kim, C.Y. Lee, M.K. Moon, S.C. Chae, I.S. Lee, S.H. Kim, K.S. Hahn and I.P. Lee, 'Potential Antiviral Effects of *Terminalis chebula, Sanguisorba officinalis, Rubus coreanus* and *Rheum palmatum* against Duck Hepatitis B Virus (DHBV)', *Phytotherapy Research*, vol. 11, issue 3, 1997, pp. 179–82; R.N. Chopra, *Glossary of Indian Medicinal Plants*, New Delhi: Council of Scientific and Industrial Research, 1956.
9. Hisashi Matsuda, Toshio Morikawa, Iwao Toguchida, Ji-Young Park, Shoichi Harima and Masayuki Yoshikawa, 'Antioxidant Constituents from Rhuharab: Structural Requirements of Stilbenes for the Activity and Structures of Two New Anthroquinne Glucosides', *Bioorganic and Medicinal Chemistry*, vol. 9, issue 1, 2001, pp. 41–50.
10. *Journal of Research Education in Indian Medicine* (*JREIM*), October–December 1991, pp. 35–9; M.S. Akhtar, M. Amin, Ahmad, Maqsood, and Alamgeer, 'Hepatoprotective Effect of Rheum Emodi Roots (Revand chini) and Akseer-e-Jigar Against Paracetamol-induced Hepatotoxicity in Rats', *Ethnobotanical Leaflets*, vol. 13, 2009, pp. 310–15.
11. Hitoshi Sato, Wakana Goto, Jun-ichi Yamamura, Masahiko Kurokawa, Seiji Kageyama, Terumi Takahara, Akiharu Watanabe and Kimiyasu Shiraki, 'Therapeutic Basis of Glycyrrhizin on Chronic Hepatitis B', *Antiviral Research*, vol. 30, issues 2–3, 1996, pp. 171–7; M. Shinada, M. Azuma, H. Kawai, K. Sazaki, I. Yoshida, T. Yoshida, T. Suzutani and T. Sakuma, 'Enhancement of Interferon-gamma Production in Glycyrrhizin-treated Human Peripheral Lymphocytes in Response to Concanavalin A and to Surface Antigen of Hepatitis B Virus', *Proceedings of the Society for Experimental Biology and Medicine*, vol. 181, issue 2, 1986, pp. 205–10.
12. *Indian Journal of Clinical Practice* (*IJCP*), vol. 7, no. 3, 1996.
13. Ramamurthy M. Sree and M. Srinivasan, 'Hepatoprotective Effect of Tephrosia Purprea in Experimental Animals', *Indian Journal of Pharmacology*, vol. 25, issue 1, 1993, pp. 34–6.
14. A.K. Saxena, B. Singh and K.K. Anand, 'Hepatoprotective effects of *Eclipta Alba* on Subcellular Levels in Rats', *Journal of Ethnopharmacology*, vol. 40, issue 3, 1993, pp. 155–61.
15. Mohammad Saleem, Aftab Alam, Salahuddin Ahmed, Mohammad Iqbal and Sarwat Sultana, '*Tephrosia Purpurea* Ameliorates Benzoyl Peroxide-induced Cutaneous Toxicity in Mice: Diminution of Oxidative Stress', *Pharmacy and Pharmacology Communications*, vol. 5, issue 7, 1999, pp. 455–61.
16. D.S. Nagarkatti, N.N. Rege, N.K. Desai and S.A. Dahanukar, 'Modulation of Kupffer Cell Activity by Tinospora Cordifolia in Liver Damage', *Journal of Postgraduate Medicine*, vol. 40, issue 2, 1994, pp. 65–7.
17. Aruna Kapil, I.B. Koul, S.K. Banerjee and B.D. Gupta, 'Antihepatotoxic Effects of Major Diterpenoid Constituents of Andrographis Paniculata', *Biochemical Pharmacology*, vol. 46,

issue 1, 1993, pp. 182–5; Rana P. Singh, S. Banerjee and A. Ramesha Rao, 'Modulatory Influence of *Andrographis Paniculata* on Mouse Hepatic and Extrahepatic Carcinogen Metabolizing Enzymes and Antioxidant Status', *Phytotherapy Research*, vol. 15, issue 5, 2001, pp. 382–90.

18. Sarwat Sultana, Shahid Perwaiz, Mohammad Iqbal and Mohammad Athar, 'Crude Extracts of Hepatoprotective Plants, Solanum Nigrum and Cichorium Intybus Inhibit Free Radical-mediated DNA Damage', *Journal of Ethnopharmacology*, vol. 45, issue 3, 1995, pp. 189–92.
19. U.M. Thatte, M.R. Kulkarni and S.A. Dahanukar, 'Immunotherapeutic Modification of Escherichia Coli Peritonitis and Bacteremia by Tinospora Cordifolia', *Journal of Postgraduate Medicine (JPGM)*, vol. 38, issue 1, 1992, pp. 13–15; H.M. Nazareth, N.N. Rege, R.D. Bapat, and S.A. Dahanukar, 'Modulation of Immunosuppression in Obstructive Jaundice by Tinospora Cordifolia', *Indian Journal of Medical Research (IJMR)*, vol. 90, 1989, pp. 478–83.
20. Muhammad Shoaib Akhtar and Muhammad Munir, 'Evaluation of the Gastric Antiulcerogenic Effects of Solanum Nigrum, Brassica Oleracea and Ocimum Basilicum in Rats', *Journal of Ethnopharmacology*, vol. 27, issues 1–2, 1989, pp. 163–76.
21. Uma Devi and A. Ganasoundari, 'Modulation of Glutathione and Antioxidant Enzymes by Ocimum Sanctum and its Role in Protection against Radiation Injury', *Indian Journal of Experimental Biology*, vol. 37, no. 3, 1997, pp. 262–8.
22. Surender Singh, D.K. Majumdar and H.M.S. Rehan, 'Evaluation of Anti-inflammatory Potential of Fixed Oil Ocimum Sanctum (Holybasil) and its Possible Mechanism of Action', *Journal of Ethnopharmacology*, vol. 54, issue 1, 1996, pp. 19–26; Surender Singh, and Shyam S. Agarwal, 'Anti-Asthmatic and Anti-Inflammatory Activity of Ocimum Santctum Linn', *Journal of Research Education in Indian Medicine (JREIM)*, 1991, pp. 23–8.
23. B.L. Pandey and P.K. Das, 'Immunopharmacological Studies on Picrorhiza Kurroa Royle-ex-Benth, part IV: Cellular Mechanisms of Anti-inflammatory Action', *Indian Journal of Physiology and Pharmacology*, vol. 33, no. 1, 1989, pp. 28–30; R.K. Halder, N.C. Neogi and R.S. Rathor, 'Pharmacological Investigations on Berberine Hydrochloride', *Indian Journal of Pharmacology*, vol. 2, issue 1, 1970, pp. 26–7.
24. Sunil Kumar and K.C. Kalus Muller, 'Medicinal Plants from Nepal; II. Evaluation as Inhibitors of Lipid Peroxidation in Biological Membranes', *Journal of Ethnopharmacology*, vol. 64, issue 2, 1999, pp. 135–9.
25. Hirohiko Akamatsu, Jinro Komura, Yasuo Asada and Yukie Niwa, 'Mechanism of Anti-Inflammaotry Action of Glycyrrhizin: Effect on Neutrophil Functions Including Reactive Oxygen Species Generation', *Planta Medica*, vol. 57, issue 2, 1991, pp. 119–21.
26. J.M. Van der Nat, W.G. Van der Sluis, L.A. 'tHart, H. Van Dijk, K.T.D. de Silva and R.P. Labadie, 'Activity-Guided Isolation and Identification of *Azadirachta indica* Bark Extract Constituents which Specifically Inhibit Chemiluminescence Production by Activated Human Polymorphonuclear Leukocytes', *Planta Medica*, vol. 57, issue 1, 1991, pp. 65–8.

15

A Brief Sketch of Anatomical Knowledge and Health in Ayurveda

Its Interactions with Modern Medicine and Outcome in India

Jayanta Bhattacharya

The practice of medicine of the ancients was an art, and not a science, and dignity it did not acquire until it was based on acquaintance with anatomy and physiology.

—Joseph Leidy, 'Lecture Introductory to the Course on Anatomy in the University of Pennsylvania for the Session 1858–9', 1859, p. 7, *A Traffic of Dead Bodies: Anatomy and Embodied Social Identity in Nineteenth-Century America*, 2002, p. 53

Knowledge of the body was, no doubt, a concern for the Ayurvedic authors. In *Caraka Saṁhitā* (*CS*)—*śarīravicayaḥ śarīropakārārthamiṣyate/ jñātvā hi śarīratattvaṁ śarīropakārakaresu bhāvesu jñānamutpadyate / tasmāt śarīravicayaṁ praśaṁsanti kuśalāḥ* // [Śā, 6.3] (Detailed knowledge of the human body is conducive to the well-being of the individual. Understanding of the factors that constitute the body provides knowledge regarding the factors which are responsible for its well-being. It is because of this, that experts extol the knowledge of the details of the body).[1] Though this passage does not vividly speak of anatomical knowledge, it does point out to the importance of bodily knowledge in Ayurveda.

Perhaps the importance of gaining anatomical knowledge cannot be better valued than the editorial of the *New England Journal of Medicine*. While

*I am deeply indebted to Deepak Kumar, Rahul Peter Das, Dominik Wujastyk and Geraldine Forbes for their generous help by providing me invaluable books, journals and other documents which could not be accessed by me at this rather marginal area.

'Looking Back on the Millennium in Medicine', the editorial comments are as follows:

> The emergence of a comprehensive understanding of the structure and function of the organ systems of the human body stands—without question—as one of the most influential advances of the past millennium. . . . Considered together, the work of Vesalius and Harvey provided the intellectual underpinnings for many advances in human anatomy, physiology, clinical medicine, and surgery that followed during the remainder of the millennium.[2]

If society and science view medicine or art of healing in an all-encompassing way, the problems, and, more importantly, the solutions will be understood following this line of thinking. If science and society view medicine as an industry and a market commodity, the problems and solutions will be understood as industrial and mercantile in nature. Because one is self-aware, the study of the human has a unique place in establishing the image one has of himself, ultimately the prosaic descriptions of the bones, muscles, blood vessels and neural pathways are the context of one's experience of life.[3]

To understand disease inside the body, one has to grapple with the knowledge of the body. The physical examination, medical imaging and other procedures, as well as the elements of the medical history, all generate clinical data that pertain to anatomical entities in the human body. Dissection-based anatomical analysis facilitated the classification of bodily components, the development of a vocabulary for describing the body with clarity and precision and mapping the bodily organs and their surface projections, which would be later used in physical diagnosis.[4] A full, or even adequate, discussion of the 'kinds' of anatomy would be in effect a history of anatomy, and a partial history of medicine, biology and natural philosophy.[5] The 'kinds' of anatomy take a different shape when looked through the window of Ayurveda. Before exploring the world of Ayurveda we might benefit from a brief journey through a part of modern medicine or, biomedicine.

Anatomical Knowledge: Modern Medicine

It is being argued that medicine may be made up of regional rationalisms that have a scientific status and also, 'medicine itself is not a science: in its epistemological spirit, it is rather a kind of ideology'.[6] Modern medicine/biomedicine has passed through paradigmatic shifts. Before the advent of anatomical knowledge the working model of the body in medicine was of two-dimensional nature—*symptom* > *illness*. Patient's history alone was the primary source of diagnosis. Though the bodily organs were described, detailed and used to explain disease causation, no pathological anatomy was known. Accurate localization of diseases inside the body was inconceivable. As an outcome of emphasis on dissection and experimentation medicine, during the late eighteenth and early nineteenth centuries, made its journey from bedside medicine to hospital medicine to laboratory medicine, and now techno-medicine. Disease appeared to being located within a three-dimensional body—*symptom* > *illness* > *sign*. Depth or volume of the body—the third dimension—was added to *symptom > illness* perception whereby the body emerged to be of three-dimensional nature. Doctors were, then, to extract sign, i.e. pathology inside the body.[7] In Indian context, Western medicine derived its 'claim to scientific objectivity and authority largely from . . . studies of morbid anatomy. . .'.[8] A new norm and epistemological structure began to emerge. Around 1800 one began to follow Bichat's (1770–1801) maxim 'open up a few corpses', as Foucault laconically remarks.[9] Illness and disease became not a matter of the whole body, but were located in body parts and their pathologies. According to Bichat, one should 'dissect in anatomy, experiment in physiology, follow the disease and make the necropsy in medicine; this is the three fold path, without which there can be no anatomist, no physiologist, no physician'.[10] According to Corvisart, the systematic study of pathological anatomy 'which had been made possible by recent establishment of hospital-based medical teaching, had revealed that organic lesions—or pathological alterations of the solid parts of the body—were "far more frequent than the majority of physicians have believed until now"'.[11]

Though till the middle of the nineteenth century, medicine was principally guided by ancient Greek humoural theory, anatomical dissection and solidism, as shown earlier, was running parallel to it and, for the first time, students were exhorted to understand the structure and function of the body by detailed dissection. Perhaps one of the most important methodological changes characteristic of early nineteenth-century medicine was the shift from *observation*

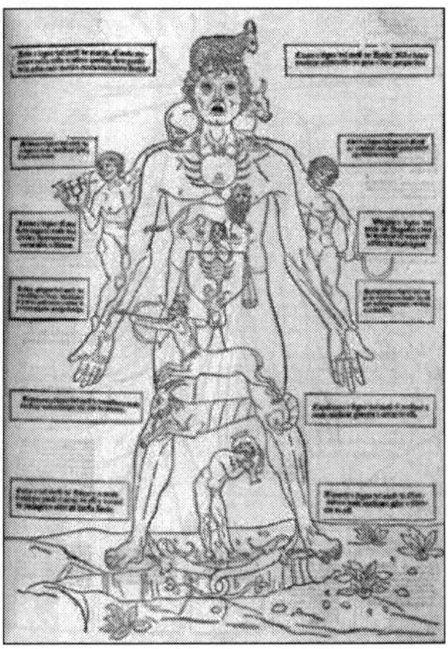

Plate 15.1: *Zodiac Man* (1493). Johannes de Ketham, *Fasiculo de medicina*, Venice: Zuane & Gregorio di Gregorii, 1494, p. 16.

Courtesy: National Library of Medicine—*Historical Anatomies on the Web.* (It is interesting to note that though a three-dimensional body image has been used in this illustration, all organs are described according to astrological medicine, much before the advent of hospital medicine.)

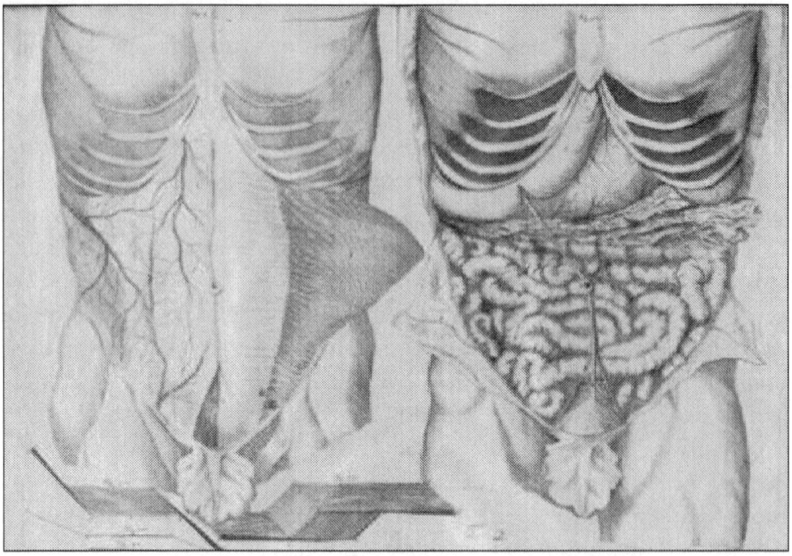

Plate 15.2: Amé Bourdon, *Nouvelles tables anatomiques*, Chez Laurens d'Houry, Paris, 1678.

Courtesy: National Library of Medicine—*Historical Anatomies on the Web*. (Unlike the previous one, change in temper and mode of representation is quite evident.)

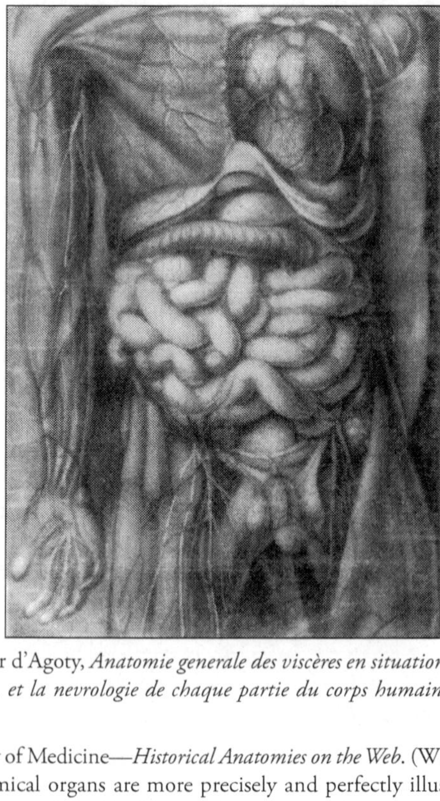

Plate 15.3: Jacques Gautier d'Agoty, *Anatomie generale des viscères en situation, de grandeur et couleur naturelle, avec l'angeologie, et la nevrologie de chaque partie du corps humain*, Gautier, Paris, 1752, Table 5.

Courtesy: National Library of Medicine—*Historical Anatomies on the Web*. (With improved technique of colour printing, anatomical organs are more precisely and perfectly illustrated. This improved ways of illustrations could be fully utilized for surgical purposes.)

to *examination.*[12] During the same period, gross anatomy held an intellectual centrality to Western medical science, surpassing anything it enjoyed before or since. Science meant empiricism, epitomized by systematic empirical correlation of symptoms observed at the bedside with lesions found at autopsy. Not only that, privileged access to the body, gained through the knowledge of anatomy, marked a social, moral, and emotional boundary crossing that conferred new knowledge and reforged sensibilities, though, the dissecting room became a site of epistemological exhaustion—fixed and unchangeable.[13] This nascent period of gaining anatomical knowledge and its successful application in surgery has been precisely described as 'a theory of surgical diseases . . . made surgery respectable by giving it an abstract foundation. In the process, the senses could not be given the free rein associated with empiricism, but had to be disciplined and ordered by a rational system'.[14] The raw materials of medical theorizing, now became the innumerable morbid events, occurring within the gross anatomical structures, which presented themselves to the clinical gaze on the crowded wards.[15] A few illustrations from different periods will clarify the issue in a more tangible way.

With all these characteristics, the European medicine through the British arrived in India. In the Indian context a new era of medicine began to emerge.

Medicine, during colonial period, was unwaveringly related with metaphors of higher civilization,[16] and also, invasion.[17] Anatomy seems to be burgeoning as a discipline of central importance, if it is viewed from the perspective of its cross-cultural nature, evolutionary history and its evolution to become universal through the advent of modern. Many a time, it has become a tool and technology for establishing superiority of Western medical culture specifically and the West in general over India. Quite apart from their excursions into trade, 'the surgeons of the Company were frequently employed on activities outside the practice of medicine.'[18] Gabriel Boughton's acquiring of *Firman* for trading rights in Bengal is the singular most example. Anatomical knowledge (and surgical excellence arising out of it) was the primary demarcating line between modern medical knowledge and Ayurveda. 'The confidence of the natives, who resort to European hospitals being greatly increased by successful surgical operations. . . .'[19] It was asserted, 'That the foundation of the Medical College of Calcutta is one of the greatest facts in the recent history of Indian Administration.'[20] The rule among the natives of Bengal were to resort to Western systems as the general belief was that the ancient Hindu system was slow in giving relief to the sufferer.[21] Mark Harrison finds that 'Western medicine was far popular with Indian aristocracy, for whom it was a mark of high social status. . . . The Raja of Farid Kot, for instance, offered a truly kingly sum of Rs. 50,000 for successful treatment of his family.'[22] Bayly notes, 'Indigenous practitioners borrowed and incorporated many Western remedies. . . . At the same time the Anglo-Indian dialectic privileged what was thought of as specifically "medical" in this branch of Shastric wisdom.'[23] However, it should be emphasized that this was not the complete scenario. There were contestations between Western and indigenous medicines. C.T. Buckland wrote to the Officiating Secretary to the Government of Bengal, Judicial (Medical) Department, on 6 July 1872 about repugnance of the natives 'to take English medicine properly and regularly, and to submit themselves to reasonable treatment. . .'. He also noted, 'how much of the effect is lost when medicine is given to a set of ignorant and doubting people in the villages, who probably do their best to destroy its valuable properties of the English drugs by combining with them (as they fancy) the prescriptions of the kabirajes or the wise and aged women of the village'.[24]

Anatomical Knowledge and Ayurveda

Importantly, *Suśruta Saṁhitā* (*SS*) emphasized, 'Śalya is pre-eminent too on account of its quick action, owing to its use of sharp and blunt instruments (śastra, yantra), caustics (ksāra), and cautery (agni).'[25] It was also stressed, 'Description of anatomy of human body upto skin is not dealt with in any part (of Ayurveda) except surgery.'[26] But how to perform the surgical procedures? It was not based on anatomical knowledge of organs. 'Experts say that surgical operations be performed after considering the measurement of *marmans* so far as to avoid them. As injury even on margin marmans leads to death, the site of vital spot should be avoided altogether.'[27] One shall shortly come to know of this uniqueness of Indian surgery.

Hence, it is not surprising at all that hitherto existing only anatomical illustration based on Ayurvedic description of organs correspond to pre-modern European illustration of bodily organs. One more point may be raised here. Surgical instruction was not part of thirteenth-century academic medicine. In the Middle Ages in Europe, quite similar to the Ayurvedic educational practice of *guru-shishya prampara* (teacher-pupil succession), 'Surgery was still taught as it traditionally had been, privately, in an association between a practitioner and his occasional disciples or apprentices in which ultimately the apprentice could hope not only to acquire his master's skills but also to inherit something of his reputation.'[28] With the advent of post-Vesalian anatomy, post-Harverian physiology and also, following experiments of Richard Lower (on transfusion and cardiopulmonary function) and William Hunter (successful surgery of aneurysm) European medicine and surgery had traversed a long and tortuous path of development within a short span, which was yet to be attained by Indians.

However, by AD 600, Indian surgery and anatomical practices were in complete disuse. 'A comparison of Suśruta and Vāgbhata I shows that the study of anatomy had almost ceased to exist in the latter's time.'[29] Hoernle comments, 'Vāgbhata I possessed no experimental knowledge of the skeleton . . . from want of anatomical knowledge . . .'.[30] P.C. Ray attributed this decline to the rise of casteism and Vedantic philosophy.[31]

Neglected state of anatomical knowledge can be found in the accounts of travellers like Bernier and Fryer. Francois Bernier wrote:

> It is not surprising that the *Gentiles* understand nothing of anatomy. They never open the body either of man or beast, and those in our household always ran away, with amazement and horror, whenever I opened a living goat or sheep for the purpose

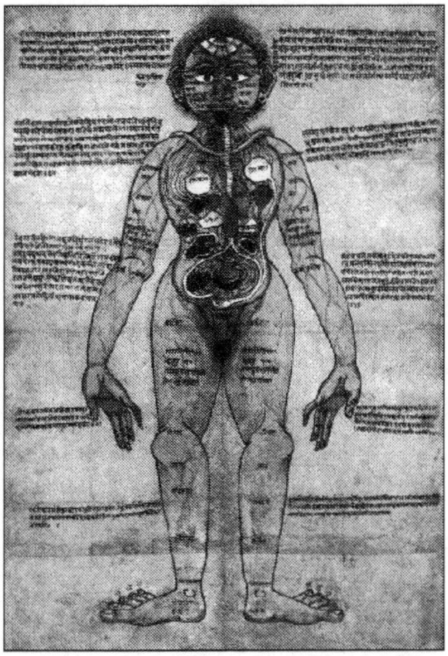

Plate 15.4: Nepalese, *c.* eighteenth/early nineteenth century, Wellcome Library no. 574912i, (Image no. V36133 or L17592).

Courtesy: Wellcome Library. (This image is entirely drawn from the Ayurvedic understanding of the human anatomy, unlike other Indian images of the human body. The channels and organs drawn on the torso are specified as in Ayurvedic literature, with organs named as receptacles for one or other of the organic fluids. However, the organs in Ayurveda, are seen in a much wider context than in the West. They are the seats of the humours (wind, bile and phlegm) and do not generally engage in the kind of processing which modern western biomedicine expects of an 'organ'.)

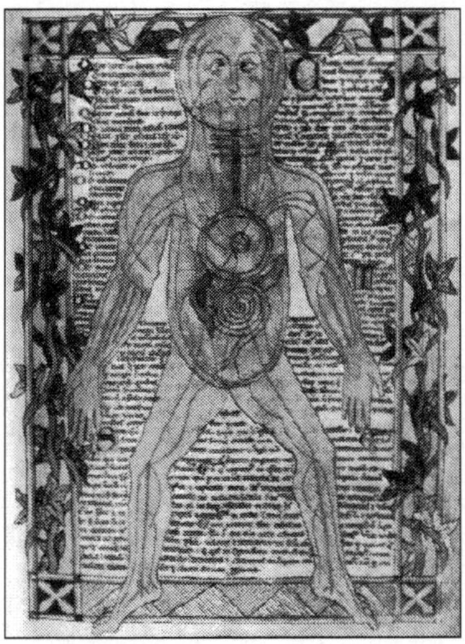

Plate 15.5: A late thirteenth-century illustration of the venous system and various systems within the body. According to Galen, the venous system was distinct from the arterial, and the blood ebbed and flowed through the body.

Courtesy: princeton.edu. URL: http://www.princeton.edu/~his291/, accessed on 10 October 2009.

of explaining to my *Agah* the circulation of the blood, and showing him the vessels, discovered by *Pecquet*, through which the chyle is conveyed to the right ventricle of the heart.[32]

In Fryer's observation, 'In Esteem among them (Indians) are principally Magick and Judicial Astrology . . . nor are they quite ignorant of Medicks, though Anatomy is not approved, wherein they lean too much on Tradition, being able to give very slender account thereof of the Rational Part thereof.'[33]

To remember, there is also mention of Indian surgical knowledge in other accounts. Manucci was possibly the first person to give a somewhat detailed account of Indian rhinopalsty. 'The surgeons belonging to the country cut the skin of the forehead above the eyebrows, and made it fall down over the wounds on the nose. . . . In a short time the wounds heal up . . . I saw many persons with such noses, and they were not so disfigured as they would have been without any nose at all. . .'.[34] Rhinoplasty may be regarded as a regular practice as Manucci saw many people undergoing this operation. Lambert observed, 'An obstruction of the spleen . . . They make a small incision over the spleen, and then insert a long needle between the flesh and skin. From this incision, by sucking thro' a horn pipe, they obtain a certain pinguous matter which resembles pus.'[35] Except such evidences in travellers' accounts are always scathing about primitive, fanciful anatomical knowledge of Indian medicine. Interestingly, Indian herbal knowledge used to be appreciated. As late as 1893, advertisement of 'The Indian Pills' was published in *The Lady's dressing-room*.[36]

Keen interest in Indian/Hindu medicine began to grow following a fascinating account of Indian rhinoplasty in 1794. Before 1794, the most remarkable work by the East India Company was *A Code of Gentoo Laws*. Its purpose was specifically stated, 'From hence, therefore, may be formed a precise idea of the Customs and Manners of these People, which, to their great injury have long been misrepresented in the Western World. . . . In a Tract so untrodden as this, *many Paths must be attempted before we can hit upon the right*.'[37]

1794: Report of Indian Rhinoplasty and Thereafter

Barak Longmate (BL) vividly reported in 1794, 'A friend has transmitted to me, from the East Indies, the following very curious, and, in Europe, I believe, unknown chirurgical operation, which has long been practiced in India with success: namely, affixing a new nose on a man's face.'[38] A Maharatta by the name of Cowasjee (though, he seems to be a Parsee) was a bullock cart driver in the employment of the English Army in the Mysore War of 1793. He was captured by Tipu Sultan's soldiers who cut off his nose for his treachery. It was deftly reconstructed by a Maharatta potter of Satara near Poona. 'Two of the medical gentlemen, Mr Thomas Cruso and Mr James Trindlay, of the Bombay presidency, have seen it performed. . . .'[39] There were also drawings on the procedure of the operation, along with a portrait of Cowasjee.

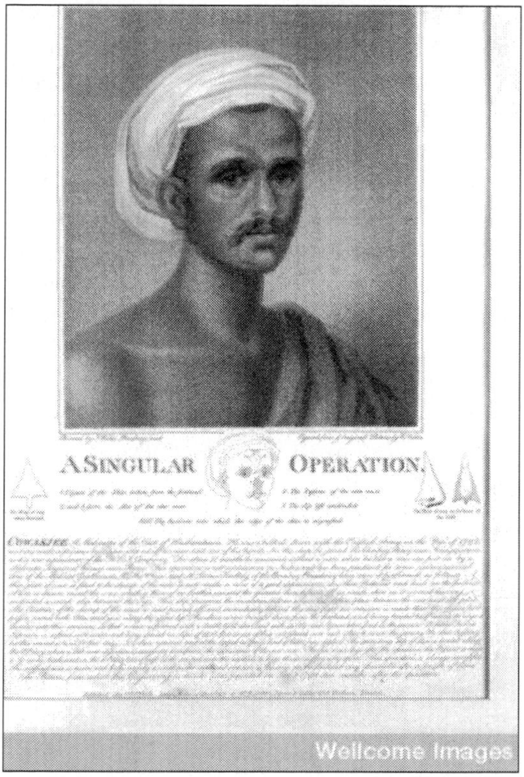

Plate 15.6: *L0007335 Credit*: Wellcome Library, London. Published: James Wales of Bombay at Mr R. Cribbs, London: Carver & Gilder (288 Holborn): 1 January 1795. Indian method of the restoration of the nose by plastic surgery, from article by B.L. to Mr Urban, concerning Cowasjee, a man who had his nose reconstructed with the aid of plastic surgery. From: *Gentleman's Magazine*, 9 October 1794, vol. 64, pt. 2, facing page 883. By: BL.

Courtesy: Wellcome Images.

All important works on Indian/Hindu medicine followed 1794. J.F. Royle found in 'Hindoo' medicine 'much fanciful Anatomy, imaginative Physiology, and absurd attention to numbers. . .'.[40] W. Ainslie published his first work on Indian materia medica in 1813. H.H. Wilson's 'On the medical surgical sciences of the Hindus' was published in 1823. The first edition of *Commentary on the Hindu System of Medicine* was published in 1845. Hence, it may not be a wild guess that the impetus to know of Indian medicine and surgery was an outcome of the report in the *Gentleman's Magazine*. Albrecht Weber realized, 'In this department European surgeons might perhaps even at the present day still learn something from them, as indeed they have already learned from them the operation of rhinoplsty.'[41] Similar view was expressed by Arthur MacDonnell too, 'In modern days European surgery has borrowed the operation of rhinoplasty . . . from India, where Englishmen became acquainted with the art in the last century.'[42] In a similar note to Bernier's observation, an American missionary doctor noted in 1856, 'The blacksmith, with his tongs, serves as dentist, and the *barber, with his razor, as surgeon*; since these are the only persons supposed to have tools adapted to the practice of these professions.'[43]

How to reconcile these two contrasting phenomena—sheer lack of anatomical knowledge of Indian practitioner on the one hand and specialized surgical practices like rhinoplasty by non-medical surgeons on the other hand? A tentative answer may be found in the previous discussions of Suśruta's text. In modern observation, 'Surgical operations demanded a knowledge of regional anatomy rather than elaborate and often unnecessary and tedious descriptions of all the structures of the body. The place of regional anatomy was supplied by concept of the *marman*.'[44] *Marman* is a junction of meeting place of the vital/lethal principles of ligaments, veins, muscles, bones and joints. Another point is high-caste practitioners were content with herbo-chemical knowledge while surgical crafts were relegated to the hands of low-caste people who used the knowledge of *marman*-s.

Place of Anatomy in Ayurveda: Epistemological Shifts in Medicine

SS teaches—*pratyaksato hi yadrstam śāstradrstam ca yadbhavet/samāsatastadubhayam bhūyo jnānavivardhanam //* (Śā, 5.48).[45] [The practical knowledge along with theoretical knowledge is very essential. Whatever is seen while doing practical study and going through Śāstra (scripture), adds the knowledge, when both are applied together.] In this text alone one finds, without a precedent or succession, 'the single and unique description of a dissection performed without a knife on a human body for the sake of instruction in the knowledge of anatomy'.[46] Moreover, Indian surgeons and physicians were able 'to study the human skeleton without the complicated procedure of a dissection'.[47]

Probable sources of gaining anatomical knowledge were primarily: (1) the bodies of the children below two years of age as their bodies were not burnt, but buried, according to Indian custom, (2) 'the anatomy of the goat, sheep, horse, and other animals used in their sacrifices',[48] and (3) bones collected after cremation of the dead as prescribed in Hindu rituals. Unlike modern European medicine, Indian conception of the body was two-dimensional—a bodily frame through which *dosa*-s, *dhātu*-s and *mala*-s flow. There was no single conception of the Indian body, but a dominant one.[49] Maas argues, 'In a diachronic perspective, however, one may safely assume that quite a number of different body concepts were current at the time of the *CS*'s composition',[50] and Suśruta's *marman* theory is a synthesis of different and partly overlapping systematic anatomical concepts among which the theory of bodily constituents served as the most comprehensive one.[51]

One meets with structures of the human body with different organs and their functions in various non-medical Vedic literatures.[52] Moreover, 'the status and condition of medicine of any age is better known by non-medical texts'.[53] There are also references to rudimentary surgical procedures in the Vedas, Brāhmanas, Aranyakas and Upanisads.[54]

The Vedic surgeons would probably use ligature (*abhiśrit*) for stopping bleeding and making incision in the neck (*Rig Veda*, viii, 1.12). He would use both knives and *mantras* for venesection (*Atharva Veda*, i.17). These ancient physicians and surgeons had some knowledge of anatomy because they slaughtered many animals for sacrifice and had to do it skilfully by the use of a 'grey knife' without displeasing the gods by mangling the limbs of the animals (*Rig Veda,* i, 162.20; *Atharva Veda*, ix, 5.4). Even a reed was also used as a catheter in cases of difficulty of micturition, but always the whole of the hymn had to be recited (Atharva Veda, i, 3.7). It has been suggested that this reed was a primitive type of catheter, called *vasti-yantra* in later Indian medicine.[55]

During this phase, disease causation was thought to exist in a space outside the body. Following the first epistemological shift from Vedic to Ayurvedic medicine disease causation was considered to be seated in the *dosa*-s within the body. It is marked 'by a distinctive change in medical thinking, indicative of an epistemology rooted in empirical observations and reasoning based on a humoural theory. . . . This theory has no antecedents in Vedic medicine'.[56]

Though epistemological shift occurred from magico-religious to empirico-rational conceptual frame (*tridosavāda*), knowledge of anatomy did not undergo any epistemological change. Not only that, there occurred dislocation and displacement of original terms connoting surgical practice by more benign medical terminologies. Zimmermann notes, '*Pañcakarman* might have been originally synonymous with *sodhana,* "the Purificatory (or Evacuant) Treatments", as categories encompassed emetics, purgatives, drastic enemas, and errhines. However, since *bloodletting* (*the fifth of the evacuant therapies*) *has fallen into disuse*, it was removed from the set of *pañcakarman*, and replaced by oily enemas. These technical changes, and shifts of meaning, involved a more fundamental change in medical philosophy, from operative medicine to more gentle methods.'[57] The same terms and notions were being used for generations till its encounter with modern medical knowledge.[58] Again, the localization of disease was much more elusive and roving in humoural medicines like Ayurveda. Following Zimmermann, it may be said that our modern categories are 'monothetic' categories, while traditional concepts have always been attractive to the layman precisely because they are polymorphous, encompassing, multifaceted, or 'polythetic' frames of thought.

Meulenbeld observes, 'Other facets of transformation of Ayurveda are the decline of surgery, and closely bound up with it, of anatomical knowledge. Surgical procedures like blood-letting and cauterization fell into disuse.'[59] The *Madhavanidāna*'s nosological, not otherwise, classification is an example of this decline.[60] *Tridosa* theory is perhaps linked with brahminization of heterodox medical practices to suit to orthodox practice. 'Statements that appeared to jeopardize the *tridosavāda* caught the eye of the commentators and gave them much food for thought in their efforts to avert any danger to the prevailing theory.'[61] The reverse may also be true—Brahmanic conceptions were changed to fit into the medical point of view.[62]

Peter Breton, the Superintendent of the Native Medical Institution of Calcutta, remarked, 'The Asiatics from being unacquainted with anatomy have no words equivalent to a number of anatomical expressions. . . . They have no distinctions for Nerve and therefore call it Nūs, asūb Shirrā &c in common with Ligaments and Tendons.'[63] In his Introductory Address delivered at Calcutta Medical College on 17 March 1836, M.J. Bramley, principal of the college, told, 'Look at the department of surgery, occupied by whom? By ignorant beings who know not a vein from an artery, and who could not secure a comparatively small blood-vessel, however alarming the hemorrhage might be.'[64] He went on to say, 'there can be no question your materia medica contains many articles of fantastic, useless, or destructive character, of which further advance in European science will point out to you the mischief and danger.'[65] One of his conclusive remarks was 'the whole aspect and temper of Native Society (at least in Calcutta) is changing; and may we not say it is changing for the best?'[66]

Such was not the scenario during the period of earlier encounter with colonial medicine. The exchange was not asymmetrical to this extent. In 1812, at the beginning of his book, John Fleming noted, 'The following catalogue is intended chiefly for the use of gentlemen of the medical profession on their first arrival in India, to whom it must be desirable to know what articles of Materia Medica this country affords, and by what names they may find them.'[67] Talking about *Puti-Caranja* or *Caesalpinia bonducella*, he found its successful use in intermittent fevers by Hindu physicians. Intermittent fevers were much formidable to the British settlers. He commented, 'This method of curing intermittents is so successful, that it has been adopted by many European practitioners, particularly in those cases which so frequently occur, in which the patients have an aversion to the Peruvian bark, or cannot retain it in the stomach.'[68]

During nationalist revival, all these inconsistencies were stripped off and efforts were made to reconstitute Ayurveda as 'modern' to fit into the tenets of modern medicine. One of the most important changes in this direction occurred in the perception of pathogenesis of disease. In Ayurveda, prodromes (*pūrvarūpa*) develop into full-fledged symptoms (*rūpa*). Secondary affections (*upadrava*) are consequences of the basic morbid process. At the end of this process, recovery takes place or fatal signs (*arista*) appear, foreboding death.[69] Efforts were made to explain this process by modern medical concept. Gananath Sen, the eminent English-trained Ayurvedic physician, who studied modern anatomy too, stated it in clear terms, 'Let us clearly understand that our Anatomy and Physiology might have been comprehensive at one time, but as we have them at present, they need to be thoroughly sifted and supplemented. Our Chemistry and Botany might have been ahead of the West but now we must recast and remodel them according to the present scientific standards.'[70]

With all these sea changes, Indian subjectivity, represented through Ayurveda to a great extent, was reconstituted forever. Moreover, as a result of such contestations between Western and indigenous medicines, there emerged a space split open—the all-powerful Western therapeutics and indigenous ontology of health. Contesting, yet vanquished, indigenous population and practitioners tried to inscribe their presence inside this space—oftentimes as 'mimicry', more often through rejection of Western medicine and resorting to indigenous healing practices, particularly in case of chronic diseases (which is till date a dark area of modern medicine).

Notes

1. *Agniveśa's Caraka Samhitā* (*Text with English Translation & Critical Exposition Based on Cakrapāni Datta's Āyurveda Dīpikā*), vol. II, tr. Ram Karan Sharma and Bhagwan Dash, Varanasi: Chaukhamba Sanskrit Series Office, 1977, p. 426.
2. Editorial, 'Looking Back on the Millennium in Medicine', *New England Journal of Medicine*, vol. 342, no. 1, 2000, pp. 42–9.
3. Lawrence H. Bannister et al., eds., *Gray's Anatomy*, 38th edn., Edinburgh and London: Churchill Livingstone, 1995, p. 2.
4. J. Older, 'Anatomy: A must for Teaching the Next Generation', *The Surgeon: Journal of the Royal College of Surgeons of Edinburgh and Ireland*, 2004, pp. 79–90.
5. Andrew Cunningham, 'The Kinds of Anatomy', *Medical History*, vol. 19, no. 1, 1975, pp. 1–19.
6. Thomas Osborne, 'Medicine and Ideology', *Economy and Society*, vol. 27, no. 2, 1998, pp. 259–73.
7. For pioneering study see, Erwin Ackerknecht, *Medicine at the Paris Hospital 1794–1848*, Baltimore, 1967; Caroline Hannaway and Ann La Berge, eds., *Constructing Paris Medicine*, Amsterdam, Atlanta and GA: Rodopi, 1999; Toby Gelfand, *Professionalizing Modern Medicine: Paris Surgeons and Medical Science and Institutions in the Eighteenth Century*, Connecticut, 1980; 'Gestation of the Clinic', *Medical History*, vol. 25, no. 2, 1981, pp. 169–80; and Ivan Waddington, 'The Role of the Hospital in the Development of Modern Medicine: A Sociological Analysis', *Sociology*, vol. 7, no. 2, 1973, pp. 211–24.
8. David Arnold, *Colonizing the Body: State Medicine and Epidemic Disease in Nineteenth-Century India*, 1993, p. 53.
9. Michael Foucault, *The Birth of the Clinic: Archaeology of Medical Perception*, tr. A.M. Sheridan Smith, New York, 1994, p. 124.
10. Quoted in Lester S. King and Marjorie C. Meehan, 'A History of the Autopsy: A Review', *American Journal of Pathology*, vol. 73, no. 2, 1973, pp. 514–44.
11. W.R. Albury, 'Corvisart and Broussais: Human Individuality and Medical Dominance', *Constructing Paris Medicine*, ed. Hannaway and Bege, pp. 221–50, see p. 226.
12. Ivan Waddington, 'The Role of the Hospital in the Development of Modern Medicine: A Sociological Analysis', *Sociology*, vol. 7, no. 2, 1973, pp. 211–24.
13. John Harley Warner and Lawrence J. Rizzolo, 'Anatomical Instruction and Training for Professionalism from the 19th to the 21st Centuries', *Clinical Anatomy*, vol. 19, no. 5, 2006, pp. 403–14.
14. Susan C. Lawrence, 'Educating the Senses: Students, Teachers and Medical Rhetoric in Eighteenth-century London', *Medicine and the Five Senses*, ed. W.F. Bynum and R. Porter, Cambridge, 1993, pp. 154–78.

15. N.D. Jewson, 'The Disappearance of the Sick-man from Medical Cosmology, 1770–1870', *Sociology*, vol. 10, no. 2, 1976, pp. 225–44.
16. Gyan Prakash, *Another Reason: Science and the Imagination of Modern India*, New Delhi, 2000; Thomas R. Metcalf, *Ideologies of the Raj*, New Delhi, 1998; Mark Harrison, *Climates and Constitutions: Health, Environment and British Imperialism in India 1600–1850*, New Delhi, 1999.
17. Laura Otis, *Membranes and Metaphors: Metaphors of Invasion in Nineteenth-Century Literature, Science and Politics*, London, 2000.
18. Donald McDonald, 'The Indian Medical Service: A Short Account of its Achievement 1600-1947', *Proceedings of the Royal Society of Medicine*, vol. 49, no. 1, 1955, pp. 13–17; J.W. Massie, *Continental India*, vol. I, London, 1840, p. 301; Charles Macfarlane, *History of British India*, London, 1858, p. 17.
19. F.H. Brett, *Practical Essay on Some of the Principal Surgical Diseases in India*, Calcutta, 1840, p. iii.
20. John William Kaye, *The Administration of the East India Company: A History of Indian Progress*, London, 1853, p. 616.
21. Uday Chand Dutt, *The Materia Medica of the Hindus* (*with a Glossary of Indian Plants by George King*), revd. edn., Calcutta, 1922, p. iii.
22. Mark Harrison, *Public Health in British India—Anglo-Indian Preventive Medicine 1859–1914*, New Delhi, 1994, p. 12.
23. C.A. Bayly, 'British Orientalism and the Indian Rational Tradition, *c.*1780–1820', *South Asia Research*, vol. 14, no. 1, 1994, pp. 1–9.
24. *Proceedings of the Lieutenant-Governor of Bengal, No. 367* (*district Burdwan*), Calcutta, Bengal Secretary Office, West Bengal State Archives, 1872, p. 46.
25. G. Jan Meulenbeld, *A History of Indian Medical Literature*, IA, Egbert Forsten, Groningen, 1999, p. 203. Also see, Girindranath Mukhopadhyaya, *The Surgical Instruments of the Hindus with A Comparative Study of the Surgical Instruments of the Greek, Roman, Arab and the Modern European Surgeons*, vol. I, Calcutta, 1909, pp. ix–x. It should be noted, though *śalya* is accepted for surgery it actually means a dart to be removed by the specially trained physician. It might have some relationship with wounds during war.
26. P.V. Sharma, *Suśruta-Saṁhitā*, vol. II, Varanasi, 2005, p. 182.
27. Ibid., p. 197.
28. Michael McVaugh, 'Surgical Education in the Middle Ages', *DYNAMIS, Acta Hisp. Med. Hist. Illus.*, 2000, vol. 20, pp. 283–304, see pp. 286–7.
29. S.N. Dasgupta, *A History of Indian Philosophy*, vol. II, Delhi, 1991, p. 433.
30. A.F. Rudolf Hoernle, *Studies in the Medicine of Ancient India: Osteology or the Bones of the Human Body*, New Delhi, 1994, p. 96.
31. P.C. Ray, *A History of Hindu Chemistry from the Earliest Times to the Middle of the Sixteenth Century, AD: With Sanskrit Texts, Variants, Translations and Illustrations*, vol. I, Calcutta, 1903.
32. François Bernier, *Travels in the Mughal Empire* (*AD 1656–1668*), tr. and revised by Vincent A. Smith, London: Archibald Constable, 1916, p. 339.
33. John Fryer, *A New Account of East India and Persia in Eight Letters being Nine Years Travels, Begun 1672. And Finished 1681*, London, 1698, p. 191.
34. Niccolao Manucci, *Storia Da Mogor or Mughal India 1653–1708*, vol. II, tr. William Irvine, London, 1907, p. 301.
35. Claude-Francois Lambert, *A Collection of Curious Observations on the Manners, Customs, Usages, different Languages, Government, mythology, Chronology, Ancient and Modern Geography, Ceremonies, Religion, Mechanics, Astronomy, Medicine, Physics, Natural History, Commerce, Arts, and Sciences, of the Several Nations of Asia, Africa, and America*, John Dunn, vol. I, London: Printed for the Translator, 1750, pp. 99–100.

36. Staffe Baroness, *The Lady's Dressing-room*, 1893, http://www.victorianlondon.org/, accessed on 22 December 2009.
37. Nathaniel Brassey Halhed, tr., *A Code of Gentoo Laws, or Ordinations of the Pundits, from a Persian Translation, Made from the Original, Written in Shanscrit Language*, London, 1776, pp. xi–xii.
38. Sylvanus Urban, ed., *The Gentleman's Magazine and Historical Chronicle. For the Year MDCCXCIV*, vol. 64, pt. 2, 1794, p. 891.
39. Ibid.
40. J.F. Royle, *An Essay on the Antiquity of Hindoo Medicine Including an Introductory Lecture to the Course of Materia Medica and Therapeutics, Delivered at King's College*, London, 1837, p. 48.
41. Albrecht Weber, *The History of Indian Literature*, tr. John Mann and Theodor Zachariae, London, 1882, p. 270.
42. Arthur A. MacDonnell, *A History of Sanskrit Literature*, New York: D. Appleton & Co., 1900, p. 437.
43. O.R. Bacheler, *Hinduism and Christianity in Orissa: Containing a Brief Description of the Country, Religion, Manners and Customs, of the Hindus, and an Account of the Operations of the American Freewill Baptist Mission in Northern Orissa*, Boston, 1856, p. 174.
44. P. Kutumbiah, *Ancient Indian Medicine*, Chennai, 1999, p. 33.
45. Jādavji Trikamji Āchārya, ed., *Suśruta Saṁhitā*, Varanasi, 2008.
46. I. Fišer and O. Fišerova, 'Dissection in Ancient India', in *History and Culture of Ancient India (for the XXVI International Congress of Orientalists)*, ed. W. Ruben, V. Struve and G. Bongard-Levin, Moscow, 1963, pp. 305–28.
47. Ibid., p. 324.
48. Bhagwat Sinh Jee, *A Short History of Aryan Medical Science*, London, 1896, p. 180; A.M. Kunte, *Astāṅgahrdaya: A Compendium of the Ayurvedic System Composed by Vāgbhata with the Commentaries (Sarvāngasundarā) of Arunadatta and (Āyurvedarasāyana) of Hemādri*, Bombay, 1902, pp. 1–15.
49. Dominik Wujastyk, 'Interpreting the Image of the Human Body in Pre-modern India', *International Journal of Hindu Studies*, vol. 13, no. 2, 2009, pp. 1–41.
50. Philipp A. Maas, 'The Concepts of the Human Body and Disease in Classical Yoga and Āyurveda', *Vienna Journal of South Asian Studies*, vol. 51, 2007–8, pp. 125–62.
51. Ibid., pp. 142–3.
52. Mira Roy, 'Anatomy in the Vedic Literature', *Indian Journal of History of Science*, vol. 2, no. 1, 1967, pp. 35–46.
53. P.V. Sharma, *Indian Medicine in the Classical Age*, Varanasi, 2000, p. 7.
54. T.A Wise, *Commentary on the Hindu System of Medicine*, London, 1860; Praphulla Chandra Ray, *A History of Hindu Chemistry. From the Earliest Time to the Middle of the Sixteenth Century AD*, Calcutta, 1903; Girindranath Mukhopadhyaya, *History of Indian Medicine: From the Earliest Ages to the Present Time*, vols. I–II, Calcutta, 1923; Chandra Chakraberty, *An Interpretation of Ancient Hindu Medicine*, Calcutta: Ramchandra Chakraberty, 1923; Meulenbeld, *A History of Indian Medical Literature*, vols. IA, IB, IIA, IIB, III, Groningen: Egbert Forsten, 1999–2002; Julius Jolly, *Indian Medicine*, tr. C.G. Kashikar, New Delhi, 1977; Jean Filliozat, *The Classical Doctrine of Indian Medicine: Its Origins and its Greek Parallels*, tr. Dev Raj Chanana, New Delhi, 1964; S.N. Dasgupta, *A History of Indian Philosophy*, vol. II, Delhi, 1991; Kenneth G. Zysk, *Asceticism and Healing in Ancient India: Medicine in the Buddhist Monastery*, Delhi, 2000; A.F.R. Hoernle, *Studies in the Medicine of Ancient India*, New Delhi, 1994; Guy Mazars, *A Concise Introduction to Indian Medicine*, tr. T.K. Gopalan, Delhi, 2006.

55. Kenneth G. Zysk, *Medicine in the Veda: Religious Healing in the Veda*, Delhi, 1998, p. 70.
56. Kenneth G. Zysk, 'Does Ancient Indian Medicine have a Theory of Contagion?', in *Contagion: Perspectives from Pre-Modern Societies*, ed. Lawrence I. Conrad and Dominik Wujastyk, London, 2000, pp. 78–95.
57. Francis Zimmermann, 'Terminological Problems in the Process of Editing and Translating Sanskrit Medical Texts', *Approaches to Traditional Chinese Literature*, ed. Paul U. Unschuld, Dordrecht, Boston and London: Kluwer Academic Publishers, 1989, pp. 141–51, see p. 149.
58. Gananath Sen, *Āyurveda Parichay* (Introduction to the Āyurveda), Calcutta, 1943; Brajendranath Seal, *The Positive Sciences of the Ancient Hindus*, Kolkata, 2001, pp. 157–61.
59. Meulenbeld, 'The Many Faces of Āyurveda', *Journal of European Āyurvedic Society*, vol. 4, 1995, pp. 1–10.
60. Meulenbeld, *The Madhavanidāna*, Delhi, 2008, p. 29 (1.3).
61. Meulenbeld, 'Some Neglected Aspects of Āyurveda or The Illusion of a Consistent Theory', *Traditional South Asian Medicine*, vol. 8, 2008, pp. 16–31.
62. Dagmar Benner, '*Samskāras* in Vagbhata's *Astāṅgahrdayasamhitā*: *Garbhādhāna, Rtusamgamana, Pumsavana*', in *Mathematics and Medicine in Sanskrit*, ed. Dominik Wujastyk, Delhi, 2009, pp. 119–38.
63. Peter Breton, *A Vocabulary of the Names of the Various Parts of the Human Body and of Medical and Technical terms in English, Arabic, Persian, Hindeee and Sanscrit for the use of The Members of the Medical Departments in India*, Calcutta, 1825, p. 1.
64. *The Calcutta Monthly Journal and General Register of Occurrences Throughout the British Dominions in the East Forming an Epitome of the Indian Press: For the Year 1836, Third Series*, vol. II, pp. 1–7.
65. Ibid.
66. Ibid.
67. John Fleming, *A Catalogue of Indian Medicinal Plants and Drugs, with Their Names in the Hindoostani and Sanskrit Language*. This book was reproduced in *Asiatic Researches or Transactions of the Society Instituted in Bengal, for inquiring into the History and Antiquities, the Arts, Sciences, and Literature, of Asia*, vol. 11, Calcutta: Cutnell, Walker, Lea, Lackington and Allen, 1812, pp. 153–96. Page number is given according to the *Asiatic Researches*.
68. Ibid., p. 160.
69. Meulenbeld, *The Mādavanidāna*, pp. 612–13. Also see P.V. Sharma, *Essentials of Āyurveda*, New Delhi: Motilal Banarsidass, 1998, pp. iii–v.
70. Gananth Sen, *Hindu Medicine: An Address on Āyurveda Delivered at the Foundation Ceremony of Benaras Hindu University*, Calcutta: Kalpatru Press, 1937, p. 15.

16

Orchid Germplasm

Its Historical Perspectives, Medicinal Importance and Possible Conservation Strategies

Nirmalya Banerjee &
Madhumita Majumdar

Orchids are one of the most diverse and widespread families of flowering plants and are also one of the few plant families that have a profile which can benefit plant conservation on a broad scale. Known for long as flower of distinction, orchids have an undeniable charm. The immense floral variations found in more than 25,000 species and 1,20,000 registered hybrids, along with their long shelf lives or longevity, make orchids one of the most important floriculture crops. The economic importance of orchids lie mainly in their ornamental value and horticultural uses. They provide cut blooms which remain fresh for long, make pretty corsages and add to the variety of floral arrangements. Many of our native species have been used for long in Europe and USA as progenitors for the production of some of the famous hybrids. There is a preference for hybrids in commercial markets. Besides ornamental beauty, a large number of orchid taxa have also proved beneficial for their traditional therapeutic uses. Several orchidaceous phytoconstituents like alkaloids, flavonoids, terpenes, carbohydrates and glycosides are employed for a variety of therapeutic uses in different systems of traditional medicine. Many species face daily threats to their survival, including habitat loss and unsustainable exploitation. Incidentally, conservation of therapeutically important orchids and their large scale cultivation using modern techniques such as tissue culture have become inevitable to meet the increasing demands of the drug industry. There is also an urgent need for building up more germplasm banks in various climatic conditions through large-scale multiplication using various conventional techniques. A number of internationally reputed plant conservation groups and organizations have a crucial role to play in countering the trend of biodiversity loss by promoting effective orchid conservation techniques, improving networking and technology transfer and educating the orchid community.

Introduction

The word orchid brings to one's mind some vision of distinctive or incredible form of flower with colour, beauty and fragrance. The family orchidaceae is among the most advanced ones of the flowering plants which are highly specialized in many ways. This is probably the largest family among all angiosperms, with an estimated 25,000 species. Orchids are well known for the great diversity displayed in their life forms and growth habits, in the contrivances of pollination and ecological adaptabilities. As a unique plant group, they are botanically quite interesting for their floral complexities, free gene flow across the specific barriers, minute seeds with undifferentiated embryos, suppressed endosperm formation, long-lived pollen tubes and dependence on a suitable mycorrhizal association for germination. They have a worldwide distribution occurring in various ecological habitats such as saprophytes, terrestrials or epiphytes, due to its geographical position, embracing so many degrees of latitude and the land often rising from sea level to heights beyond the limits of vegetation.[1] India also harbours a varied flora comprising both temperate and tropical species. According to Atwood, more than 70 per cent of orchid species are epiphytic that mostly inhabit the tropics.[2] In India alone, about 1,100 species have been found that are distributed in 163 genera. Among them, more than 300 species are endemic.[3] The major orchid-rich phytogeographical regions of India are peninsular India, north-eastern India and the eastern and western Himalayas.

Due to their attractive flowers, orchids comprise of a major group of horticultural crops. Their unmatched ornamental value accounts for multimillion dollar cut-flower industries in several countries. They are also important indicators of environmental degradation because of their habitat specificity. The essence of vanilla, which is obtained from the seed capsule of the climbing orchid *Vanilla planifolia* is also well known.

History of Medicinal Orchids

Notwithstanding their ornamental value, orchids are well known for their medicinal usage especially in the traditional folk medicine. The medicinal use of orchids was first reported by the Chinese scientists[4] (Bulpitt 2005). The Chinese pharmacopoeia 'Sang Nung Pen Tsao Ching', illustrated *Dendrobium* as a source of tonic, astringent, analgesic and anti-inflammatory compounds which is known as far back as 200 BC and since the Vedic period in India. Acharya Charak, crowned as the Father of Indian medicine, brought Indian orchids to the notice of the world as early as AD 100. He had described the medicinal qualities and functions of 1,00,000 herbal plants and had specially emphasized on the influence of diet and its activity on mind and body. Orchids are the major source of important secondary metabolites like dendrobine, nobiline, and erianin. Several medicinally important orchids have therapeutic potential as antioxidant, antiangiogenic and antitumour agent.

'Ashtavarga' is a group of 8 drugs in the Ayurvedic system which are used for the preparation of tonic, such as 'Chyavanprash', which consists of four orchid species, viz., *Malaxis muscifera, Malaxis acuminate, Habenaria intermedia* and *Habenaria edgeworthi.*

The use of orchids in herbal medicines has a very long history. There is not a single ailment for which therapeutic and curative elements are not found in one or the other orchid species. It is also reported that orchids held a great repute as a medicine with strengthening and demulcent qualities. Orchids are used in traditional medicine as they are rich in active compounds including several alkaloids.[5] Dried pseudo-bulbs of *Malaxis acuminate* serve as important source of Ashtavarga utilized in the preparation of the Ayurvedic tonic, which has most promoting effect on human health and preventing disease.[6] The rich orchid diversity has provided an initial advantage to its inhabitants for observing and scrutinizing the orchid flora for developing their own traditional knowledge for importance of valuable orchid diversity and their conservation [Plates 16.1(A–F)]:

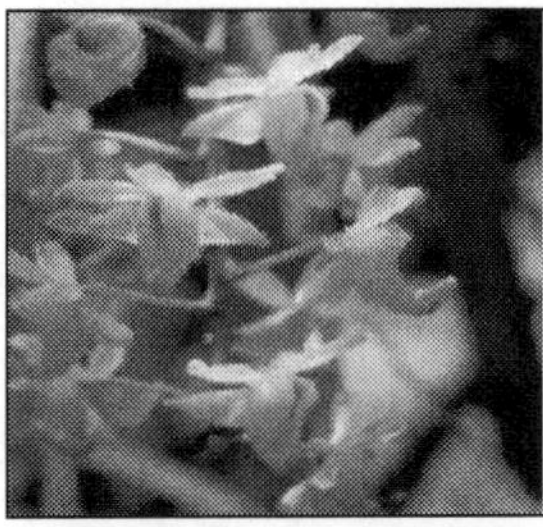

Plate 16.1(A): *Aerides*

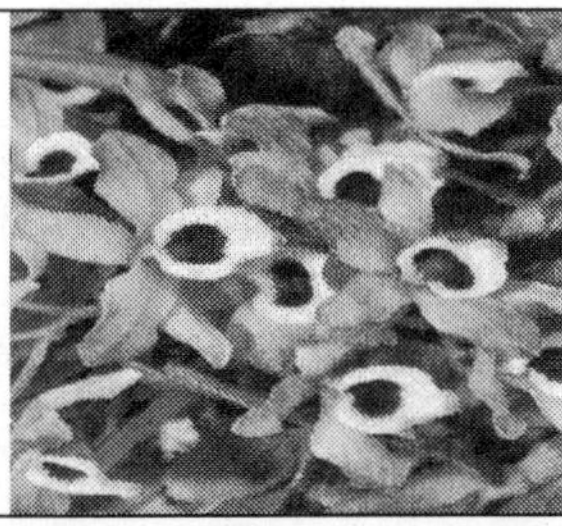

Plate 16.1(B): *Dendrobium*

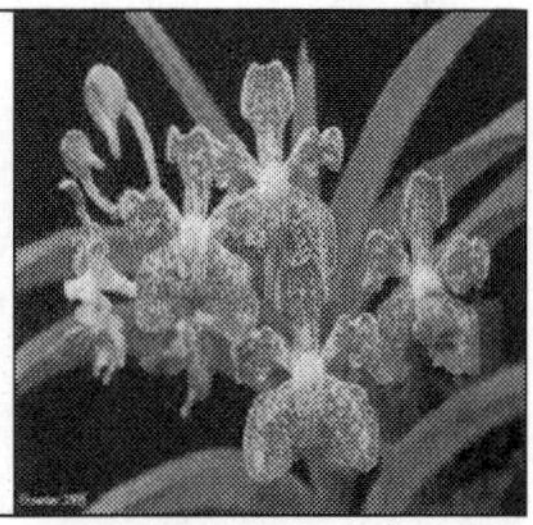

Plate 16.1(C): *Vanda*

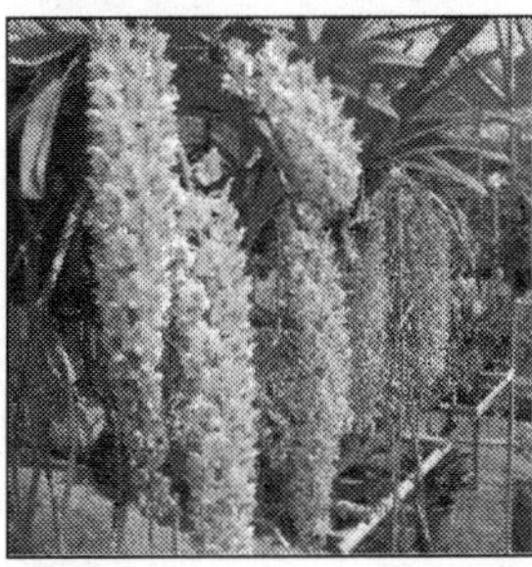

Plate 16.1(D): *Rhyncostylis*

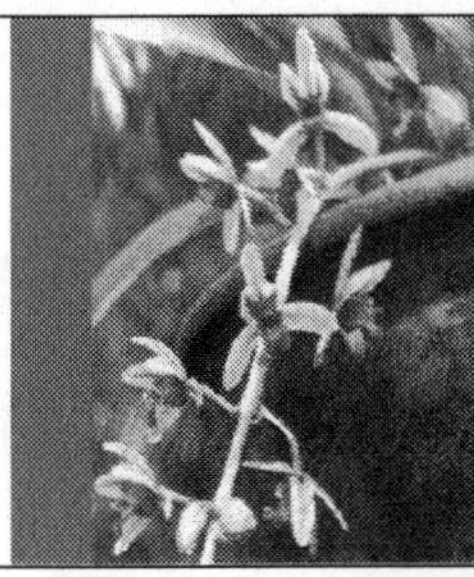

Plate 16.1(E): *Cymbidium*

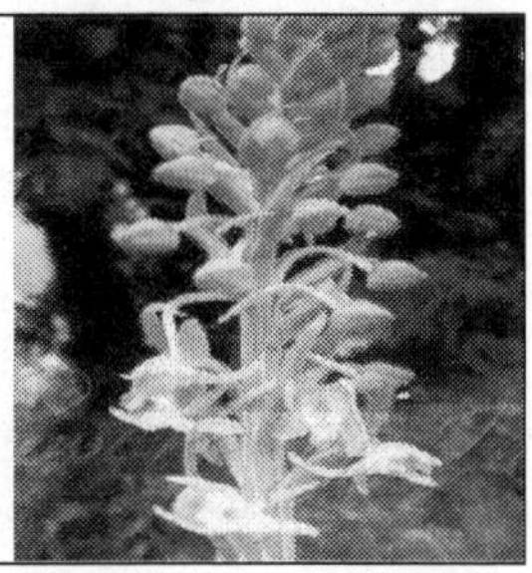

Plate 16.1(F): *Habenaria*

Plates 16.1(A–F): Photograph of Some Medicinally Important Orchids

Phytochemicals Present in Orchids

Alkaloids

A large number of alkaloids have been reported from the family Orchidaceae.[7] Liining screened about 525 orchid species for their alkaloid contents. As many as 77 of these contained more than 0.01 per cent and another 21 more than 0.1 per cent of alkaloid concentration. Most of the orchid alkaloids are either pyrrlizidine or dendrobine derivatives, whereas the remaining exhibit mainly unrelated structure. Significantly, a large number of alkaloids are met within the genus *Dendrobium* which contains many alkaloid-rich species. Beside dendrobine, nobiline is isolated from *D. nobile* and *D. gracile*. Another Chinese drug, known as 'Chukanso' was derived from *D. lohohense*, where an alkaloid shihunine was isolated. Several alkaloids like denramine, dendroxine, 6-hydroxydendroxine, hygrine, phalaenopsin, malaxin, cholin are widespread in the several orchidaceous members.

Flavonoids and Related Phytoconstituents

The orchid-leaf flavonoids have been studied by Williams and Jorapur.[8] Anthocyanins which range from yellow to red and magenta in colour play a major role in orchid flower pigmentation. Three predominant anthocyanins are cyanidine, pelargonidine and petunidine. For their chemical complexity, structural variability, physiological stability, comparative ease of isolation and identification, serve as good chemotaxonomic characters.

Fragrance

The leaves and rhizomes of *Spiranthes michuacana* and flowers of *Dendrobium farmeri* are fragrant and are known to maintain their fragrance for a long time. Gas chromatographic analysis showed that flower fragrance contains methyl benzonate, β-caryophylene, and α-tepinene as main essence materials. The other most prominent fragrances in orchids include α-β-pinene, 1,8-cinacol, methyl benzoate, benzyl acetate, citronellol and eugenol.

Carbohydrates and Glycosides

Polysaccharides and oligosaccharides have been reported from various orchids.[9] The pseudobulbs of *Microstylis wallichii*, an Indian drug used in 'Ashtavarga', contains sugar besides basic compounds.[10] The well known orchid glucosides are loroglossin, cis- and trans-erassinodin isolated from many orchid species. The latter one is isolated from *Dendrobium crassinode.* Some therapeutically important orchid species used as medicine by the people are mentioned in Table 16.1.

Conservation Strategies of Orchid Germplasm

Despite their many-fold utilities, commercial cultivation of orchids was considered highly difficult, due to the lack of knowledge on orchid seed germination as well as their slow rate of vegetative propagation. Therefore, to meet the commercial demand for the orchids, illegal collection of the plants from their natural habitats became a common practice among many orchid traders. As a result, a large number of orchids have become rare, threatened or endangered in their natural habitat either as indirect or direct effect of human activities.[11]

Table 16.1: Some Therapeutically Important Orchids Used in Medicine

Name of plant	*Habitat*	*Plant parts used*	*Therapeutic uses*
Aerides odorata	Epiphytic	Tb*	Sources of important phytochemical 'Aeridin'.
Acampe carinata	Epiphyte	Rt*	Used in acute rheumatism, sciatica and also beneficial for uterine disease.
Bletia purpurea	Epiphyte	Cm*	As tonic and antidote to fish poisoning.
Cymbidium aloifolium	Epiphyte	Tb*	Used to reduce paralysis.
Dendrobium nobile	Epiphyte	Tb*	Important source of alkaloid dendrobine which is used in the treatment of pulmonary tuberculosis, general debility, night sweats and anorexia.
D. macraei	Epiphyte	Lv*	Herb juice used to cure redness of eyes, increase strength, vigour and vitality.
D. alpestre	Epiphyte	bulb	For treating pimples, boils and other skin eruptions.
Dactylorhiza hatagirea	Terrestrial	Rt*	Used as tonic and also aphrodisiac.
Habenaria intermedia	Terrestrial	Tb*	Used as general tonic.
H. acuminata	Terrestrial	Tb*	As tonic.
Malaxis muscifera	Terrestrial	Pseudo-bulb	Used in bleeding, burning, sensation and fever.
M. acuminata	Terrestrial	Pseudo-bulb	Dried bulbs serve as important sources of Astavarga utilized in the preparation of the Ayurvedic tonic 'Chyavanprash'.
Grammatophyllum speciosum	Terrestrial	Tb*	Used in Thailand to prepare an herbal elixir against inflammation.
Orchid latifolia	Epiphyte	Rt*	As tonic and expectorant.
Polystachya concreta	Epiphyte	Tb*	Used in arthritis and rheumatism.
Rhyncostylis retusa	Epiphyte	Lv*	Leaf juice used to cure rheumatic disease.
Spiranthes divretica	Epiphyte	Rt*	As diuretic.
Vanda criststa	Epiphyte	Lv*	As expectorant.

*Tb—Tuber, Rt—Root, Lv—Leaves, Cm—Cambiu

Direct threat to plant survival includes climate change, pollution, habitat loss through clearing and fragmentation of natural habitat for urban development, shifting cultivation and various natural calamities. Moreover, for orchid, a critical factor undoubtedly is the decrease or loss of the fungi, required for seedling development and other life-history stages.[12] Therefore, it has become an immediate need to take appropriate measures to conserve such precious orchid germplasm.

Biological conservation aims at maintaining the diversity of living organisms, their habitats and the interrelationships between organisms and their environment.[13] According to International Union for Conservation of Nature (IUCN) red list of threatened plants, 1,779 species of orchid are reported to be threatened with extinction. The main purpose of the IUCN red list is to catalogue and highlight those taxa that are facing a higher risk of global extinction[14] (i.e. those listed as critically endangered, and vulnerable). Such categorization is based on biological factors related to extinction risk and includes rate of decline, population size and area of geographic distribution. In India, out of 1,100 species, 215 species have been declared as endangered and 14 nearly extinct, which comprise more than 20 per cent of the total orchid flora.[15] There are two conventional approaches for conservation of plant genetic resources, viz., in situ and ex situ conservation.

In situ conservation, the most efficient way to conserve orchids, is to ensure that they continue to exist as an integral part of the intact ecosystem. Efficient management of natural habitat like formation of sanctuaries and national parks are some of the most important objectives of in situ conservation. Implementation of the Convention on International Trade in Endangered Species of Wild Fauna and Flora (CITES) regulation is also an important tool for the conservation of threatened taxa in situ.

Ex situ conservation is primarily aimed at creation and maintenance of germplasm pool outside the natural habitat. Two major approaches to create germplasm pools is the development of orchidorium and seed bank. Ex situ techniques can be used to complement in situ methods and in some instances, may be the only option for some species.[16]

In many cases, in vitro technologies are used as alternative strategies for conservation where safety measures of the living collections are ensured. There are three basic approaches of in vitro conservations, which are described as follows:

In Vitro Propagation

Apart from the difficulties of seed germination, vegetative propagation of orchids is an extremely slow process. Therefore, mass scale production of orchids depends heavily on different in vitro methods. Such methodologies could be effectively used for conservation purposes in both direct and indirect ways. In vitro raised seedlings could be used for supplementing natural orchid population which has been reduced to a critical size, and thereby is a way of preventing inbreeding depression amongst such populations. Both in vitro seed culture and different clonal propagation methods could be used for commercial production of economically important species, which has an indirect role in preventing collection of wild plants. All possible pathways for plantlet regeneration through in vitro technique occur in two primary ways [Plates 16.2(A) and 16.2(B)].

Methods

According to Debergh and Maene: which are commercial micropropagation involves five stages:

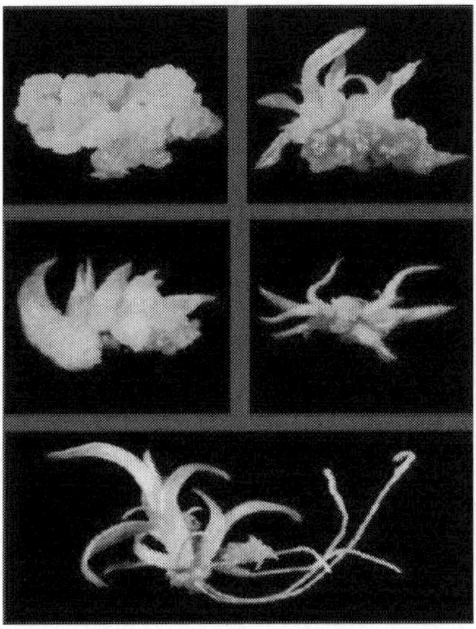

Plate 16.2(A): In vitro propagation from shoot-tips through direct and callus-mediated pathway

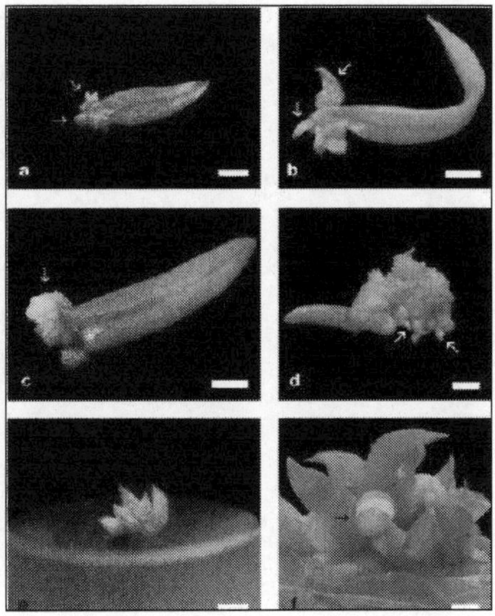

Plate 16.2(B): In vitro propagation from leaf explants

- Direct plant regeneration through shoot tip culture and meristem culture.
- Indirect plant regeneration via callus mediated organogenesis and somatic embryogenesis

Stage	0	Preparative stage.
Stage	I	Initiation and establishment of aseptic culture.
Stage	II	Proliferation of shoots and shoot buds (axillary and adventitious buds).
Stage	III	Rooting of in vitro formed shoots.
Stage	IV	Acclimatization of plants and field transfer.[17]

In Vitro Storage

In vitro storage in reduced or minimal growth condition and using growth inhibitors is highly useful as a means for medium-term conservation of plant germplasm. Both these methods could be carried out either using agar medium or through the employment of gel-encapsulation techniques [Plates 16.3(A) and 16.3(B)]. Slow growth or reduced growth procedures allow plant materials to be stored for 1–15 years under tissue culture condition with periodic subculturing, depending on species.[18] In vitro conservation requires preservation of genetic information, maintenance of maximal survival rate and the reduction of subculturing frequency. Increasing the subculture period to every 6 or 12 months saves money and reduces the contamination rate and also the accidental substitution of genotypes.[19] This approach of in vitro storage is useful primarily because it could be utilized to maintain the valuable germplasm in in vitro condition. This approach also could be efficiently implemented in

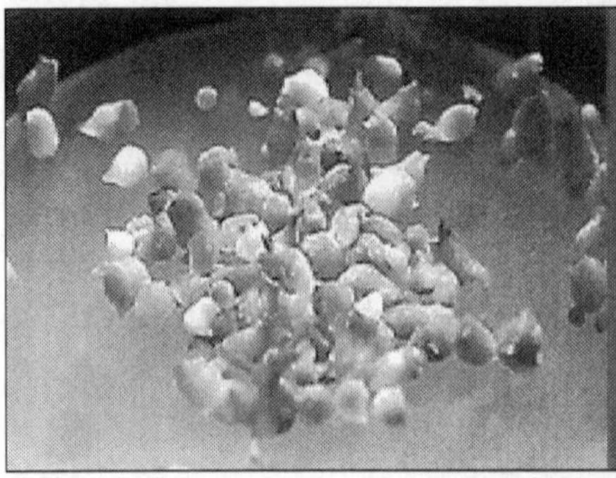

Plate 16.3(A): Conservation in agar medium

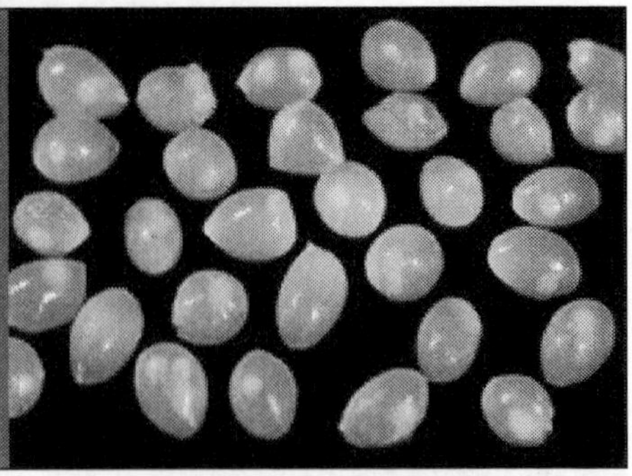

Plate 16.3(B): Conservation through alginate-encapsulation (artificial seed technology)

the industrial arena, so that whenever required, the seedlings stored at reduced growth condition could be transferred to suitable regrowth media and plantlets could be generated as per the requirement within a short duration. Although there are several reports on in vitro storage of several crops and several fruit-yielding plants, reduced growth maintainance for orchids has been reported by only few workers.[20]

Cryopreservation

Seeds, shoot meristems, protocorms and protocorm-like bodies could be stored in liquid nitrogen at –196° C under in vitro condition. During this storage period, all the metabolic processes of the cells and tissues are completely arrested and seed aging is also completely inhibited. Cryopreservation can be used for storing of tissues for unlimited period. Several successesful attempts have been made to cryopreserve the cells and tissues of orchids and at present about 20 species of orchid appear as promising for germplasm storage.

Conclusion

Substantial information is available about the folklore therapeutic uses and phytoconstituents of orchids, but biological evaluation of these plants or of their derived products has not been systematically undertaken so far. Thus, this particular area of research on orchids requires more in depth attention so that the drugs and phytochemicals may be suitably utilized on the basis of modern scientific evaluation. Traditional knowledge has been used for centuries by indigenous and local communities and plays a vital role in the area of medicinal treatment. India is expected to boost the production of traditional drugs from the well represented medicinally important orchids. Today, the local as well as tribal populations of north-eastern region of India use many orchids as folk medicines and many diseases are cured as orchids are rich in alkaloids, flavonoids, glycosides, carbohydrates and other photochemical which have great importance in medicinal fields. People have gathered a great deal of knowledge regarding the use of plants and plant products in curing various ailments which, in turn, enriches the wealth of traditional knowledge of the local people on orchid diversity and herbal healthcare. Conservation of wild orchids is now a matter of universal concern. However, there is an urgent need to protect the valuable orchid species in their natural habitat as orchids are very sensitive to ecological disturbances. Incidentally, conservation of therapeutically important orchids and their cultivation on a large scale using modern techniques such as tissue culture are absolutely essential to meet the increasing demands of the drug industry, otherwise through their excessive use in the manufacture of traditional drugs, such orchids may get depleted.

Notes

1. J.T. Atwood, 'The Size of the Orchidaceae and the Systematic Distribution of Epiphytic Orchids', *Selbyana*, vol. 7, 1986, pp. 171–86; J.V. Freudenstein and F.N. Rasmussen, 'What does Morphology Tell us about Orchid Relationship?: A Cladistic Analysis', *American Journal of Botany*, vol. 86, no. 2, 1999, pp. 225–48.
2. J.T. Atwood, op. cit.
3. S.N. Hegde, 'Orchid Wealth of India', *Arunachal Forest News*, vol. 14, 1996, pp. 6–19.
4. C.J. Bulpit, 'The Uses and Misuses of Orchids in Medicine', *QJM: An International Journal of Medicine*, vol. 98, issue 9, 4 September 2005, pp. 625–31.
5. M. Elander, K. Leander, J. Rosenbloom and E. Ruusa, 'Studies on Orchidaceae Alkaloids', in *Crepidine, crepidamine and dendrocrpine from Dendrobium crepidatum Lindl. Acta Chemical Scandinevica*, vol. 27, 1973, pp. 1907–13; L.J. Lawler and M.L. Slytor, 'The Distribution of Alkaloids in New South Wales and Queensland Orchidaceae', *Phytochemistry*, vol. 8, issue 10, October 1969, pp. 1959–62.
6. M.R. Uniyal, 'Astavarga Sandigdha Vanaushadhi', *Dhanwantri Partrika*, Aligarh, India: Sri Jwala Ayurved Bhawan, 1975; R. Govindarajan, D.P. Singh and A.K.S. Rawat, 'High-performance Liquid Chromatographic Method for the Quantification of Phenolics', in 'Chyavanprash' a potent Ayurvedic drug, *Journal of Pharmaceutical and Biomedical Analysis*, vol. 43, issue 2, 17 January 2007, pp. 527–32.
7. B. Liining, 'Studies of Orchidaceae for Alkaloids I: Screening of Species of Alkaloids', vol. 18, 1964, pp. 1507–16.
8. C.A. Williams, 'The Leaf Flavonoids of the Orchidaceae, Phytochemistry', *Photochemistry*, vol. 18, issue 5, 1979, pp. 803–13; S.M. Jorapur, 'Flavonoids in Relation to Chemotaxonomy of Orchidaceae from Western Ghats (India)', Paper presented at the Nationl Seminar on the Biology, Conservation and Culture of Orchids, Chandigarh, 1997; S.M. Jorapur, 'Flavonoids in Relation to Chemotaxonomy of Orchidaceae from Western Ghats (India)', Paper presented at the Nationl Seminar on the Biology, Conservation and Culture of Orchids, Chandigarh, 1997.
9. D. Mahmoud, P. Fahrettin and E. Jean, 'Polysaccharides of Orchids', *Bull. Soc. Chim. Biol*, vol. 45, 1963, pp. 1247–54; H. David, Harold A. Swenson and Steldom F. Kurenth, 'Configuration and Hydrodynamic Properties of Fully Acetylated Salep Glucomannes', *Journal of Polymer Science, Part A-2: Polymer Physics*, vol. 5, issue 2, March 1967, pp. 361–75; R. Ernst, J. Arditti and P.L. Healey, 'Biological Effects of Surfactants. I. Influence on the Growth of Orchid Seedlings', *New Phytologis.*, vol. 70, issue 3, May 1971, pp. 457–75.
10. J.K. Bhatnagar, S.S. Handa and S.C. Duggal, 'Chemical Investigations on Microstylis Wallichii', *Planta Medica*, vol. 20, 1971, pp. 156–61.

11. A.L. Batty, K.W. Dixon, M.C. Brundrett and K. Sivasithamparam, 'Orchid Conservation and Mycorrhizal Associations, Chapter 7', in *Microorganisms in Plant Conservation and Biodiversity*, ed. K. Sivasithamparam, K.W. Dixon and R.L. Barrett, Kluwer Academic Publishers, 2002, pp. 195–226.
12. D.F. Whigham, J.P. O'Neilla, H.N. Rasmussen, B.A. Caldwell and M.K. McCormick, 'Seed Longevity in Terrestrial Orchids: Potential for Persistent in situ seed Banks', *Biological Conservation*, vol. 129, issue 1, 2006, pp. 24–30.
13. I.F. Spellerberg and S.R. Hardes, *Biological Conservation*, New Delhi: Cambridge University Press, 1992.
14. K.S. Walter and H.J. Gillett, eds., '1997 IUCN Red List of Threatened Plants', World Conservation Monitoring Centre, IUCN—The World Conservation Union, Gland, Switzerland and Cambridge, UK, 1998.
15. Hegde, op. cit., p. 15; T. Okamoto, M. Natsume and T. Onaka, 'The Structure of Dendroxine', *Chem. Pharm. Bull*, vol. 14, 1966, pp. 672–5.
16. V. Sarasan, R. Cripps, M.M. Ramsay, C. Atherton, M. McMichen, G. Prendergast and J.K. Rowntree, 'Conservation in vitro of Threatened Plants Progress in the Past Decade', in *Vitro Cellular & Developmental Biology Plant*, vol. 42, 2006, pp. 206–14.
17. P.C. Debergh and L.J. Maene, 'A Scheme for Commercial Propagation of Ornamental Plants by Tissue Culture', *Scientia Horticulture*, vol. 14, issue 4, April 1981, pp. 335–45.
18. N.K. Rao, 'Plant Genetic Resources: Advancing Conservation and Use through Biotechnology', *African Journal of Biotechnology*, vol. 3, no. 2, 2004, pp. 136–45.
19. L.A. Withers, '*In vitro* Conservation and Germplasm Utilization', in *Use of Plant Genetic Resources*, ed. A.D.H. Brown, O.H. Frankel, D.R. Marschall and J.T. Williams, Cambridge: Cambridge University Press, 1989, pp. 309–34; A. Bertrand-Desbrunais, M. Noirot and A. Charrier, 'Minimal Growth *in vitro* Conservation of Coffee (*Coffea spp*.), *Plant Cell*, vol. 27, issue 3, December 1991, pp. 333–9.
20. D.C. Agrawal, G.C. Morwal and A.F. Mascarenhas, '*In vitro* propagation and slow growth storage of shoot cultures of Vanilla walkeriae wight-an endangered orchid', *Lindleyana*, vol. 7, no. 2, 1992, pp. 95–9; F. Kishi and K. Takagi, 'Efficient Method for the Preservation and Regeneration of Orchid Protocorm-like Bodies', *Scientia Horticulture*, vol. 68, October 1997, pp. 149–56; M. Divakaran, K.N. Babu and K.V. Peter, 'Conservation of *Vanilla* Species', *in vitro*. *Sci Hort*, vol. 110, 2006, pp. 175–80; K.P. Martin and A.K. Pradeep, 'Simple Strategy for the in vitro Conservation of *Ipsea Malabarica* an Endemic and Endangered Orchid of the Western Ghats of Kerala', *India Plant Cell, Tissue and Organ Culture*, vol. 74, issue 2, 2003, pp. 197–200.

17

Tribal Medicine

Traditional Therapeutic Uses of Plants among the Tribes of Birbhum District, West Bengal

HABIBUR RAHAMAN

SINCE THE DAWN of the civilization, man is dependent upon plants, primarily for its food, shelter and health care. From the history of mankind it is observed that plants are closely related with the life of human beings and have been playing a very important role in shaping the human society since its primordial stage. The branch of plant science which deals with the scientific study of the relationship between man and plant is known as ethnobotany. This term was first coined by Harshberger in 1895. Ethnobotany can be defined as the total natural and traditional relationship and the interactions between men, domesticated animals and their surrounding plant wealth. Ethnobotany, a multidisciplinary subject, deals with the studies among the tribal and rural people for recording their unique knowledge about plant wealth and for search of new resources of herbal drugs, edible plants and other aspects of plants (Mudgal and Jain 1983). Ethnomedicine is the interdisciplinary subject of ethnobotany which involves the study of plant uses as crude drug by various ethnic communities including tribal people for curing different diseases and ailments. So tribal medicine is a part of the discipline ethnomedicine which includes the systems of medicine of various tribal communities in the world. Like other global indigenous systems of medicine (Chinese, Egyptian, Tibetan, Ayurveda, Unani, etc.), tribal medicine is also an age-old therapeutic system which is traditionally practised among different tribal communities for their primary health care needs worldwide. It is a traditional knowledge of preserving health through the practise of using medicinal plants and magical incantations. This tribal knowledge of medicine has been established as a system through trial and error method over time and it has a history of oral transmission. For this, global awareness is created among the scientists and academicians to document and conserve this traditional herbal knowledge before it is going to be lost due to cultural erosion of tribal society. Like other traditional systems of medicine, tribal medicine is also considered as an alternative one because it is cost effective—not so expensive like modern medicine, easily available to all, safe and natural and have no or negligible side effect, and moreover culturally acceptable to the people.

About 80 per cent of the population of developing countries rely on traditional herbal medicine for their primary health care. Traditional medicine systems of different countries in the world are doing wonderfully in the field of health care of common people. The Chinese herbal system—oldest system in the world—includes nearly 5,700 plant species which are traditionally used in treating the diseases and ailments since 6,000 years. Some other noteworthy traditional systems in the world are Japanese, Tibetan (Amchi), Indonesian, Malayasian, Thai, Indian, etc. Among the Indian traditional systems of medicine, Ayurveda is the oldest one, which originated in the ancient period nearly 4,500 years ago, contributing a great role in Indian health care service. Similarly, the other systems like Siddha (originated in ancient period), Unani (introduced into India in medieval period) and Yoga and Naturopathy (originated in ancient period) have also significantly contributed to the health care of Indian people. From an old estimate published in a report of Indian System of Medicine, Ministry of Health and Family Welfare, New Delhi (Satyavati 1990), it is found that a substantial number of traditional practitioners, dispensaries, hospitals, graduate and postgraduate training colleges and institutes of Ayurveda, Siddha and Unani are working in the health sector of our country (Satyavati 1990) (Table 17.1). Like other countries of the world, in India too these traditional systems are being popularized as an alternative system of medicine which is reflected in a database of registered medical practitioners and licensed pharmacies of Ayurveda, Siddha and Unani that was published in a report of Department of AYUSH, New Delhi (Natesh 2001) (Table 17.2). It is interesting to note that the Department of AYUSH, Ministry of Health and Family Welfare, New Delhi did not include ethnomedicine or tribal medicine in their list of Indian Systems of Medicine. But the traditional knowledge related to folklore or ethnomedicine available in public domain is being documented by creating the Traditional Knowledge Digital Library (TKDL) by the Department of Indian Systems of Medicine and Homoeopathy and National Institute of Science Communication, Government of India (Mukherjee 2004).

The systematic study on tribal medicine in India had been initiated by P.O. Bodding. Bodding carried out an extensive monographic work on Santhal medicine and connected folklore and published it in two volumes (1925 and 1927).This is the first organized documented work in the field of tribal medicine in India. Later on, Bressers (1951) did a great job in this area of traditional medicine and documented it in the form of a book which contains the valuable information on ethnomedicine of various ethnic groups of Ranchi district of then Bihar state. Recently a detailed scientific study on tribal medicine

Table 17.1: Number of Hospitals/Dispensaries/Teaching Institutes in Traditional Systems of Medicine in India

	Ayurveda	*Unani*	*Siddha*
Traditional practitioners	2,510,71	28,382	11,532
Dispensaries	12,111	867	316
Hospitals	1,460	100	105
Graduate training colleges	97	18	1
Postgraduate training institutes/Department	23	2	1
Approximate annual out-tern of the Institutes	2,400	210	35

Source: Indian Systems of Medicine, Ministry of Health and Family Welfare, New Delhi, April 1984.

of four major ethnic groups of India (Lodha, Munda, Oraon and Santhal) has been done by two eminent ethnobotanists of India—Dr S.K. Jain and Dr D.C. Pal—documenting 2,000 prescriptions of tribal medicine including introductory notes on basic characteristic features of tribal medicine, its pharmacology, tribal concept of disease diagnosis, treatment, magico-religious belief, taboos, etc. (Pal and Jain 1998). Another gigantic database on tribal medicine or ethnomedicine of 550 ethnic communities all over India has been developed in recent time with financial assistance from Ministry of Environment and Forests, New Delhi which embodies the data of 1,75,000 drug preparations made from about 7,500 plant species (Anonymous 1998). Subsequently, a large volume of research works in the field of ethnomedicine as well as ethnobotany has been published in the form of books or research articles from different geographical areas of India. Among them, some of the works are on specific ethnic or tribal groups of the particular geographical areas of our country

Table 17.2: Number of Medical Practitioners and Pharmacies in Traditional Systems of Medicine in India

Registered Medical Practitioners	*Total Number*
Ayurveda	427,504
Unani	42,445
Siddha	16,599
LICENSED PHARMACIES	
Ayurveda	8,533
Unani	462
Siddha	385

Source: Department of AYUSH, Ministry of Health and Family Welfare, New Delhi (S. Natesh, 2001).

(Goel et al. 1987; Jain 1965; Jamir 1997; Maheshwari et al. 1981; Varghese, 1996; Varghese and Hembrom 2000). Now there is an utmost need to compile and compare those vast data on ethnomedicine by using statistical and ethnobotanical tools and to make a concise scientific documentation of it for each tribe or ethnic group in India. Through scientific validation of those documented information, the tribal medicine may then be established as a recognized system of Indian medicine.

There is a worldwide resurgence of interest in ethnobotanical as well as ethnomedicinal studies now, to meet the growing needs of agro-industries, herbal drug industries, conservation and development of plant genetic resources. This branch of ethnobotany is now getting more importance in the field of pharmacognosy for its basic information regarding medicinal plants, their various traditional uses, mode of preparation, doses and ways of administration of crude drugs, clinical studies, new drug discovery, etc. In India, organized studies in ethnobotany have been initiated long ago and during the last 50 years, scientific studies have been proceeded on various lines like ethnobotany of certain regions, of specific tribes, of particular plant groups or diseases and on many other miscellaneous sub- or interdisciplinary approaches (Jain 1965, 1981, 1991, 1997; Maheshwari 2000; Mandal 1988; Mandal and Yonzone 1987; Rahaman and Mandal 1998; Rahaman et al. 2007, 2008, 2009; Singh and Pandey 1998; Trivedi and Sharma, 2004; Yonzone and Mandal 1982; Yonzone et al. 1981).

Tribal people believe that diseases and death are caused by certain spirits or supernatural powers. Tribal attitude towards disease diagnosis and treatment is a very typical one. As discussed earlier, according to the philosophy of tribal medicine the diseases in general are of two types. The first type of disease is developed due to physical problem which is cured by crude drugs obtained from locally available plant and animal sources. The next type is developed due to bad effect of certain hostile spirits or supernatural powers that is treated by some magico-religious rituals, magical incantation, charms, amulets, witchcraft, etc. The diseases common among the tribal men, women and children are fever, colic, diarrhoea, dysentery, dyspepsia, hepatic disorder, skin diseases, influenza, pneumonia, etc. The diseases commonly found in the male community are apoplexy, eczema, orchitis, venereal diseases, etc. Females of the tribal groups are generally prone to the diseases like anaemia, menorrhagia, dysmenorrhagia, hysteria, leucorrhoea, etc. Children generally suffer from anaemia, bronchitis, intestinal parasites, measles and mumps, night blindness, rickets and scurvy, dysentery, jaundice, etc. Various studies on food, nutrition, health of the tribal people identified some causes of the diseases. Among them, the main causes are malnutrition, excess liquor consumption, lack of personal hygiene, etc. Erosion of tribal culture is also a supportive cause as in most of the cases it is found that lifestyle of tribal people has totally been changed.

The pharmacology of tribal medicine includes the preparation of drug or medicine, its forms and doses, route of application of medicine, duration of treatment, harvest of the plant parts used and some belief and taboos attached with medicinal plants. Generally preparation of medicine is of two types—monoherbal, a single drug preparation and polyherbal, a compound or multiple drug preparation. Prepared medicine or drugs are administered by the tribals in a variety of forms like infusion, decoction, syrup, paste, powder, pills, extract (water and alcoholic), burning ash, plaster, etc. Doses are prescribed according to the age of the patients; thus, it varies in cases of adult males, females and children. Application of drug or medicine is done through the external and internal routes. Again, duration of treatment varies from disease to disease. It takes 2–3 days in cases of diarrhoea, cold and cough, etc., 5–7 days for fever, dysentery, etc., and it may take 1–3 months for treatment of paralysis, gouts, etc. Belief and taboos attached with medicinal plants and its collection are very unique in tribal pharmacology. Tribal people consider latex (a milky secretion of plant) containing plants to have medicinal value; fresh plant before flowering are more effective than dried one; root parts of plant are more effective than shoots; violation of any taboo makes the medicine ineffective (Pal and Jain 1998).

Number of medicinal plants is steadily being increased in the herbal inventory of ethnomedicine of India through extensive research work in the field of ethnobotany. In India, about 7,500 plant species are used as ethnomedicine by 550 different ethnic communities for curing the diseases and ailments. Many of such ethnomedicinal plants represent a major potential source of crude drugs for management of different diseases and ailments. In India, only a small portion of these ethnomedicinal plants has scientifically been evaluated till date (Anonymous 1998).

A brief discussion on tribal medicine of Birbhum district, West Bengal is as follows. Literature on tribal medicine of the district Birbhum and a long personal experience of this author on the subject (Das and Rahman 2014; Mondal and Rahaman 2012; Rahaman and Pradhan 2011; Rahaman and Saha 2011; Rahaman et al. 2007, 2008, 2009), revealed that the basic characteristics of tribal medicine of the district are, in many aspects, similar with that of tribal medicine of other parts of the state of West Bengal as well as India (Chatterjee et al., 1989; Pal and Jain 1998). Similarities found in some aspects of tribal medicine are—use of some typical herbs for curing some specific diseases and ailments, the tribal concept of disease development and its cure through magico-religious belief, mode of preparation and administration of crude drugs, etc. It is estimated that about 200 plants are used in herbal medicine by the tribal people of the district Birbhum for their primary health care (Rahaman 2011).

Birbhum is one of the smallest districts of West Bengal which is full of natural resources. The district extends over about 4,528.61 sq. km. and is situated between 87°10′ and 88°2′ East longitude and between 23°33′ and 24°35′ North latitude. On the north, the district is bounded by Murshidabad district, on the west by Santhal Parganas (presently Dumka district of Jharkhand) and in the south by Burdwan district. A large number of tribal people migrated from adjoining tribal belt of Santhal Parganas had settled permanently in different areas of the district. The tribal population of the district is 2,03,127 and it is 6.7 per cent of the total population of the district (Census of India 2001). Many tribal communities like Santhal, Kora, Munda, Kherwal, Birhore, etc., are found in the district. Among them, Santhal community dominates the district. The tribal people here are mainly dependent on the forest resources for their subsistence and use plant resources in various ways like in curing the diseases and ailments, for food, fruits, tubers, fibres, shelter, etc. Some of the significant information regarding the ethnomedicinal uses of plants by the Santhal tribe of Birbhum district, West Bengal have been provided here, most of which have not been reported earlier from the district (Das et al. 2009; Ghosh et al. 2011; Mandal 1988; Mondal et al. 1998; Rahaman and Pradhan 2011; Rahaman et al. 2007, 2008, 2009).

Material and Methods

The data regarding the therapeutic uses of the plants by the tribal people of Birbhum district provided in this essay is the outcome of a decade-long scientific observation made by the author during the survey in different tribal pockets of the district. For collection of ethnomedicinal information and its scientific analyses, the standard methods of ethnobotany have been followed (Cotton, 1996; Cunningham 2001; Jain 1987, 1989; Jain and Mudgal 1999; Martin 1995). Regular field trips have been made in various tribal pockets of the district including forest areas in different seasons to collect the information. During the field survey, tribal people and herbal medicine men of the district have thoroughly been interrogated to collect the information regarding their medicinal uses of the plant wealth. To confirm the authenticity of the collected data, they were cross checked by interviewing other persons of the same and different localities. The plant specimens collected during the field survey have thoroughly been examined in the laboratory and identified botanically with the help of different floras (Maheshwari 1963; Manilal and Sivarajan 1982; Panigrahi and Murti 1989; Saldanha and Nicolson 1976; Sanyal 1994; Varma 1981). The collected plant specimens have been preserved as herbarium specimens following the standard method of Jain and Rao 1977 and kept in the Visva-Bharati Herbarium (VBH), Department of Botany, Visva-Bharati, Santiniketan for future references.

Results and Discussion

Altogether 34 medicinal plants have been included here in this discussion which are used as ethnomedicine by the tribal people of Birbhum district, West Bengal. These 34 plants are used in preparation of 34 types of ethnomedicine that cure 26 types of diseases and ailments. Among the 34 ethnomedicinal preparations—five preparations are administered as polyherbal ones (where more than one plant material are involved), 26 preparations are used as monoherbal (only one plant is involved) and remaining three types are used as charm, incantation, etc., which are employed by the tribal people out of their magico-religious belief in curing the diseases and ailments. In polyherbal preparations, plants like *Acacia nilotica, Achyranthes aspera, Hibiscus rosa-sinensis, Ziziphus oenoplia* and *Bombax ceiba* are used in the treatment of leucorrhoea and menstrual problem. In another preparation, *Aristolichia indica* and *Cynodon dactylon* are administered to relieve the stomach ache. *Adhatoda vasica* is used along with *Ocimum sanctum* in preparation of a polyherbal drug for curing cold and cough. The barks of *Shorea robusta* and other plants like *Madhuca indica, Terminalia arjuna, Buchanania lanzan* are used in preparation of a polyherbal tribal drug that is administered in any type of burn. Tribal people of the district treat the skin diseases by using a polyherbal preparation of *Achyranthes aspera* and *Phyllanthus emblica*. The monoherbal preparations are of 26 types where only one plant is used as the ingredient and are administered to cure 22 types of diseases and ailments like fever, skin diseases, dysentery, diarrhoea, constipation, rheumatism, leucoderma, asthma, septic wounds, cholera, etc. Like the tribal people of other parts of the world, there is also a strong magico-religious belief with respect to the development of diseases and its cure among the tribals of Birbhum district. Here, 3 types of magico-religious uses of plants have been recorded which are employed by the tribal people in the district for curing the diseases and ailments. The root and stem of *Achyranthes aspera*, roots of *Tamarindus indica* and *Aegle marmelos* and seeds of *Semecarpus anacardium* are employed in a typical way as charms to cure fever, to facilitate delivery (childbirth) and to save the children from evil eyes respectively.

The 34 recorded plant taxa spread over 33 species, 29 genera and 25 families of dicotyledons and 1 species, 1 genus and 1 family of monocotyledons (Table 17.3). Habitually the investigated plant taxa fall under 4 groups—Trees (22 in number), Shrubs (6 in number), Herbs (3 in number) and Climbers (3 in number), and their respective percentage has been defined (Table 17.4). Considering the individual plant parts used, it is found that roots are used in 11 cases (32.35 per cent), leaves in 11 cases (32.35 per cent), barks in 11 cases (32.35 per cent), stem and others in 3 cases (8.82 per cent), fruits and seeds in 5 cases (14.7 per cent), flowers in 2 cases (5.88 per cent) (Table 17.5). The information have been collected from different herbal medicine men and other knowledgeable persons of the district. Names and addresses of some of the informants are presented here: (1) Name: Manik Hembram,Vill.: Sarpukur, Dist.: Birbhum, West Bengal (Plate 17.33); (2) Name: Madan Baski, Vill.: Khairdanga, Dist.: Birbhum, West Bengal (Plate 17.34); (3) Name: Kali Murmu,

Table 17.3: Percentage composition of different types of plant species and their groups

	Dicot Plants		*Monocot Plants*	
Taxa	*No.*	*Percentage*	*No.*	*Percentage*
Families	21	91.30	2	8.69
Genus	29	90.62	3	9.37
Species	30	90.90	3	10.0

Table 17.4: Incidence of plants based on habit

Habit	*Total number*	*Percentage (%)*
Trees	15	45.45
Shrubs	4	12.12
Herbs	9	27.27
Climbers	5	15.15

Vill.: Fuldanga, Dist.: Birbhum, West Bengal (Plate 17. 35); (4) Name: Paru Murmu, Vill.: Sarpukur, Dist.: Birbhum, West Bengal (Plate 17.36), etc.

All 34 plant species have been listed in a tabular form providing botanical names, tribal and local names, habit, parts used, names of the diseases and ailments and occurrence (Table 17.6). From the occurrence of the plant taxa in the district, it is understood that the plants are available in the district and the tribal herbal persons are making a good use of those locally available plant resources. Finally, the recorded plants have been enumerated alphabetically depending upon their botanical names along with local and tribal names, parts used, distribution in the world, occurrence in the district, their medicinal uses and chemical constituents.

Enumeration of the Investigated Plant Taxa

1. **Botanical name:** *Acacia nilotica* (Lam.) Willd. ex Del. subsp. *indica* (Benth.) Brenan (Mimosaceae) (Plate 17.1).

Local name: Babla.

Tribal name: Kikar.

Botanical characters: Tree; branches with axillary stipular spines; leaves bipinnate, entire, glabrous; inflorescence head; flowers yellow, numerous; pod stalked, compressed, moniliform; seeds 8–12.

Distribution: Hotter parts of the world and all over India.

Occurrence: Common in the district; grown in fallow lands, along roadsides and on the borders of cultivated fields.

Table 17.5: Percentage composition of plant parts used in tribal medicine

Sl. No.	*Plant parts*	*Total number*	*Percentage*
1.	Roots and rhizomes	7	21.21
2.	Barks	11	33.33
3.	Shoots and stems	4	12.12
4.	Fruits and seeds	4	12.12
5.	Leaves	7	21.21
6.	Flowers	2	6.06

Table 17.6: List of investigated ethnomedicinal plants with brief information

Sl. No.	*Botanical name and family*	*Local/ Tribal Name*	*Habit*	*Parts used*	*Diseases*	*Occurrence*
1.	*Acacia nilotica* (Lam.) Willd. ex Del. subsp. *indica* (Benth.) Brenan (Mimosaceae)	Babla/Kikar	Tree	Root	White discharge and irregular mensturation	Common
2.	*Achyranthes aspera* Linn. (Amarantaceae)	Apang/ Circhirip	Herb	Root, stem leaves fruit	Fever and skin disease, white discharge	Common
3.	*Adhatoda vasica* L. (Acanthaceae)	Basak/ Arandi-ba	Shrub	Leaves	Cold and cough	Uncommon
4.	*Aegle marmelos* (L.) Corr. ex Roxb. (Rutaceae)	Bel/Bel	Tree	Roots	To facilitate delivery	Common
5.	*Annona reticulata* L. (Annonaceae)	Nona ata/ Gom	Small tree	Fruits, leaves	Dysentery and fever, insect repellent	Uncommon
6.	*Aristolochia indica* L. (Aristolochiaceae)	Ishwarmul	Climber	Root	Stomach ache	Common
7.	*Artocarpus heterophyllus* Lam. (Moraceae)	Kanthal	Tree	Root and leaves	Diarrhoea and skin disease	Common
8.	*Azadirachta indica* A. Juss. (Meliaceae)	Neem/ Bokom-dare	Tree	Bark	Ear pain and pus formation	Common
9.	*Basella alba* L. (Basellaceae)	Puin shak	Climber	Leaves	Constipation	Common
10.	*Butea monosperma* (Lam.) Kuntze (Fabaceae)	Palas/Palas-baha	Tree	Root	Urinary problem	Common
11.	*Calotropis gigantea* (L.) R.Br. ex Ait. (Asclepiadaceae)	Akanda/Ark, Parkha	Shrub	Latex and leaves	Toothache and muscular pain	Common
12.	*Cassia fistula* L. (Caesalpiniaceae)	Bandarlathi/ Bero-Hari	Tree	Gum of fruit	Hooping Cough	Common
13.	*Cassia occidentalis* Linn. (Caesalpiniaceae)	Kalkasunda/ kasunda	Shrub/ under-shrub	Leaves and root	Hysteria and fever	Common
14.	*Cassia tora* L. (Caesalpiniaceae)	Chakunda, Panevar	Herb	Seeds	Ringworm and other diseases	Very common

(*Contd.*)

Table 17.6 (*Contd.*)

Sl. No.	*Botanical name and family*	*Local/ Tribal Name*	*Habit*	*Parts used*	*Diseases*	*Occurrence*
15.	*Clitoria ternatea* L. (Fabaceae)	Aparajita	Climber	Root	Leucorrhoea	Uncommon
16.	*Curculigo orchioides* (Amaryllidaceae)	Talmuli/ Tarmuli	Herb	Rootstock	Leucorrhoea, asthma	Uncommon
17.	*Ficus racemosa* L. (Moraceae)	Jaggya Dumur	Tree	Bark	Septic wounds	Uncommon
18.	*Gmelina arborea* L. (Verbenaceae)	Gamar, Gumbar	Tree	Root bark	Septic wounds	Uncommon
19.	*Hibiscus rosa-sinensis* L. (Malvaceae)	Jaba/Jaba batha	Shrub	Flowers	White discharge and irregular menstruation	Common
20.	*Holarrhena antidysenterica* (Lam.) Wall. (Apocynaceae)	Kurchi/Hot	Tree	Leaves, stem bark	Menstrual problem, Dysentery	Common
21.	*Mangifera indica* L. (Anacardiaceae)	Aam/Ulidaru	Tree	Bark	Dysentery	Very Common
22.	*Mimusops elengi* L. (Sapotaceae)	Bakul/Bohur	Tree	Bark	Ulcer in mouth	Common
23.	*Morinda citrifolia* L. (Rubiaceae)	Al/Chaili	Tree	Roots and root bark	Septic wound and Rheumatism	Uncommon
24.	*Moringa oleifera* Lamk. (Moringaceae)	Sajina/Doro	Tree	Stem bark	Cholera	Common
25.	*Nyctanthes arbor-tristis* L. (Oleaceae)	Sheuli/ Saparom	Small Tree	Leaves	Fever and intestinal worm	Common in garden
26.	*Phyllanthus emblica* L. (Euphorbiaceae)	Amlaki/ Miral daru	Tree	Leaves	Skin disease	Common
27.	*Phyllanthus reticulatus* Poir. (Euphorbiaceae)	Pansheuli Panjeli-lata	Shrub	Young Leaves	Muscular pain	Common
28.	*Psidium guajava* L. (Myrtaceae)	Peyara/ Tamras	Tree	Bark	Loose motion	Common
29.	*Punica granatum* L. (Punicaceae)	Dalim, Bedana	Shrub/ small tree	Flower	Asthma	Uncommon

(*Contd.*)

Table 17.6 (*Contd.*)

Sl. No.	*Botanical name and family*	*Local/ Tribal Name*	*Habit*	*Parts used*	*Diseases*	*Occurrence*
30.	*Semecarpus anacardium* Linn.f. (Anacardiaceae)	Bhela/ Bhelwa	Tree	Seed	As a charm against evil eye	Common
31.	*Shorea robusta Gaertn.* f. (Dipterocarpaceae)	Sal/Sakhu Sal	Tree	Bark	Any type of burn, Dysentery	Common
32.	*Tamarindus indica L.* (Caesalpiniaceae)	Tentul/Imli	Tree	Root	To facilitate delivery	Common
33.	*Terminalia bellirica* Roxb.(Combretaceae)	Bahera/ Michra	Tree	Bark	Dysentery	Very common
34.	*Terminalia chebula* Retz. (Combretaceae)	Haritaki/ Rola-daru	Tree	Fruits	Leucoderma	Common

Parts used: Root.

Uses: Root of this plant and barks of *Bombax ceiba* and *Ziziphus oenoplia*, fruit of *Achyranthes*, flower of *Hibiscus*—all are made into paste, mixed with warm water and taken in the morning in empty stomach to cure irregular menstruation and leucorrhoea (white discharge).

Chemical constituents: Tannins (12.19–20 per cent), galloylated and tetrahydroxyflavan–3, 4-diols, amino acids and ascorbic acids.

2. Botanical name: *Achyranthes aspera* L. (Amaranthaceae) (Plate 17.2)

Local name: Apang, charcharey

Tribal name: Chir-chirip

Botanical characters: Slightly woody herbs or under-shrubs; leaves opposite, simple, ovate or elliptic, obtuse or acuminate, short petioled; flowers in terminal spikes, minute, greenish white or pink, deflexed; fruits urticles; seeds oblong, brown.

Distribution: Tropical and subtropical regions of Asia, Africa and Australia. Commonly grown throughout India.

Occurrence: Very common in bushes, thickets, waste places and along roadsides.

Parts used: Root and stem, leaves and fruits.

Uses: In magico-religious belief: (1) A piece (2–2.5 cm.) of root tied with red cotton thread around the neck as magical cure for fever. (2) Small piece of (about 4 cm. long) stem laced in a chain with white thread and wear it around the neck. Leaves are made into paste and applied in skin disease. Fruits of the plant and bark of *Bombax ceiba* and *Ziziphus oenoplia*, root of *Acacia nilotica* and flower of *Hibiscus rosa-sinensis* are made into paste, mixed with warm water and taken in the morning in empty stomach to cure irregular menstruation and leucorrhoea (white discharge).

Chemical constituents: Whole plant contains betaine, a water soluble alkaloid achyranthine. Seeds contain achyranthes saponins A and B. In roots, oleanolic glycoside is found.

3. **Botanical name:** *Adhatoda vasica* L. (Acanthaceae) (Plate 17.3).

Local name: Basak.

Tribal name: Arandi-ba.

Botanical characters: Stout shrub; leaves elliptic—lanceolate, glabrous; inflorescence axillary dense spike; flowers medium sized; fruits capsules; seeds orbicular, oblong.

Distribution: Sri Lanka, tropical Africa, Java, Philippines and throughout hotter parts of India.

Occurrence: Uncommon in the district; found in thickets and hedges.

Parts used: Leaves.

Uses: Leaves of this plant and Basil leaves are made into paste, juice is extracted and taken twice daily in morning and evening to cure cold and cough.

Chemical constituents: Vasicine, vasicinine, vasicinol, vasicinone, vasicol, essential oil (0.076 per cent), etc.

4. **Botanical name:** *Aegle marmelos* (L.) Corr. ex Roxb. (Rutaceae) (Plate 17.4).

Local and Tribal name: Bel.

Botanical characters: Tree; leaves trifoliolate; leaflet elliptic or ovate-lanceolate; flowers greenish-white, sweet scented; fruits globose or ellipsoid with a woody; seeds embedded in mucilage and orange or yellow sweet pulp.

Distribution: Throughout the tropics and widely distributed in India.

Occurrence: Common in the district; grown in forests, fallow lands and gardens.

Parts used: Roots.

Uses: In magico-religious belief: Root pieces (2–3 cm. long) of this plant along with *Tamarindus* root are tied to woman's hair in such a way that she can inhale the smell of the roots to facilitate the delivery. The root should be removed immediately after childbirth.

Chemical constituents: A number of alkaloids, amino acids, anthocyanins, lecoanthocyanins, carbohydrates, carotene, essential oils, fatty acids, sterols, tannic acid, tannins and vitamins.

5. **Botanical name:** *Annona reticulata* L. (Annonaceae).

Local name: Nona ata.

Tribal name: Gom, Nag-hawa.

Botanical characters: Small tree; leaves alternate, simple, oblong–lanceolate, acuminate, glabrous; flowers 2–3 together, axillary, tomentose, scented; fruits syncarpus, sub-globose, reddish purple when ripe; seeds many, black smooth.

Distribution: Throughout the tropical America and India.

Occurrence: Uncommon; found near the tribal habitation and in thickets both as self sown and cultivated one.

Parts used: Fruits and leaves.

Uses: Fruits used in the treatment of dysentery and fever. Leaves and unripe fruits are used as insect repellent.

Chemical constituents: Alkaloids, diterpenoids, catechin, epicatechin, hyperoside, rutin, etc.

6. **Botanical name:** *Aristolochia indica* L. (Aristolochiaceae) (Plate 17.5).

Local name: Iswarmul.

Tribal name: Gad.

Botanical characters: Climbing herbs; leaves opposite, simple, oblong—obovate, entire, acuminate; flowers in axillary racemes; fruits capsules, 6-valved; seeds triangular, flat, winged.

Distribution: Tropical and temperate regions of the world; grown throughout the plains of India.

Occurrence: Uncommon; grown in forest floor, in thickets and hedges.

Parts used: Root.

Uses: Roots of this plant and leaves of the grass *Cynadon dactylon* are made into paste and juice of the paste is taken in the morning in empty stomach to cure stomach ache.

Chemical constituents: Roots contain an alkaloid aristochine, tetracyclic sesquiterpenes like ishwarone, ishwarane, aristolochene, etc.

7. **Botanical name:** *Artocarpus heterophyllus* Lam. (Moraceae) (Plate 17.6).

Local name and Tribal name: Kanthal.

Botanical characters: Tree with milky latex; leaves dense elliptic, thickly coriaceous; stipules scaly brown; inflorescence terminal or axillary spikes; fruits large, sharply tubercled, stalked; seeds oblong or reniform.

Distribution: Indo-Malayan region, China, and throughout India.

Occurrence: Common; grown in gardens, near the human settlements.

Parts used: Root and leaves.

Uses: Roots used as antidiarrhoeal. Paste of tender leaves is administered as poultice in case of skin disease.

Chemical constituents: Cycloarten group of tetracyclic triterpenoids, rich source of carbohydrates and essential amino acids, carotenes, ursolic acid, sitosterol and flavonoids.

8. **Botanical name:** *Azadirachta indica* A. Juss. (Meliaceae) (Plate 17.7).

Local name: Neem.

Tribal name: Bokom-dare.

Botanical characters: Tree with bitter scent; leaves imparipinnate, arranged in sub-opposite pairs; inflorescence panicles of racemes; flowers fragrant, bracteate; fruits ellipsoid, 1-seeded berry.

Distribution: Throughout the Indo-Malayan region, Africa and all over India.

Occurrence: Common along the roadsides, in village surroundings and fallow lands.

Parts used: Bark.

Uses: Bark of Nim (5 gm.), roots of *Coccinia grandis* (2 gm.) and *Datura* metel (2 gm.) are made into paste, juice is extracted and after warming it is administered 3 drops in the ear daily for ear pain and pus formation.

Chemical constituents: Rich source of diterpenoids notably nimbin, nimbidine, azadirachtin and their derivatives, flavonoids, sterols, triterpenoids, tannins, proteins, etc.

9. **Botanical name:** *Basella alba* L. (Basellaceae).

Local name and Tribal name: Puin shak.

Botanical characters: Perennial herb; stem climbing succulent, angled, glabrous; leaves broadly ovate, thick, glabrous and shining; flowers many in axillary spikes; fruits ovoid.

Distribution: Throughout India; grown as wild or cultivated.

Occurrence: Common in the district.

Parts used: Leaves.

Uses: Juice of the leaves is given 1–2 teaspoonful once daily in cases of constipation.

Chemical constituents: Iodine, fluorine, carotenoids, several vitamins, calcium, iron, oxalates, zinc, magnesium, sodium, manganese, sulphur and bi-flavonoids, etc.

10. **Botanical name:** *Butea monosperma* (Lam.) Kuntze (Fabaceae) (Plate 17.8).

Local name: Palas.

Tribal name: Palas-baha.

Botanical characters: Tree; leaves pinnately 3-foliolate, leaflets obovate, rhomboid, coriaceous, silky tomentose beneath; flowers orange-red in panicle of racemes, bracteates; pods flattened, thickened at sutures, silvery tomentose when young.

Distribution: Throughout the hotter parts of world and widely distributed in India.

Occurrence: Common in the forest, fallow lands, near human habitation

Parts used: Root.

Uses: Root (3–4 cm. long) decoction is given once in a day in the morning for 7 days to cure urinary problem.

Chemical constituents: Chalcone and aurones, imidazole derivatives, anthocyanidin, monospermin, fatty acids, sitosterol and amyrin.

11. **Botanical name:** *Calotropis gigantea* (L.) R. Br. ex Ait. (Asclepiadaceae) (Plate 17.9).

Local name: Akanda.

Tribal name: Ark, Parkha.

Botanical characters: Shrubs; leaves opposite, ovate-cordate, coriaceous, subsessile; flowers white or pale purple in umbel, simple or compound; follicle short, recurved.

Distribution: Tropical and subtropical regions of Africa and Asia, and throughout India.

Occurrence: Common in waste lands, along roadsides, river bank.

Parts used: Latex and leaves.

Uses: Latex is applied on the affected teeth to get relieve from toothache. Leaf dorsal side smeared with mustard oil, after warming it is put over the affected area to get relieve from any type of chest or muscular pain.

Chemical constituents: Cardiac glycosides, e.g. calotropin, a-calatinic acid, b-calotropol, b-amyrin, calcium oxalate and gigantin.

12. **Botanical name:** *Cassia fistula* L. (Caesalpiniaceae) (Plate 17.10).

Local name: Bandarlathi.

Tribal name: Bero-Hari.

Botanical characters: Medium-sized deciduous tree with whitish grey bark; leaves paripinnate; leaflets 8–16, ovate, petiolated; flowers bright yellowish in long lax racemes; pods brownish, cylindrical, pendulous, 25–50 seeded.

Distribution: Tropical regions of the world and all over India.

Occurrence: Common along roadsides, in gardens and forest.

Parts used: Gum of the fruit.

Uses: Gum of the fruit soaked in water for 1–2 hours and administered 5 teaspoonful thrice daily for 5 days to treat children's hooping cough.

Chemical constituents: Sugars, anthocyanidins, anthraquinones, glucosides, bi- and tri-flavonoids, tannins (3.18 per cent), etc.

13. **Botanical name:** *Cassia occidentalis* L. (Caesalpiniaceae) (Plate 17.11).

Local name: Kalkasunda.

Tribal name: Kasunda.

Botanical characters: Slightly woody under-shrubs, or shrubs, erect, branches often purplish; leaves alternate, compound, paripinnate, petiolated; leaflets 3–5 pairs, ovate-lanceolate, apex acute; flowers yellow in short peduncled racemes, corymbose; petals 5; stamens 10; pods thick, recurved, compressed, distinctly torulose; seeds 20–30, ovoid, smooth, dark olive green.

Distribution: Tropical regions of the world and all over India.

Occurrence: Common in waste places, in open and fallow lands, along roadsides.

Parts used: Leaves and root.

Uses: Decoction of leaves and root is used in relieving spasm of hysteria patient. Root juice is used in scorpion sting. Leaves are given to cure fever, as purgative.

Chemical constituents: Plant extracts contain emodin, physcion (anthraquinone), chrysophanol, sitosterol, cassiolin (xanthone), etc. Seeds contain fatty matter, tannic acid, gum, sugar, starch, iron silica, malic acid, etc.

14. **Botanical name:** *Cassia tora* L. (Caesalpiniaceae) (Plate 17.12).

Local name and Tribal name: Chakunda, Panevar.

Botanical characters: Gregarious annual woody herb; leaves pinnate; leaflets 6, ovate-oblong; flowers usually in nearly sessile pairs in axils of leaves; pods subtetragonous; seeds uniseriate.

Distribution: Tropical regions of the world and throughout India.

Occurrence: Very common in waste places and open field, along roadsides.

Parts used: Seeds.

Uses: Seed powder mixed with lime (3 : 1) is administered to cure ringworm and other skin diseases.

Chemical constituents: Anthraglucosides, chrysophanol, rhein, kaempferol, glycosides, tigonellene, choline, euphol, auraphrol and anthocyanidin.

15. **Botanical name:** *Clitoria ternatea* L. (Fabaceae) (Plate 17.13).

Local name and Tribal name: Aparajita.

Botanical characters: Perennial scandent climber; leaves stipellate; leaflets 5–7, ovate or oblong, subcoriaceous, petioluled; flowers bright blue with an orange centre, rarely white, spoon-shaped, solitary; pods linear, flattish, 6–10 seeded.

Distribution: Common in India; also occurs among hedges all over the tropical region from the Himalayas to Ceylon.

Occurrence: Uncommon; grown in private gardens and in hedges.

Parts used: Root.

Uses: Root of the plant and 5 pieces of black pepper are made into paste, prepare 21 tablets, 3 tablets given once in a day for 7 days to cure leucorrhoea (Ghosh 2009).

Chemical constituents: Flavonoids and their glycosides, anthocyanins, triterpenoids, sterol and fatty acids.

16. **Botanical name:** *Curculigo orchioides* Gaertn. (Amaryllidaceae) (Plate 17.14).

Local name: Talmuli, Kali mushli.

Tribal name: Tarmuli,Tarmuri, Ketal.

Botanical characters: Small dwarf herbs with stout tuberous rootstock; leaves simple, sessile, long, linear-lanceolate; scapes short, clavate; flowers small, bright yellow, male and bisexual; stamens 6; fruits capsules, densely villose with slender beak; seeds 3–4, oblong, black, shining.

Distribution: Found tropical regions of the world. In India it is grown in subtropical Himalayas; Kumaon to Assam and in Western Ghats from Konkan southwards.

Occurrence: Uncommon; found in forest floors, orchards as under growth.

Parts used: Root stock.

Uses: One teaspoonful of rootstock is given once a day for 7 days to cure leucorrhoea. One tablet made from root paste is taken daily in empty stomach for 15 days to cure asthma.

Chemical constituents: Resin, tannins, mucilage, fat, starch, and ash containing oxalate of calcium.

17. **Botanical name:** *Ficus racemosa* L. (Moraceae) (Plate 17.15).

Local name: Jaggya Dumur.

Tribal name: Loa.

Botanical characters: Tree with smooth, brownish-grey bark; leaves broadly ovate, entire, membranous, petiolate; flowers minute, unisexual, numerous, collected on receptacles; fruits purplish red when ripe, sub-globose or pyriform, in dense clusters.

Distribution: In tropical countries of the world and throughout India.

Occurrence: Uncommon; grown in village thickets, fallow lands and near tribal habitation.

Parts used: Bark.

Uses: The paste of stem bark is administered in cases of septic wounds.

Chemical constituents: Glycosides, tannins, psoralen, cerylbehenate, lupeol and its acetate, stigmasterol, gluanol acetate, phytosterols, etc.

18. **Botanical name:** *Gmelina arborea* L. (Verbenaceae) (Plate 17.16).

Local name: Gamar.

Tribal name: Gumbar.

Botanical characters: Moderate sized deciduous tree; leaves alternate, simple, broadly ovate, slightly decurrent at base; flowers in racemes, long, brownish, yellow; fruits drupes, succulent, yellow when ripe; seeds oblong.

Distribution: Tropical and subtropical regions of the world and throughout the India.

Occurrence: Uncommon; planted along the roadsides, in forest and fallow lands.

Parts used: Root bark and Fruits.

Uses: Decoction of root bark is used for washing septic wounds. Fruit paste is applied on the baby's head to make the skull bone strong.

Chemical constituents: Butyric acid, tartaric acid, resinous substances and saccharine.

19. **Botanical name:** *Hibiscus rosa-sinensis* L. (Malvaceae) (Plate 17.17).

Local name: Jaba.

Tribal name: Jaba-batha.

Botanical characters: Shrubs; leaves alternate, simple, lanceolate, dentate; flowers axillary solitary, big, tubular bellow, generally reddish in colour; plants do not produce fruits,in general.

Distribution: China, Japan and planted in the gardens throughout India.

Occurrence: Common in private gardens.

Parts used: Flowers.

Uses: Flowers of the plant and bark of *Bombax ceiba* and *Ziziphus oenoplia*, root of *Acacia nilotica* and fruit of *Achyranthes* are made into paste, mixed with warm water and taken in the morning in empty stomach to cure irregular menstruation and white discharge.

Chemical constituents: Cyanidin diglycoside, tetraxeryl acetate, calcium oxalate, vitamins, flavonoids and their glycosides.

20. **Botanical name:** *Holarrhena antidysenterica* (Lam.) Wall (Apocynaceae) (Plate 17.18).

Local name: Kurchi.

Tribal name: Kurchi, Hot.

Botanical characters: Small trees; leaves opposite, simple, ovate-elliptic; flowers in axillary and terminal corymbose cymes, white or cream coloured; corolla lobes 5, contorted; fruits follicles in pairs, long cylindrical; seeds linear oblong, tipped with hairy comas.

Distribution: Tropical Asia. Grown in all parts of India.

Occurrence: Common in forest areas, occasionally found in private gardens.

Parts used: Leaves and stem bark.

Uses: One teaspoonful of leaf decoction is administered twice daily in case of menstrual disorder. Infusion of stem bark with one teaspoonful of honey given as cure for dysentery.

Chemical constituents: Bark contains various types of alkaloids like conessine, conissimine, holarrhidine, kurchamine, etc., and terpenes.

21. **Botanical name:** *Mangifera indica* L. (Anacardiaceae) (Plate 17.19).

Local name: Aam.

Tribal name: Uli-daru, Amati.

Botanical characters: Large evergreen trees; leaves alternate, simple; flowers in racemes, greenish-white; fruits drupe, fleshy; seeds stony flat.

Distribution: Throughout the hotter parts of the world and all over India.

Occurrence: Very common in the gardens and village surroundings.

Parts used: Bark.

Uses: Barks of *Mangifera indica*, *Terminalia arjuna*, *Spondias pinnata*, *Shorea robusta*, *Streblus asper* and *Terminalia bellirica* in equal proportion are made into paste, mixed with a small amount of lime and then administered one teaspoonful twice a day for 7 days to cure dysentery.

Chemical constituents: Potassium and vitamin A, carotine, xanthophylls, carbohydrates, sucrose, glucose, fructose, acids (0.18–3.66 per cent), etc.

22. **Botanical name:** *Mimusops elengi* L. (Sapotaceae) (Plate 17.20).

Local name: Bakul.

Tribal name: Bohur.

Botanical characters: Trees; leaves alternate, simple, elliptic; flowers fascicled, white, fragrant; fruits berries, yellow when ripe; seeds ovoid, compressed, brown, shining.
Distribution: Tropical regions of the world and throughout the hotter parts of India.
Occurrence: Common in private gardens and in the village surroundings, near the tribal habitation.
Parts used: Stem bark.
Uses: Stem bark decoction is used by Santhal as washing agent for curing the ulcer in mouth (Pal and Jain 1998).
Chemical constituents: Triterpenoid saponins and essential oils.

23. **Botanical name:** *Morinda citrifolia* L. (Rubiaceae) (Plate 17.21).
Local name: Al.
Tribal name: Chaili.
Botanical characters: Small trees; leaves opposite, rarely verticillate, broadly elliptic; flowers in dense ovoid heads, white; fruits drupes.
Distribution: Throughout the tropics and greater parts of India.
Occurrence: Uncommon; grown in forest and villages; sometimes along the roadsides.
Parts used: Root and root bark.
Uses: Root decoction is used by Santhal for washing septic wounds. Root bark paste with paste of garlic (3 : 2) used by Lodhas for curing rheumatism (Pal and Jain 1998).
Chemical constituents: Anthraquinones, asperulside, carotenes and glucose, etc.

24. **Botanical name:** *Moringa oleifera* Lamk (Moringaceae) (Plate 17.22).
Local name: Sajina.
Tribal name: Doro.
Botanical characters: Trees; leaves alternate, pinnately compound; flowers in axillary panicles, white, fruits pods, cylindrical; seeds 3-angled, winged.
Distribution: Throughout the tropics of the world and planted throughout India.
Occurrence: Common in village surroundings and near the houses of tribal people.
Parts used: Stem barks.
Uses: Stem bark decoction with table salt is given 2–3 teaspoonful twice a day for 7 days to treat cholera.
Chemical constituents: Vitamin C, flavonoids, e.g. quercetin, kaempferol, polysaccharides, amino-acids and minerals, etc.

25. **Botanical name:** *Nyctanthes arbor-tristis* L. (Oleaceae) (Plate 17.23).
Local name: Seoli, Sephalika.
Tribal name: Saparom.

Botanical characters: Small trees; branches quadrangular; leaves opposite, simple ovate, rough; flowers in trichotomous cymes, white, with bright orange tubes, fragrant; fruits capsules, flat, broad at apex; seeds flat.

Distribution: Throughout the world and widely distributed in India.

Occurrence: Common in gardens; occasionally found in the tribal habitations.

Parts used: Leaves.

Uses: One teaspoonful of leaf juice is given twice a day to treat fever. It is also used along with honey or sugar in cases of children having intestinal worms.

Chemical constituents: d-manitol, tannin, glucose, oil consist of glycerides, sitosterol, etc.

26. **Botanical name:** *Phyllanthus emblica* L. (Euphorbiaceae) (Plate 17.24).

Local name: Amlaki.

Tribal name: Miral daru.

Botanical characters: Large deciduous trees; leaves pinnately compound, pinna-oblong-elliptic; flowers unisexual, green; fruits berries; seeds hard, angular, brown.

Distribution: Planted throughout the world; both wild and planted all over India.

Occurrence: Common in the forest; occasionally found in private gardens.

Parts used: Leaves.

Uses: Leaves of this plant and *Achyranthes aspera* are made paste and applied in any type of skin disease.

Chemical constituents: Ascorbic acid, phyllembelic acid, gallic acid, indole acetic acid and other auxins, etc.

27. **Botanical name:** *Phyllanthus reticulatus* Poir. (Euphorbiaceae) (Plate 17.25).

Local name: Pansheuli.

Tribal name: Panjeli-lata.

Botanical characters: Shrubs; leaves alternate, pinnately compound, flowers in fascicles, unisexual, minute; fruits capsules, trilobed; seeds trigonous.

Distribution: Tropical and subtropical regions of the world; throughout the warmer parts of India.

Occurrence: Common in hedges and thickets.

Parts used: Young leaves.

Uses: The paste of young leaves is administered for treatment of muscular pain.

Chemical constituents: glucosides of gibberellins, proteins, fatty acids, carbohydrates, etc.

28. **Botanical name:** *Psidium guajava* L. (Myrtaceae) (Plate 17.26).

Local name: Peyara.

Tribal name: Tamras.

Botanical characters: Trees; leaves opposite, simple, lanceolate, finely pubescent; flowers in axillary, solitary, sometimes 3-chotomous cymes, white, fragrant; fruits berry, vary in shape; seeds small, stony.

Distribution: Cultivated all over the world including India.

Occurrence: Common in orchards and house gardens.

Parts used: Bark.

Uses: Barks of *Psidium guajava* and *Shorea robusta* (1 : 2) are made into paste and it is mixed with very small amount of lime. Then, it is administered 2 and ½ teaspoonful once daily for 3 days in case of loose motion.

Chemical constituents: Leucocyanidin, flavonoids, e.g., quercetin, phytosterols, carotenes, tannins, saponins, vitamin C and B_6, carbohydrates, diethoxy alkanes as flavour component.

29. Botanical name: *Punica granatum* L. (Punicaceae) (Plate 17.27).

Local name and Tribal name: Dalim, Bedana.

Botanical characters: Shrub or small deciduous trees; leaves sub-opposite, oblong or obovate, entire; flowers usually scarlet red, rarely yellow, axillary, solitary or somewhat clustered; fruits globose with coriaceous rind, crowned by persistent calyx; seeds numerous embedded in white or ruby coloured pulp.

Distribution: Throughout the tropics and widely distributed in India.

Occurrence: Uncommon; grown in private gardens.

Parts used: Flowers.

Uses: Flowers of the plant and root of *Ocimum sanctum* (2 : 1) are made into paste, mixed with sugar candy, prepare 7 tablets and 1 tablet given in a day for 7 days to treat asthma.

Chemical constituents: Alkaloids, e.g., pelletierine, estrone, tannins, fatty acids, carbohydrates, triterpenoids, phytosterols, etc.

30. Botanical name: *Semecarpus anacardium* L.f. (Anacardiaceae) (Plate 17.28).

Local name: Bhela.

Tribal name: Bhela, Bhelwa.

Botanical characters: Medium sized trees; leaves alternate, simple, large, oblong or ovate-oblong, leathery, densely grey pubescent, obtuse or rounded at apex; flowers small green, sub-sessile in terminal panicles; fruits drupes, obliquely ovoid or oblong, smooth, black when ripe, present on yellow fleshy receptacles; seed one.

Distribution: Found in Indo-Malayan regions of the world. Grown throughout India.

Occurrence: Common in forest areas, sometimes found near the habitation of the tribal people.

Parts used: Seed.

Mode of administration: In magico-religious belief, one seed is tied with red or black thread and hanged around the neck of children as charm against evil eyes.

Chemical constituents: Pericarp of the fruit contains a bitter and astringent principle, a phenolic compound semecarpol; a dark viscous oil that contains bhilawanol and other compounds.

31. Botanical name: *Shorea robusta* Gaert n.f. (Dipterocarpaceae) (Plate 17.29).

Local name: Sal.

Tribal name: Sakhu, Sal.

Botanical characters: Deciduous trees; leaves alternate, simple, ovate, oblong; flowers small, yellowish white, in terminal and axillary lax panicles; fruits samaroids, winged with persistent sepals; seeds fleshy with unequal cotyledons.

Distribution: Tropical regions of the South-East Asian countries and Philippine islands. All over India in dry deciduous forest.

Occurrence: Very common in forest areas, tribal villages and open land.

Parts used: Bark.

Uses: Barks of this plant and *Spondias pinnata, Terminalia arjuna, Mangifera indica, Terminalia bellirica, Streblus asper* (in equal proportion) are made into paste and mixed with lime then administered one teaspoonful daily for 7 days to treat dysentery.

32. Botanical name: *Tamarindus indica* L. (Caesalpiniaceae) (Plate 17.30).

Local name: Tentul.

Tribal name: Imli.

Botanical characters: Large trees; leaves unipinnately compound paripinnate; flowers in racemes, yellow coloured; stamens 3, monadelphous; fruits pods, lomentum indehiscent, pulp sour; seeds orbicular, compressed, shining blackish brown.

Distribution: Tropical regions of Old and New world; all over India.

Occurrence: Common in forest areas, village surroundings, fallow lands and along the roadsides.

Parts used: Root.

Uses: In magico-religious belief, root pieces (2–3 cm. long) of this plant along with *Aegle marmelos* root, are hanged with the hair of woman's head in such a way that she can inhale the smell of the roots to facilitate the delivery. The root should be removed immediately after child birth.

Chemical constituents: Tamarind pulp contains tartaric acid, citric acid, malic acid, invert sugar, gum, and pectin. Seeds contain albuminoids, fat, carbohydrate, fibre, and ash.

33. Botanical name: *Terminalia bellirica* Roxb. (Combretaceae) (Plate 17.31).

Local name: Bahera.

Tribal name: Michra.

Botanical characters: Trees; leaves alternate, simple, elliptic-obovate; flowers in axillary spikes, pale, greenish-yellow; fruits drupe, ovoid, grey, soft hairy; seeds stony.

Distribution: Tropical and subtropical regions of the world and all over India.

Occurrence: Very common in the forests, fallow lands and along roadsides.

Parts used: Bark.

Uses: Barks of this plant and *Shorea robusta, Spondias pinnata, Terminalia arjuna, Mangifera indica, Streblus asper* (in equal proportion) are made into paste and mixed with lime, then administered one teaspoonful daily for 7 days to treat dysentery.

Chemical constituents: Tannin (25 per cent), gum, a green fixed oil, phyllembin and gallic acids.

34. **Botanical name:** *Terminalia chebula* Retz. (Combretaceae) (Plate 17.32).

Local name: Haritaki.

Tribal name: Rola-daru.

Botanical characters: Trees; leaves alternate, simple, hairy, elliptic-oblong; flowers in spikes, dull white; fruits drupes, ellipsoid, yellowish-green; seeds stony, 5-angled.

Distribution: Throughout the tropics and widely distributed in India.

Occurrence: Common in the forest and occasionally found in fallow lands, along roadsides.

Parts used: Fruits.

Uses: Fruit pulp paste is used for treatment of leucoderma.

Chemical constituents: About 30 per cent of astringent substances, e.g. chebulinic acid, tannic acid, gallic acid, chebulagic acid, resin, anthraquinone and sennoside.

Conclusion

Tribal medicine is one of the most valuable traditional knowledge systems in the world. A worldwide awareness has now developed among the people to conserve and document any sort of traditional knowledge system before it is lost from the respective traditional society. It is now a priority issue to the people for documentation, preparation of database and conservation of knowledge on tribal medicine. The Government of India has also initiated digital documentation of various types of knowledge systems existing in different ethnic or traditional society through the preparation of the Traditional Knowledge Digital Library (TKDL) and documentation of many of the knowledge systems has already been completed. This precious folk knowledge on herbal medicine is also being scientifically documented in the country just to save it from its gradual eroding oral form and for preservation of Intellectual Property Right (IPR) of tribal people that are attached with these knowledge systems.

The information documented in this study will enrich the database of tribal medicine for the district of Birbhum which will finally be helpful in preparation of state as well national level inventories of tribal medicine. Digital inventory on tribal medicine of this district is to be prepared urgently covering information on botanical, local and tribal names of the plants, their medicinal uses, details of mode of administration of crude drug with special emphasis on magico-religious belief attached with religio-cultural sentiment of the tribal people. For revitalization of tribal medicine and its health care practices, the awareness about the importance of tribal medicine among the tribal people should be created through various programmes like workshops, trainings, exhibitions, festivals, etc., on tribal medicine. In different tribal pockets of the district, herbal gardens of typical tribal medicinal plants are to be established with the help of different government and non-government organizations as part of the awareness as well as tribal welfare programmes. A steady supply of seedlings, seeds and other propagules of medicinal plants has to be ensured through establishment of nurseries to the local people for their home or back yard herbal gardens. Finally, it is understood that without scientific validation of the knowledge of tribal medicine, it would not get any concrete basis to be considered as a recognized system like other Indian systems of medicine. For this, multidisciplinary research programme on efficacy, safety and development of drug has to be performed keeping active collaboration between botanists, ethnobotanists, phytochemists, pharmacologists, folklorists, historians and medical doctors.

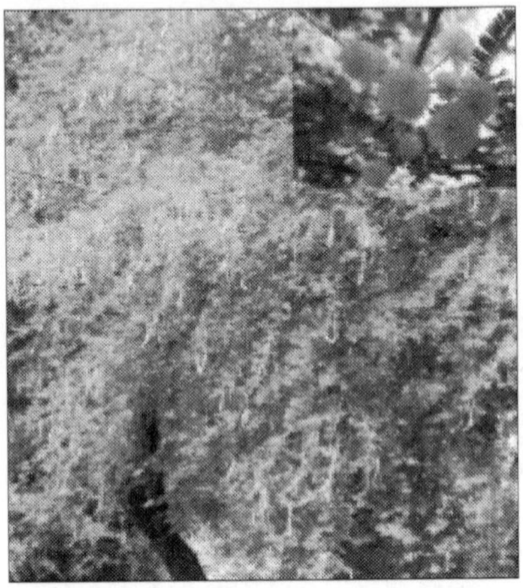

Plate 17.1. *Acacia nilotica* (Lam.) Willd. ex Del.

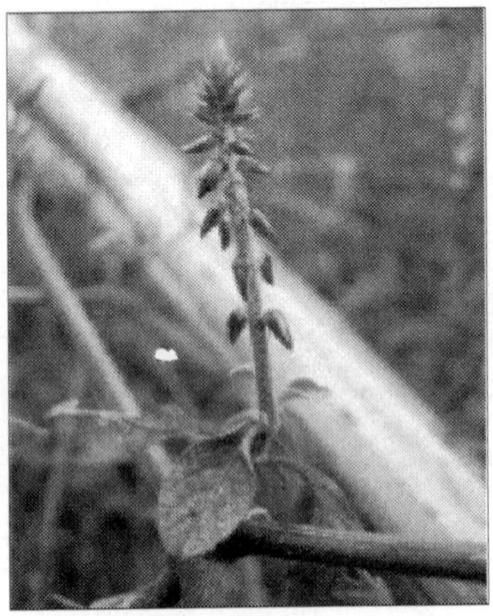

Plate 17.2. *Achyranthes aspera* L.

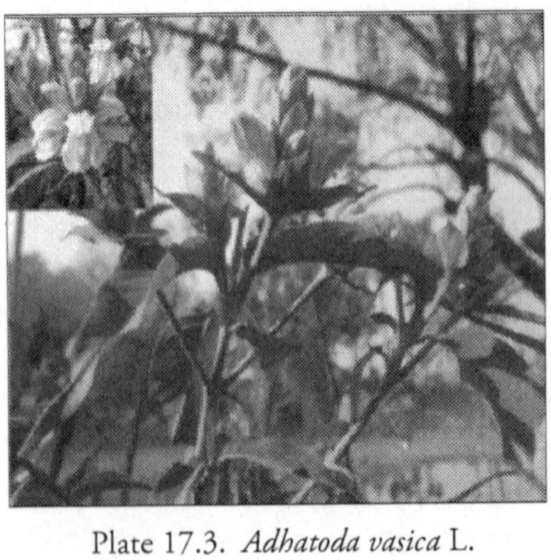

Plate 17.3. *Adhatoda vasica* L.

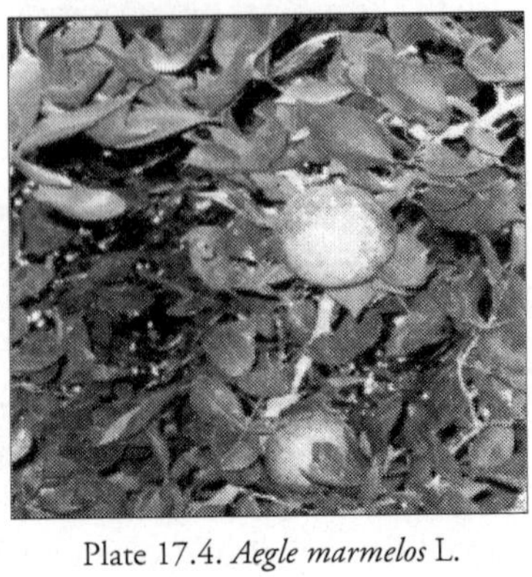

Plate 17.4. *Aegle marmelos* L.

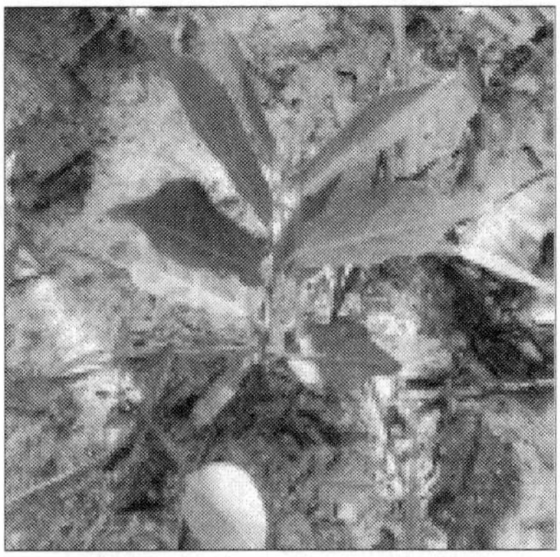

Plate 17.5. *Aristolochia indica* L.

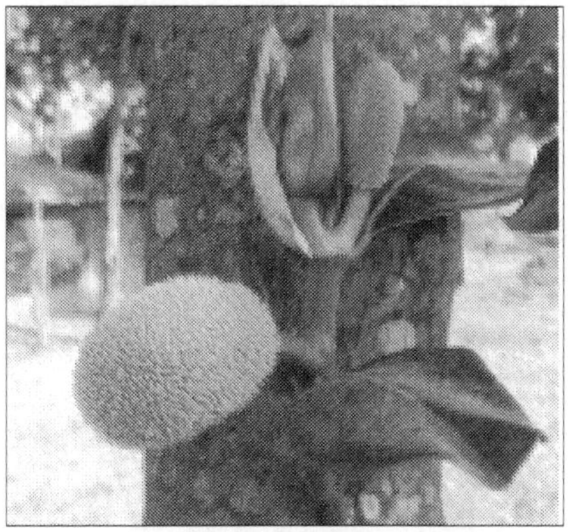

Plate 17.6. *Artocarpus hetrophyllus* Lam.

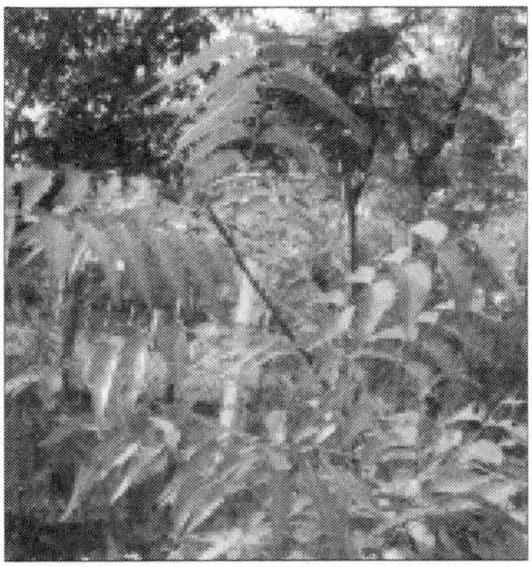

Plate 17.7. *Azadirachta indica* A. Juss.

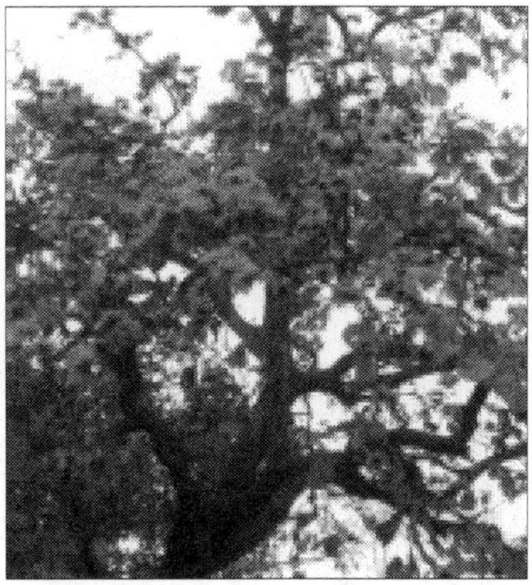

Plate 17.8. *Butea monosperma* (Lam.) Taub.

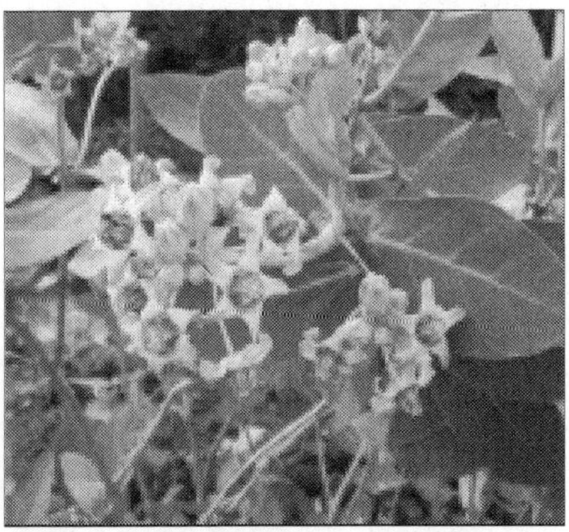

Plate 17.9. *Calotropis gigantea* (L.) R. Br. ex Ait.

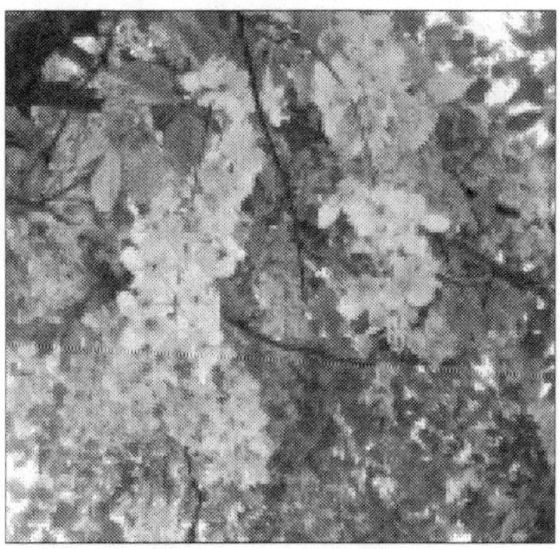

Plate 17.10. *Cassia fistula* L.

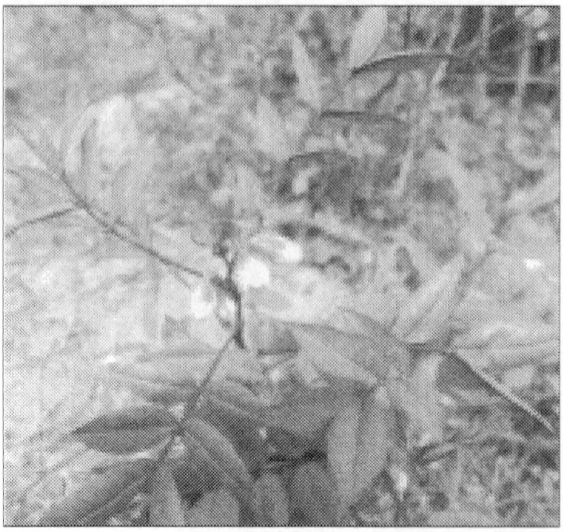

Plate 17.11. *Cassia occidentalis* L.

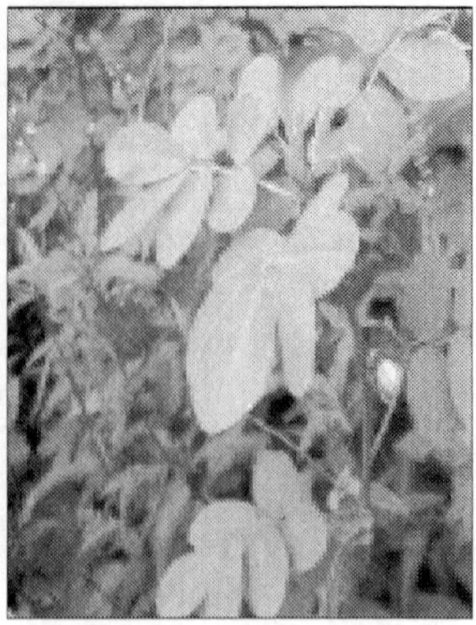

Plate 17.12. *Cassia tora* L.

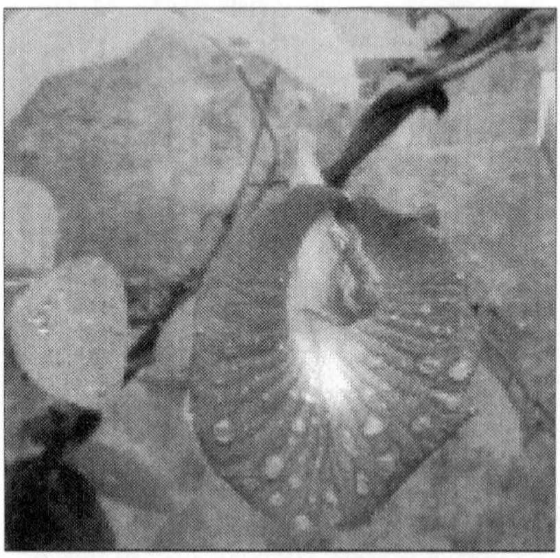

Plate 17.13. *Clitoria ternatea* L.

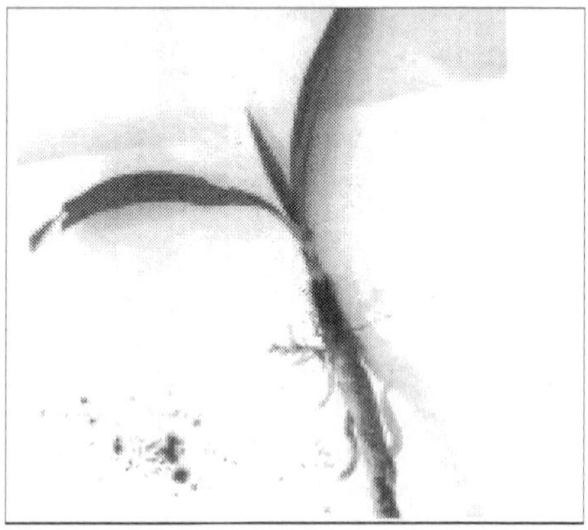

Plate 17.14. *Curculigo orchioides* Gaertn.

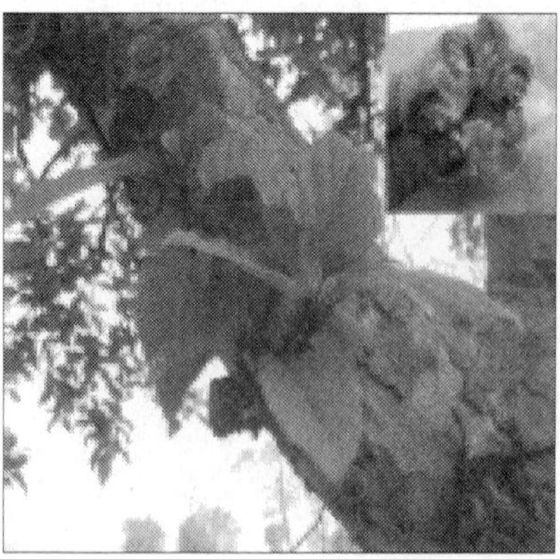

Plate 17.15. *Ficus racemosa* L.

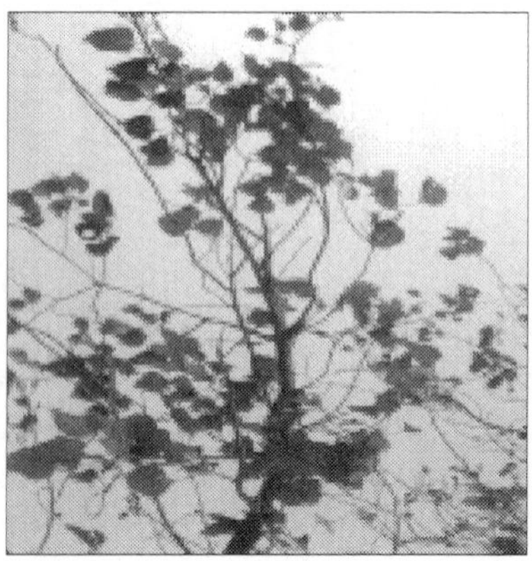

Plate 17.16. *Gmelina arborea* L.

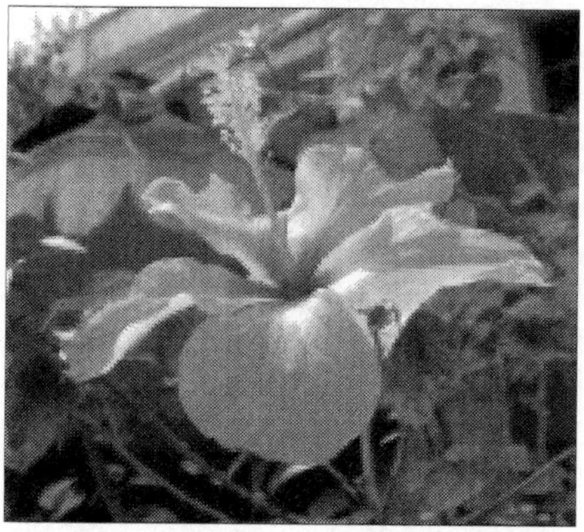

Plate 17.17. *Hibiscus rosa-sinensis* L.

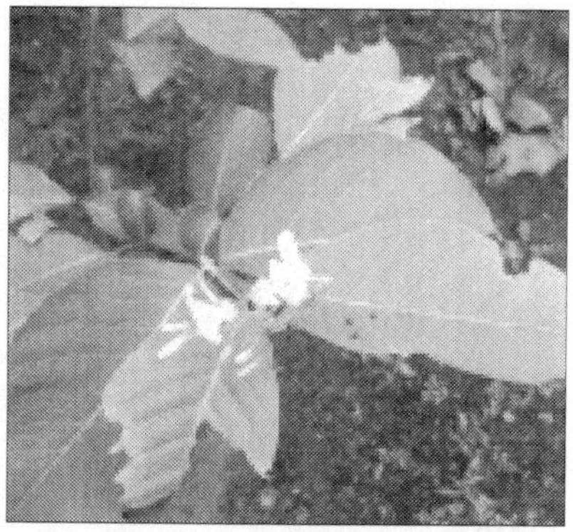

Plate 17.18. *Holarrhena antidysenterica* (Lam.) Wall.

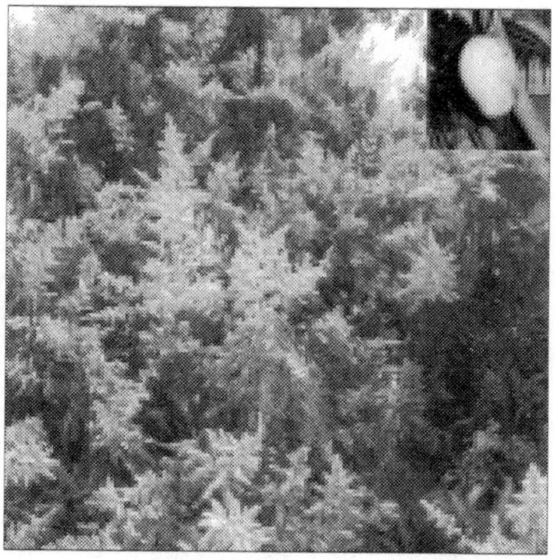

Plate 17.19. *Mangifera indica* L.

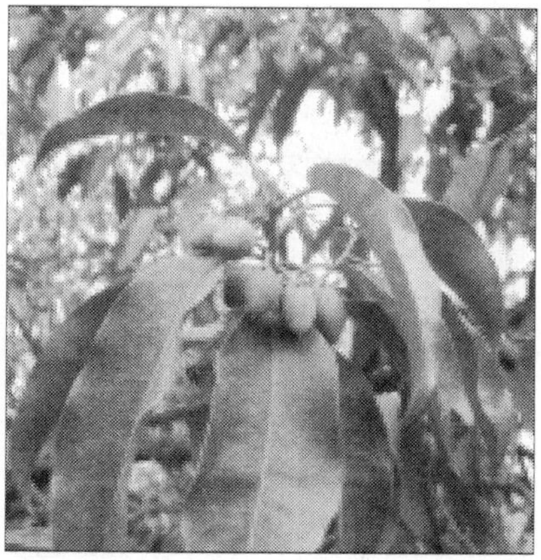

Plate 17.20. *Mimusops elengi* L.

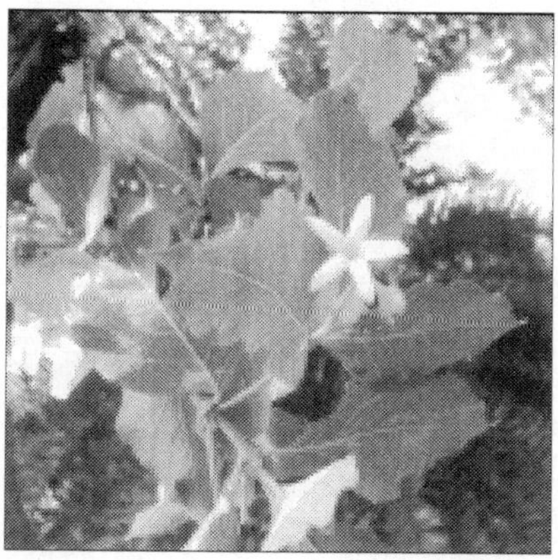

Plate 17.21. *Morinda citrifolia* L.

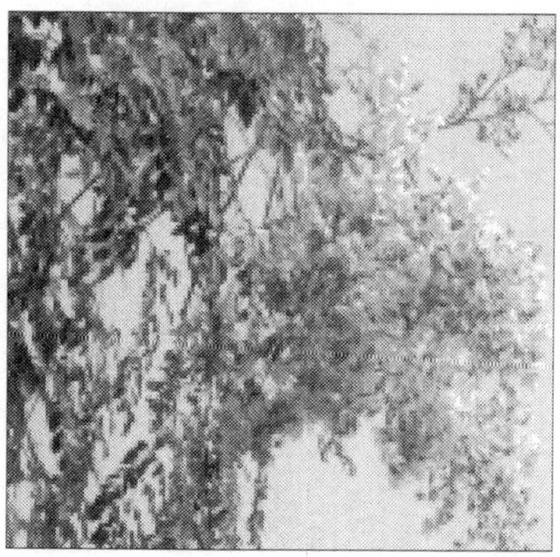

Plate 17.22. *Moringa oleifera* Lamk.

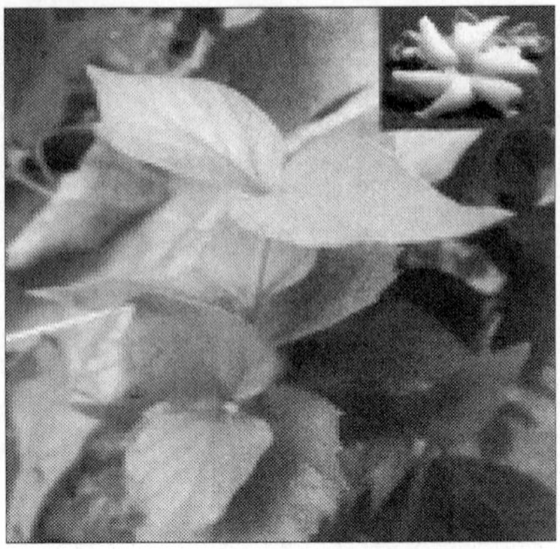

Plate 17.23. *Nyctanthes arbor-tristis* L.

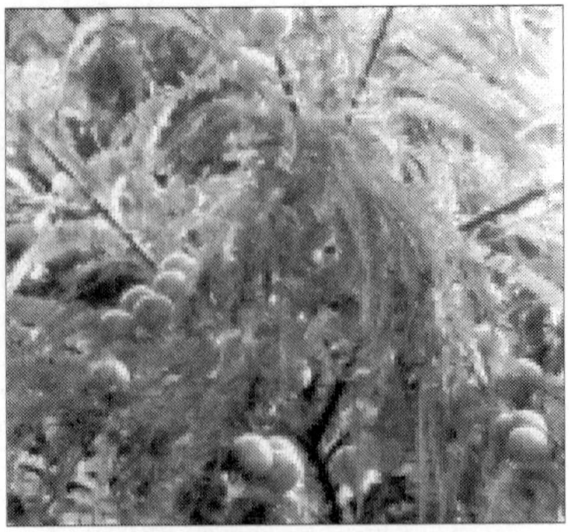

Plate 17.24. *Phyllanthus emblica* L.

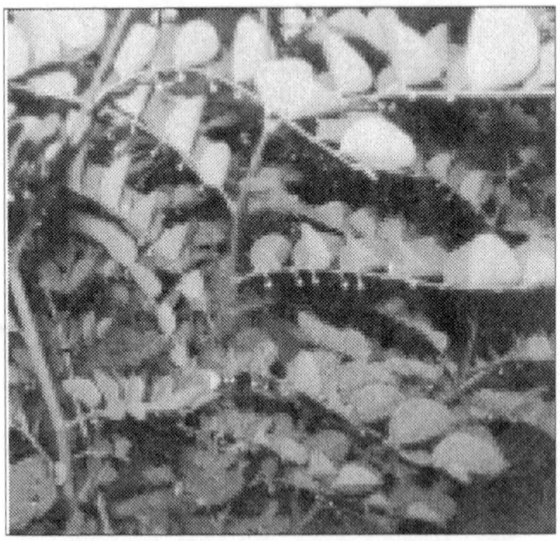

Plate 17.25. *Phyllanthus reticulatus* Poir

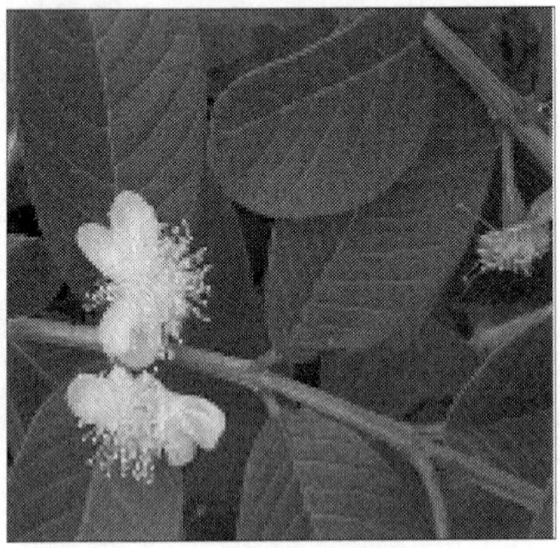

Plate 17.26. *Psidium guajava* L.

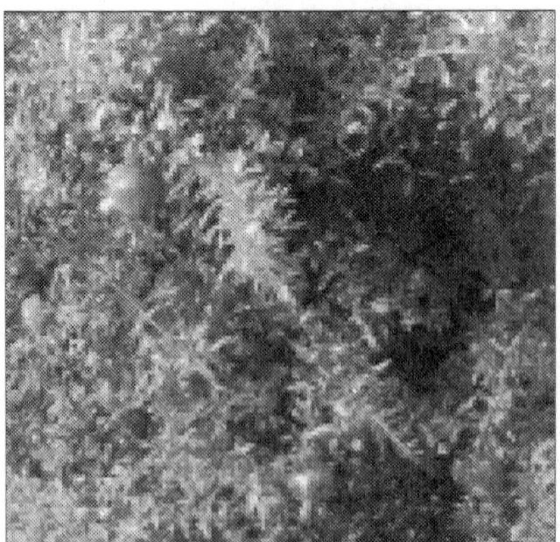

Plate 17.27. *Punica granatum* L.

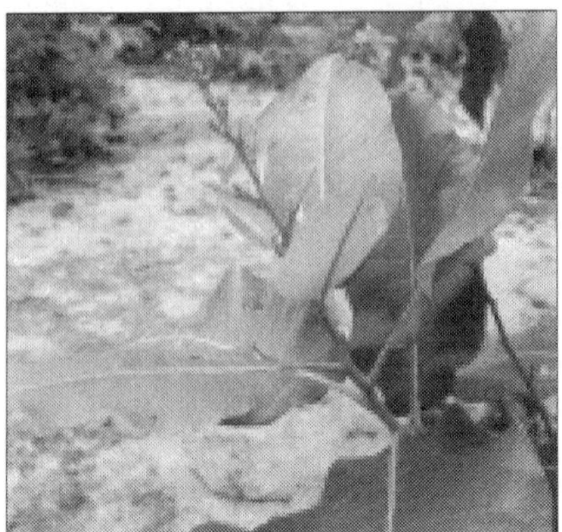

Plate 17.28. *Semecarpus anacardium* L.f.

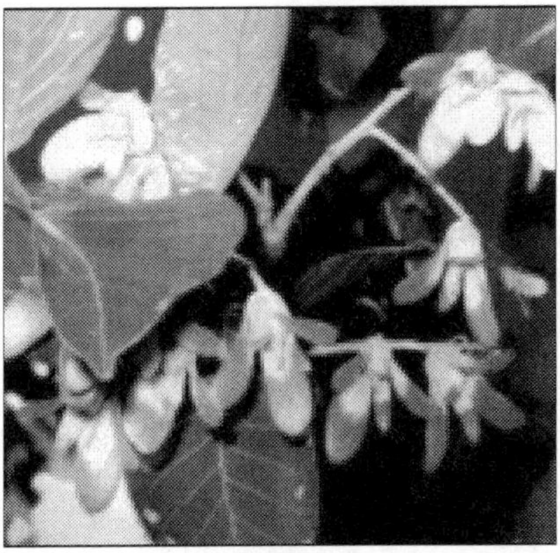

Plate 17.29. *Shorea robusta* Gaert n.f.

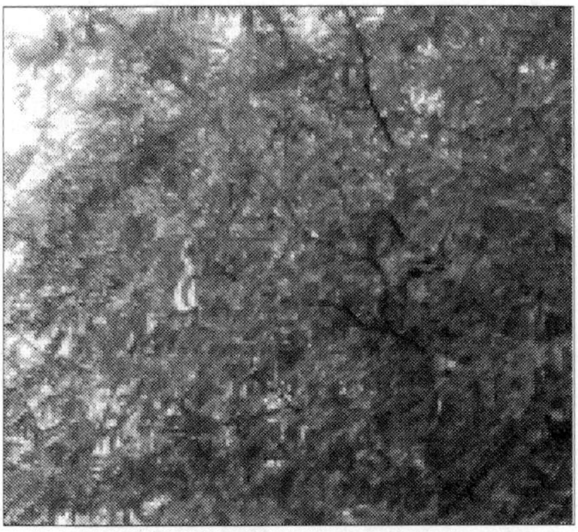

Plate 17.30. *Tamarindus indica* L.

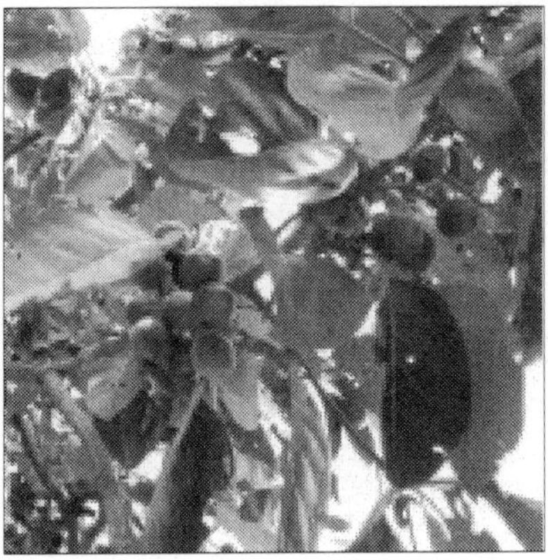

Plate 17.31. *Terminalia bellirica* Roxb. (Gaert n.)

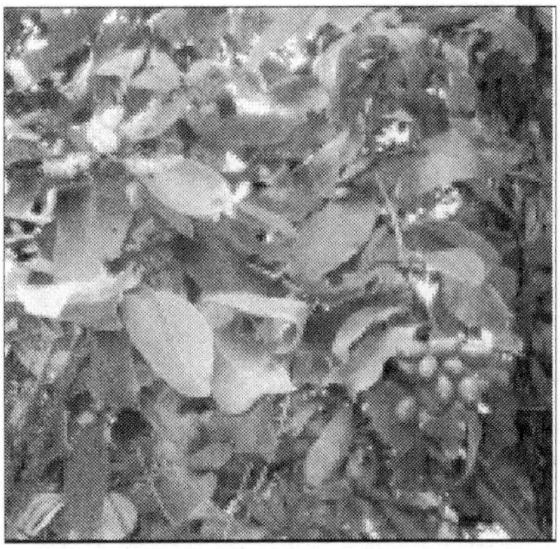

Plate 17.32. *Terminalia chebula* Retz.

Herbal Medicine Men

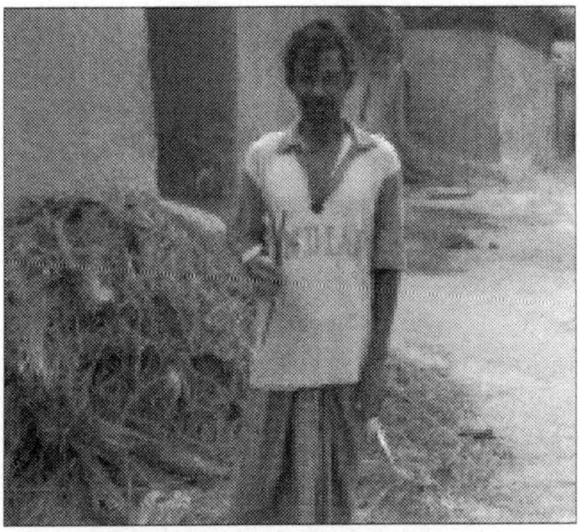

Plate 17.33. Manik Hembram

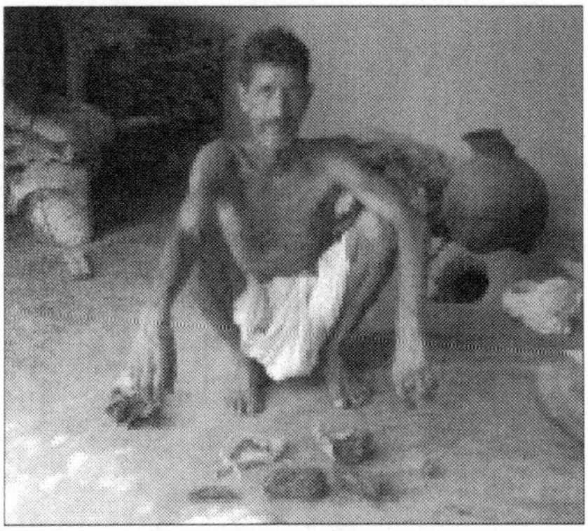

Plate 17.34. Madan Baski

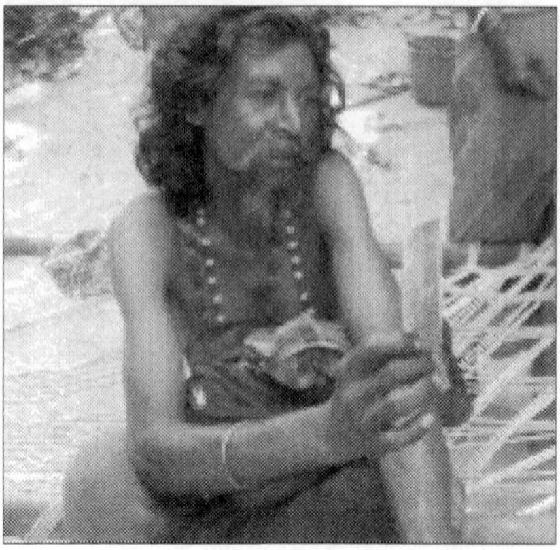

Plate 17.35. Kali Murmu

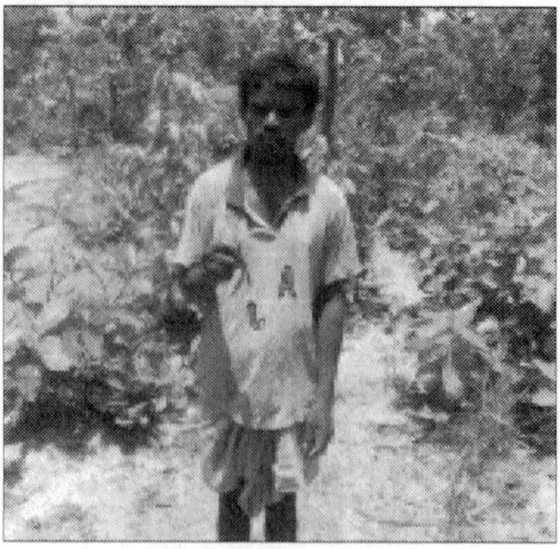

Plate 17.36. Paru Murmu

References

Anonymous, 1998. Project report: All India Co-ordinated Research Project on Ethnobiology, Ministry of Environment and Forests, Government of India, New Delhi.

Bodding, P.O., 'Studies in Santhal Medicines and Connected Folklore: Part I, Santhals and Disease', *Mem. Asiatic Soc. Bengal*, vol. 10, no. 1, 1925, pp. 1–132.

———. *Santal Medicine*, Calcutta: The Book Trust, 1927.

Bressers, J., *The Botany of Ranchi District*, Bihar, 1951.

Chatterjee, K.K., B. Chaudhuri and D. Dasgupta, eds., *Tribal Medicine*, Regional Research and Study Centre, Midnapore, West Bengal, 1989.

Cotton, C.M., *Ethnobotany: Principles and Applications*, New York: John Wiley, 1996.

Cunningham, A.B., *Applied Ethnobotany: People, Wild Plant Use and Conservation*, London and Sterling: Earthscan Publications, 2001.

Das, U. and C.H. Rahaman. 'An observation on the phytotherapeutic uses of plants by the tribal people of some forest areas in Birbhum and Burdwan districts, West Bengal, India, *J. App. Pharm. Sci.*, vol. 4, no. 4, 2014, pp. 72–8.

Das, U., C.H. Rahaman and S. Mandal, 'Traditional Uses of Plant Wealth in Herbal Medicine by the Tribal People of Birbhum District, West Bengal, India', in S. Mandal and S. Bhattacharya, eds. *Advances in Plant Biology (Debidas Bhattacharya Birth Centenary Commemorative Volume)*, Binapani Educational and Welfare Trust, Sriniketan, West Bengal, pp. 400–10.

Ghosh, A., C.H. Rahaman and S. Madal, 'Observation on the Ethnomedicinal Uses of Plants for Gynaecological, Urinogenital and Other Related Problems by the Tribal People of Birbhum and Murshidabad Districts,West Bengal, India', *J. Econ. and Taxon. Bot.*, vol. 35, no. 1, 2011, pp. 17–26.

Goel, A.K., A.K. Sahoo and V. Mudgal, *A Contribution to the Ethnobotany of Santal Pargana*, Calcutta: Botanical Survey of India, 1984.

Jain, S.K., 'Medicinal Plant Lore of Tribals of Baster', *Eco. Bot.*, vol. 19, no. 3, 1965, pp. 236–50.

———, ed., *Glimpses of Indian Ethnobotany*, New Delhi: Oxford and IBH Publ. Co., 1981.

———, ed., *A Manual of Ethnobotany*, Jodhpur: Scientific Publ., 1987.

———, ed., *Methods and Approaches in Ethnobotany*, Society of Ethnobotanists, Lucknow, 1989.

———, *Dictionary of Indian Folk Medicine and Ethnobotany*, New Delhi: Deep Publishers, 1991.

———, ed., *Contribution to Indian Ethnobotany*, Jodhpur: Scientific Publ., 1997.

Jain, S.K. and V. Mudgal, *A Handbook of Ethnobotany*, Dehradun: Bishen Singh Mahendra Pal Singh, Dehradun, 1999.

Jain, S.K. and R.R. Rao, *A Handbook of Field and Herbarium Methods*, New Delhi: Today and Tomorrows, Publ., 1977.

Jamir, N.S., 'Ethnobiology of Naga Tribe in Nagaland: Medicinal Herbs', *Ethnobotany*, vol. 9, 1997, pp. 101–4.

Maheshwari, J.K., *Flora of Delhi*, New Delhi: Council of Scientific and Industrial Research, 1963.

———, ed., *Ethnobotany and Medicinal Plants of Indian Subcontinent*, Jodhpur: Scientific Publ., 2000.

Maheshwari, J.K., K.K. Singh and S. Saha, *The Ethnobotany of Tharus of Kheri district, Uttar Pradesh*, Lucknow: National Botanical Research Institute, 1981.

Mandal, S., 'Ethnobotanical Studies on the Flora of Birbhum District, West Bengal—Some Reports on Herbal Medicine', *Environ. & Ecol.*, vol. 6, 1988, pp. 558–62.

Mandal, S. and R. Yonzone, 'Ethnobotanical Notes on Some Plants used by the Lepchas of Kalimpong, West Bengal, India', *Environ. & Ecol.*, vol. 5, 1987, pp. 741–6.

Manilal, K.S. and V.V. Sivarajan, *Flora of Calicut*, Dehradun: Bishen Singh Mahendra Pal, 1982.

Martin, G.J. *Ethnobotany: A Methods Manual*, London: Chapman and Hall, 1995.

Mondal, S. and C.H. Rahman, 'Medicinal plants used by the tribal people of Birbhum district of West Bengal and Dumka district of Jharkhand in India', *Ind. J. Tradi. Knowledge*, vol. 11, no. 4, 2012, pp. 674–9.

Mondal, S., P. Mukhopadhyay and S. Mandal, 'A Contribution to Some Ethno-medicinally Important Plants of Birbhum District', *Environ. and Ecol.*, vol. 16, 1998, pp. 397–404.

Mudgal, V. and S.K. Jain, *Ethnobotany in India*, Calcutta: Botanical Survey of India, 1983.

Mukherjee, T., 'Medicinal Plants: Need for Protection', in *Medicinal Plants Utilization and Conservation*, ed. P.C. Trivedi, Jaipur: Avishkar Publishers Distributors, 2004, pp. 391–404.

Natesh, S., 'The Changing Scenario of Herbal Drugs: Role of Botanists', *Phytomorphology*, Golden Jubilee, vol. 51, 2001, pp. 75–96.

Pal, D.C. and S.K. Jain, *Tribal Medicine*, Calcutta: Naya Prakash, 1998.

Panigrahi, G. and S.K. Murthy, *Flora of Bilaspur (Madhya Pradesh)*, vol. 1, Calcutta: Botanical Survey of India, 1989.

Rahaman, C.H., *Medicinal and Aromatic Plants of Birbhum District, West Bengal*, Project Report, WBSCS&T, Department of Science and Technology, Government of West Bengal, India, 2011.

Rahaman, C.H. and S. Mandal, 'Ethnomedicinal Studies of Some Plants of Purnea District, Bihar', *Ind. J. Landcape Sys. and Ecol. Studies*, vol. 21, 1998, pp. 173–9.

Rahaman, C.H. and B. Pradhan, 'A Study on Ethnomedicinal Uses of Plants by the Tribal People of Birbhum District, West Bengal', *J. Econ. and Taxon. Bot.*, vol. 35, no. 3, 2011, pp. 24–34.

Rahaman, C.H. and S. Saha, 'Traditional phytotherapies for gynaecological, urine-genital and other related problems practiced among the rural people of Bolpur Subdivision under Birbhum District, West Bengal, India', Columban, *J. Lfe Sci.*, vol. 12, nos. 1&2, 2011, pp. 73–8.

Rahaman, C.H., A. Ghosh and S. Mandal, 'Non-Timber Forest Products: Used by Tribal People with Reference to Ethnomedicine', in *Natural Resource Management and Sustainable Development in North-East India*, ed. N. Ali, New Delhi: Mittal Publ., 2009, pp. 173–82.

———, 'Studies on Ethnomedicinal Uses of Plants by the Tribals of Birbhum District, West Bengal', *Indian J. Environ. and Ecoplan*, vol. 15, nos. 1–2, 2008, pp. 71– 8.

———, 'Studies on the Ethnoveterinary Medicinal Plants used by the Tribals of Birbhum District, West Bengal', *J. Econ. Taxon. Bot.*, vol. 33, 2009, pp. 333–8.

Saldanha, C.J. and H. Dan Nicolson, *Flora of Hassan District*, New Delhi, 1976.

Sanyal, M., *Flora of Bankura District*, Dehradun: Bishen Singh Mahendra Pal Singh, 1994.

Satyavati, G.V., 'Use of Plant Drugs in Indian Traditional Systems of Medicine and their Relevance to Primary Health Care', in *Economic and Medicinal Plant Research: Plants and Traditional Medicine*, ed. H. Wagner and N.R. Farnsworth, London: Academic Press, London, 1990, pp. 39–56.

Singh, V. and R.P. Pandey, *Ethnobotany of Rajasthan, India*, Jodhpur: Scientific Publishers, 1998.

Trivedi, P.C. and N.K. Sharma, *Ethnomedicinal Plants*, Jodhpur: Pointer Publishers, 2004.

Varghese, E., *Applied Ethnobotany: A Case Study among the Kharia of Central India*, New Delhi: Deep Publishers, 1996.

Varghese, E. and P.P. Hembrom, *Ethnomedicinal Lore of the Paharias*, Mumbai: Centre for Human Ecology, 2000.

Varma, S.K., *Flora of Bhagalpur (Dicotyledons)*, New Delhi: Today and Tomorrows Printers and Publishers, 1981.

Yonzone, R. and S. Mandal, 'A Preliminary Report on the Ethnobotanical Survey of Kalimpong in the Darjeeling District, West Bengal', *J. Beng. Nat. Hist. Soc.*, n.s., vol. 1, 1982, pp. 96–9.

Yonzone, R., S. Mandal and S. Chanda, 'A Contribution to the Ethnobotany of Darjeeling Hills', *Trans. Bose. Res. Inst.*, vol. 44, 1981, pp. 75–81.

18

Issues Relating to Ontology Design for Indian Medical System

S.N. OJHA

HEALTH IS ESSENTIALLY an equilibrium between the challenges of nature to the body and the body's ability to resist them, survive and even become stronger. Significant changes have taken place in the twenty-first century in the spectrum of human diseases. The morbidity and mortality of some chronic diseases, such as cardiovascular diseases, cancer and chronic respiratory diseases are significantly trending upwards in increasingly younger patients (Yach et al. 2004). The key question relating to health seems to be whether prevailing scientific methods can describe the entirety of living beings or not. If one assumes that science, in principle, is able to give a complete 'solution' of a living being, and if it is furthermore true that science uses as a conceptual frame some mechanistic form of 'organicism', then (and only then) do we have good reasons to believe that living beings are such organisms and nothing further. If one does not assume that science will ever give a complete solution of a living being, then there is space for a richer form of heuristics than that which comes from an extrapolation from the organism concept which is used on scientific biology.

For many centuries, biology and medicine have been organized principally as descriptive sciences, with much less emphasis on elaborate theories and deduction than on remembering and applying the right chunks of knowledge and experience to experimental or clinical problems. However, now a new era of biomedical science is here. Essential to this new discipline is the application of formal ideas such as logic, probability, and computational methods for organizing and manipulating large-scale repositories of both data and knowledge. Objective support of computer-based aiding tools that store, retrieve, communicate, select, emphasize, analyse, recognize, understand and visualize image-based diagnostic content can make significant improvements in the process of diagnosis and treatment of illness. The data and knowledge take both numerical and symbolic forms. The organizational structure of data and knowledge is an essential part of the enterprise, not just a convenience.

India has its own indigenous medicine systems such as, Ayurveda, Siddha and Unani-tibb which, in stark contrast to the Western medicine system, incorporate religion and spirituality. Indigenous medicine system recognizes that the Western medicine has largely concentrated almost exclusively on growth of complexity in human physiological system. However, the growth in complexity of organism goes hand-in-hand with a concurrent growth in complexity of environment and thus of organism-environment relations. The resurgence of yoga, meditation, etc., in the form of Complementary and Alternative Medicine (CAM) has been enhancing the quantum of information (knowledge) by many-folds.

Western interest in Asian medicine has a long history, dating back to classical times. Western scholars showed little interest in this subject. Even those who cultivated a global perspective on Asian medicine considered it in the shadow of Asian religion, art and philosophy, which is the *locus classicus* of Western interest in Asian conceptions of self, the body, and the world. The Asian art of healing, its scientific theories and epistemologies was overtaken by the cultural wave of 'modernization' and 'Westernization' (Leslie and Young 1992). Now, another acculturation adjustment in attitudes, interpretation, and theories which is bunched together under the tag 'globalization' seems to be causing resurgent interest in biotic healing theories of Asian origin, Ayurveda and Yoga being at the highest priority.

Integration of indigenous knowledge and ethnoscientific approach to contemporary frameworks for management of health and disease will become increasingly important in policies on an international and national level, both in countries that are industrialized and those that have a developing status. This paper attempts to set the scene on how this can be done by exploring the key conditions and dimensions of a dialogue between 'ontologies' and the roles, which ethnosciences could play in this process.

Socio-historical Setting of Western Medical System

If one has to understand the role and utility of Indian medicine system, it is pertinent to understand and contrast it with the Western medicine system which has grown in to the discipline of 'biomedicine'. Recall of some momentous events in the history of biomedicine may help to delineate three interrelated ontological spheres (concepts of existence), viz., scientific enterprise, symbolic-cultural expression and expression of social power within capitalistic society (Baronov 2008).

The scientific aspect of biomedicine states that it is based on strict empirical norms of the experimental sciences. Its development may be correlated with eighteenth-century rise of the physical sciences. Its scientific-material content is attuned for universal beliefs and practices. The prevailing utilitarian, instrumentalist ethics lead to a belief in progress and the ability to control nature by replacing the fatalistic reliance upon god's will. Observation, measurement, and experimentation, modelled after the investigative techniques of Galileo and Newton, lead to epistemological shift for assuring truth and objectivity. The biomedicine also represents a versatile social edifice that encapsulates the nineteenth century material-ideological format of Western capitalist societies and hence is a symbolic-cultural expression of that period. This differentiates it from culture-bound ethnomedicine from medical systems in other, non-Western, cultural settings. Biomedicine appeared in Western world during an era of social and political upheavals unleashed by industrial capitalism leading to concentrated economic power and a long chain of social dislocation (Hobsbawm 1989). Obviously, biomedicine is considered to have born at the intersection of competing social forces in the late nineteenth century. 'Medicine's burst of development came with the displacement of the criterion of truth from tradition and rationality to 'look and see' (Gordon 1988).

Western advancements in medical knowledge met with success by succeeding taking medicine forward humoural pathology through Thomas Sydenham's doctrine of specificity to the current genome mapping that were made possible by dramatic shifts in how medical science was conducted and understood. This history is marked by major moments of advance (e.g. bacteriology) and also long periods of stagnation. The primary task of scientific medicine, thus, shifted to mapping the variety of distinct diseases and their causes. After Sydenham helped find nosology (the science of classifying diseases), Linné, Boissier de Sauvages, Cullen and others went on to create the grand nosological systems of the eighteenth and nineteenth centuries based on symptom clusters that classified diseases into orders, families, genera, and species. Pathological anatomy, however, required the observation of conditions within the body and therefore, the physician had to rely on a patient's description of symptoms. The situation changed greatly after the mid-eighteenth century with the introduction of Auenbrugger's percussion technique and Laennec's stethoscope about 60 years later. Yet, the diagnosis of disease continued to be an art and only partially a science. This changed from mid-nineteenth century with successive inventions of ophthalmoscope, otoscope, and laryngoscope to examine the eye, ear, and throat, respectively, as also Röntgen's X-rays. The set of medical gadgetry created a superlative sense of detached objectivity and greater certainty in measurement of physiological phenomena, akin to the methods in physics and chemistry. The widespread use of precision equipment set the stage for 'germ theory' embedded in Robert Koch's discovery of *tubercle bacillus* and Louis Pasteur's rabies vaccine. The germ theory put forward that diseases have specific and definite causes and therefore, organized medical research relating to microbes, infection and its transmission became the primary focus. For biomedicine, the body as a whole (the person) was less and less a primary point of reference. The Western medicine shaped a worldview for most of the developed and several developing countries at the turn of twentieth century and it became a standard against which the indigenous ethnomedicines were compared.

The world view of Western medicine endorsed the scientific objectivity of detached, impersonal and technocratic approach (organicism) in medical care. The physician started to set himself apart from the human patient like an engineer repairing the machinery. 'The Cartesian schema was a stroke of scholastic genius. It legitimated the study of the body as a mechanism by the science of physiology and preserved the soul as the domain of theology' (Eisenberg 1977). The standard metaphor of a machine in need of occasional fine-tuning and repair remains the most common biomedical image of the human body and stands as a lasting testament to biomedicine's eighteenth-century Enlightenment roots. Harvey's description of the circulation of blood, to take just one example, was celebrated as a direct application of Newton's mechanical physics (Wightman 1971). Biomedicine's objectivity and its foothold in germ theory led to least priority consideration for broader social, cultural and institutional contexts in its approach. Further, the treatment remedied the physiological abnormalities arising from the socio-cultural stress and not the stress itself.

However, adoption of biomedicine across the Western nations is not uniform. Payer studied some extreme difference and opined that the actual disease diagnoses can be a function of one's nationality. The same clinical signs may even receive different diagnoses. Often, all one must do to acquire a disease is to enter a country where that disease is recognized—leaving the country will either cure the malady or turn it into something else' (Payer 1988: 25).

Baronov (2008) has pointed out that biomedicine emerged in a specific place (Western Europe and North America), at a unique time (the later nineteenth century), under particular social conditions (industrial capitalism and the consolidation of monopoly corporate power). Therefore, its institutionalization is an expression of social power shaped through interplay of a particular set of social, economic, and political forces. It received favour from a group of powerful social classes who chalked out its growth by deciding on the practitioners, the medicine, the earnings, as well as the conditions for medical practices.

Porter (1997) and Baer (1989) have reported that allopaths' methodologies of 'bleeding, blistering, purging and high-dosage medication' were often looked down due to physical inconvenience and low success rate and common man had a dreary and fear-provoking image of allopathic physicians. The authors argue that the process by which allopathic physicians overtook the medical care in the US (in league with a powerful national lobby, a core group of elite medical schools and major corporate sponsors) helps to explain, in part, the story of how biomedicine came to control US medical care by the early twentieth century.

Incorporation of Advanced Digital Technologies

Obviously, the fledgling field of Information Technology could not have been a mute spectator. Information Technology not only supports the medical practice of today, but also makes new challenges and opportunities stimulating the progress in medicine. The Holter ECG recorders, Computed Tomography or the rapidly evolving abilities to manipulate images during pre-operative planning to increase accuracy of surgical treatment may be evoked as direct examples of such inventions. Medical image perception is a very complex activity involving interplay between vision and cognition, and requiring detection, classification and actionable decision tasks performed on highly variable objects (lesions, for example). However, humans are limited in their ability to detect and diagnose disease during image interpretation due to their non-systematic search patterns and to the presence of structured noise-masking normal and abnormal anatomical background. Observer variation is due to many factors—the degree of individual training, experience, interest, imaging equipment and the quality of technical work performed. The remark that an experienced physician usually sees a visible lesion clearly but there are times when he does not, is still up to date. This is a baffling problem, apparently partly visual and partly psychological. It constitutes the still unexplained human equation in diagnostic procedures. Two most prominent reasons for essentiality of new technology should be recalled. First, there has been data deluge in biomedicine, especially after genomics emerged. Second, the emphasis on evidence-based care demanded exploration of empirical data from across the global biomedicine laboratories. The responses have been to put more reliance on internet-based technologies, online bibliographic databases and electronic publication practices.

The 'Evidence-Based Medicine' (EBM) paradigm (Fig. 18.2) is centred on the concept of 'best evidence' and clinical studies based on this approach are more likely to be considered by physicians in their practice. In the following sections, the concept and use of ontology under the computational field of 'Artificial Intelligence' or simply AI, for representing the core theory involved in integrative medicine and meta-analysis have been discussed. It has already been argued as to how an ontological approach can be applied both for reviving the foundations of ethnomedicine and for allowing a more effective knowledge-based information retrieval in literature (Pisanelli et al. 2003).

Sharing and reusing large subsets of the medical terminology has become a necessity in various areas, such as knowledge-based systems, information retrieval, standardization, etc. The main obstacle to sharing and reusing medical terminologies is the lack of conceptual integration of terms across various medical systems and diverse politico-socio-cultural units. Actually, the intended meaning of terms is different according to the context in which they appear and to the context of use. Interdisciplinary research in ontology provides good evidence that use of generic ontologies specified from the literature is the grounding matter for conceptual integration of terminologies. Detailed generic theories require rich languages and tools as well as collaborative effort to be extensively used.

Impact of Modern Technology

The modern computing paradigm gave rise to further innovation which spreads rapidly, creates a circular relation of means to ends, and in its lap progress is not just an ideology, but an 'inherent drive of technological society'.

The rise of biomedicine in tandem with modern technologies has somewhat led to re-conceptualization in medical system. For example, yesterday's slow learner is today the one who suffers from a disease called attention-deficit/hyperactivity disorder and is treated with drugs and senility has become alzheimer's disease. New diagnostic processes have enabled observers to make clinico-pathological correlations, thereby increasing efforts to improve quality of care, decrease in healthcare costs, and implementation of more efficient and productive means. Simultaneously, there has been incidence of accented scholarship in integration, application, and teaching of knowledge.

The information overload entreats knowing how to organize information and how to conduct effective information searches. This has asked for interdisciplinarity as a norm in not just biomedicine but also in Complimentary and Alternative Medicine (CAM) studies. Research is required in three critical areas, namely, organizational systems-level research into the design of health care systems processes and workflow; computable knowledge structures and models for medicine needed to make sense of available patient data including preferences, health behaviours, and so on; and human-computer interaction in a clinical context.

This has created a new breed of experts, Health Information Management (HIM) professional, who are inclined to take up and imbibe new kind of research and scholarship as opportunities arise. A more daunting task for the health professions, however, was building a body of knowledge based on sound, systematic research that validated the discipline's scope of practice.

The health professionals require dealing with the data deluge through codified unification of health informatics emerging from the global researches. Consequently, there has been evolution of miscellaneous classification systems (Codification Standards) such as ICD-10-CM, CPT, SNOMED CT and a few more.

C03	**Malignant neoplasm of gum** *Includes:* alveolar (ridge) mucosa gingiva *Excludes:* malignant odontogenic neoplasms (C41.0–C41.1)
C03.0	**Upper gum**
C03.1	**Lower gum**
C03.9	**Gum, unspecified**
C04	**Malignant neoplasm of floor of mouth**
C04.0	**Anterior floor of mouth** Anterior to the premolar-canine junction

Fig. 18.1: Examples of WHO's International Classification of Diseases (ICD-10), which is used for all general epidemiological, health management and clinical purposes

What is Ontology under Artificial Intelligence

Several philosophers—from Aristotle (fourth century BC) to Leibnitz (1646–1716), and more recently the nineteenth-century major ontologists like Bolzano, Brentano, Husserl and Frege have provided criteria for distinguishing between different kinds of objects (e.g. concrete *vs.* abstract) and the relations between them. In the late twentieth century, Artificial Intelligence (AI) adopted the term and began using it in the sense of a 'specification of a conceptualization' in the context of knowledge and data sharing (Gruber 1995). In Artificial Intelligence, ontology is specification of a conceptualization, a body of knowledge, describing facts assumed to be always true by a community of users. The conceptualization is 'an abstract, simplified view of the world that wish to represent for some purpose'. Given a domain, its ontology forms the heart of any system of knowledge representation for that domain.

Guarino and Welty (2000) provide the following definition for an ontology: 'A set of logical axioms designed to account for the intended meaning of a vocabulary', whereas Sowa (2000) proposes the following: 'The subject of ontology is the study of the categories of things that exist or may exist in some domain. The product of such a study, called an ontology, is a catalog of the types of things that are assumed to exist in a domain of interest D from the perspective of a person who uses a language L for the purpose of talking about D.'

From an AI perspective, therefore, ontology is not only a discipline, but also the outcome of the activity of ontological analysis and modelling. In this sense, one can speak of 'ontology of cardiac valves' or 'ontology of inflammation'. Such ontologies are examples of the so-called 'domain ontologies', whereas 'foundational ontologies' represent domain-independent concepts like objects, events, processes. Ontology-based applications have also been built in the field of Medical Natural Language Processing. Gómez-Pérez et al. (2004) propose the following list of ontology types:

1. Knowledge representation (KR) ontologies
2. General or common ontologies
3. Top-level ontologies or upper ontologies
4. Domain ontologies
5. Task ontologies
6. Domain-task ontologies
7. Method ontologies
8. Application ontologies

Not all of these types of ontology can be found in the field of medical informatics, and some are more relevant to the understanding than others.

The use of ontologies in medicine is mainly focused on the representation and reorganization of medical terminologies. Physicians developed their own specialized languages and lexicons to help them store and communicate general medical knowledge and patient-related information efficiently. The rationale for clinical coding is that it will make it possible to associate with the terms used by humans in expressing patient data, the sorts of uniform syntax and precise meanings that can be interpreted by software. There are 12 current terminology projects: Galen, the Unified Medical Language System (UMLS), the Medical Entities Dictionary (MED), SNOMED-CT, LOINC, the Foundational Model of Anatomy (FMA), the Gene Ontology (GO), ISO Reference Terminology Model for Nursing Diagnosis, NDF-RT, RxNorm, the NCI Thesaurus, and DOLCE+. Such terminologies, optimized for human processing, are characterized by a significant amount of implicit knowledge. Medical information systems need to be able to communicate complex and detailed medical concepts (possibly expressed in different languages) unambiguously. This is obviously a difficult task and requires a profound analysis of the structure and the concepts of medical terminologies. But it can be achieved by constructing medical domain ontologies for representing medical terminology systems.

An integration of information should incorporate a theory of the reality to which both coding systems and electronic health records may be connected. The last two decades have seen considerable efforts directed towards making electronic health records interoperable through improvements in medical ontologies, terminologies and coding systems. Unfortunately, these efforts have been hampered by a number of influential ideas inherited from the work of Eugen Wüster, the father of terminology standardization and the founder of ISO TC 37 (Smith et al. 2005). Wüster's influence led to a pervasive confusion between concepts and entities in reality. In contrast, the author proposes that applying a pragmatic ontology to coding systems and to EHR architectures (Gordana and Susan 2006) means, in the first place, ensuring that the latter are calibrated to such mundane things as—particular patients, diseases, therapies, surgical acts, and the universals which they instantiate—which form the subject matter of healthcare. In this way, one can make coding systems more coherent, both internally and in their relation to the EHRs which they are designed to support, and externally in relation to the patients, physicians, nurses, etc., toward whom they are directed.

Why Ontology

Elicitation and application of the medical expert knowledge using his willing expression may not be accepted as the objective measure. Although assumed not to be biased intentionally, it is influenced by several mental factors. Two principal factors are: memorization and verbalization.

Memorization uses the short-term memory and a part of human attention to capture his own behaviour. The behaviour is, thus, not spontaneous as it were naturally and the auto-observation usually implies subconscious auto-restriction. As a result the memorized facts are altered and not complete.

Verbalization is necessary to express the memorized knowledge with a limited set of tokens belonging to a specified vocabulary. Such dictionary depends on the language used, but is also influenced by subjective preferences of the speaker. Therefore, the output of an interview with an expert concerning his own reasoning may not be considered more seriously as discrete, rather it could lead to incomplete and inaccurate impressions.

Observer performance improvement, i.e. increased stability, perfection, repeatability and reliability, is the main purpose of computer assistance. It starts with clarification (standardization and normalization) in more objective description of normal and abnormal findings including variability of symptoms regardless of acquisition parameters and technical conditions.

Knowledge Sharing

Biomedical data arising from various medical systems are heterogeneous, highly variable in size as well as type and structure, but from molecules to humans to populations, there are some common themes. The varieties of biomedical data have some biological and technical aspects in common. Some of the technical aspects include how to encode something that is not a numeric measurement (gene and protein sequences, organ names and relationships, descriptions of clinical findings, names of diseases, etc.), how to organize both numeric and non-numeric data for easy retrieval and interpretation, and how to represent hierarchical relationships or groupings of data that have an *a priori* relationship (e.g. a collection of genes whose expression levels are being measured or a set of related blood tests). Some of the biological aspects include how to represent higher level phenomena (e.g. phenotypes, diseases, and therapies) in relation to lower level ones (e.g. genotypes, cellular and organ level processes, and body structure), and how to systematically and consistently assign names and classifications to all the entities, processes, and relationships.

The International Medical Informatics Association WG6 has made recommendations for development of conceptual models and ontologies in medicine. This section relates the recommendations to the nature of biomedical concepts as illustrated in Fig. 18.2.

Interoperability

It denotes capability of information systems to exchange (functional interoperability) and meaningfully use (semantic interoperability) the data units. The diversity of goals, approaches, and achievements across the different medical systems (indigenous or Western) and communities according to their main orientation, which may be patient's care, research or public health, make it difficult to get an overall picture of the scope of medicine in order to agree on generally accepted medical terminologies. Often, medical terms and definitions differ between groups, with different groups not infrequently using identical terms with different meanings. Interoperability is essential when it comes to moving information from one system to another, be it in the same hospital, between different hospitals, or even across national borders. Systems need to have similar (or even the same) 'conceptualizations' of the world described by the software for enabling free movement of information. Interoperability is obviously essential to ensure that ontological systems are safe for the patients.

Reusability of Software Components

Building medical knowledge-based systems or patient databases has entailed, until now, constructing new conceptual representation from scratch. It could instead incorporate reusable external components. Ontologies can be used to bridge the different notions in both patient databases and medical knowledge bases, and thus, participate in making databases and knowledge bases manageable as parts of a large information infrastructure for both health care and research. Thus, a new medical system would interoperate with existing systems and could be used for clinical decision since declarative knowledge, problem-solving techniques, and reasoning services could be shared among systems. This approach would facilitate building larger and more accurate systems for patient's health care and research.

Global Models for Knowledge

Biological knowledge bases (ontologies) such as GO, EcoCyc, the FMA, and others are collections of information about classes of biological entities, in contrast to the data from individuals (electronic medical records). The terms in medical terminology systems such as Galen and the UMLS refer to classes of phenomena and entities. For example, a frame called 'pneumonia' refers to the disease phenomenon in general, not to particular occurrences in individual patients.

Description of Huge Amounts of Information

Ontologies use a chosen construct of software logic, such as 'description logic' or DL to create the data repositories which can be manipulated for knowledge extraction. The basic idea of a DL is that entities (individuals and classes) are defined by their *descriptions*, i.e. what properties they have. A description is a formula made up of terms and connectors or operators. There are many DLs, each with its own sets of connectors from which it builds descriptions. The entities represented by the terms in a DL formula are *Concepts*, *Roles*, and *Individuals*. They are related by connectors and qualifiers, but the collection of connectors may vary from one DL to another. Some DL implementations even leave out individuals and represent only concepts and roles. The concepts and roles are kept together (both abstractly and in typical implementations) in a container called the *TBox*. The TBox consists of all the *terminological* descriptions. DL systems that support descriptions about individuals have another container called the *ABox*. The ABox consists of all these *assertional* descriptions, so-called because they assert facts about individuals.

On the basis of the experience in genomics, some additional criteria for medical ontologies may be suggested as follows:

A Common Framework: There are several systems/natural languages for various ethnomedicines. A translation framework for semantic compatibility is required to be the part of medical ontologies.

Knowledge-Based (KB) Systems: Such a system would be based on the principle of formal knowledge representation. This will ensure semantic cross-verification by the practitioner-users of the ontologies.

Mechanism: Interoperability across several medical groups would make it mandatory to associating several components. For example, the Ayurveda system will be more dependent on the pulse-rate rather than blood examination report. The opposite may be true in allopathy. Hence, both the components, clinical symptoms as well as pathological descriptions, must be included for interoperability.

Annotated KB Models: The quantitative description may be associated with symbolic knowledge for unambiguity. For example, in large data stores such as Genbank, the sequences are often thought of as the primary data, and are the subject of much computation (sequence comparisons, sequence searching for small patterns like motifs). However, there is a lot of knowledge in the annotations, the text information that accompanies each sequence. This is generally not in an easily computable form, but it is computationally powerful material. For example, information about which protein(s) a gene encodes, and what the function(s) and pathways in which it participates is useful for reasoning about cellular metabolism. Projects like GO are a step towards making these pieces of knowledge the basic elements of a computational scheme. Another example is the EcoCyc ontology of metabolic pathways in *E. coli* and its generalization to many other organisms.

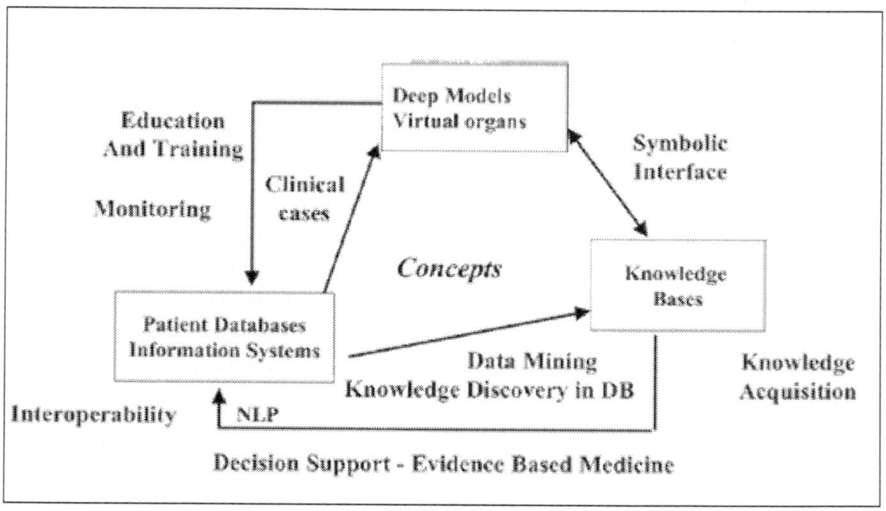

Fig. 18.2: Ontologies as core of medical system (Burgun et al. 2001)

Information Indexing: It involves organization of huge repositories of encyclopedic knowledge, expert knowledge and epidemiologic knowledge for availability across the user community. The search results should provide answer to the queries on defined principles. In other words, meticulous indexing of information is essential to render it usable by the partially computer literate audience.

Principles and Design Criteria

Exact application of the design principles of bio-ontologies poses certain constraints. Difficulties in the biomedical domain arise from the fact that medical concepts are empirical rather than perfectly defined, leading to semantic and conceptual adaptation.

Parsimony

As a general principle, bio-ontologies contain enough concepts but only those concepts that are strictly necessary. However, the ADM system, developed in France since the 1970s and containing information on more than 15,000 diseases or syndromes, contains 1,859 items for pain. For example, Fig. 18.3 depicts a table enlisting a subset of those items for facial pain. This shows the use of adjectives and qualifiers in medical objects, which arises from richness of meticulous patients observations, described by subtle attributes.

Clarity

Ontologies are required to communicate the intended meaning. If possible, logical axioms should be used for definitions to enhance the clarity. However, in medicine, it constitutes a difficult proposition. For example, Couinaud classification of liver anatomy divides the liver into eight independent segments, but traditional English-speaking authors, described liver in terms of segments, lobes, etc., but differently. In effect, ontologies seek that definitions should be objective and independent of human or computational context.

Categories Versus Terms

Ontologies should not aim at the specification of the terms, because there is a vast quantity of rather loosely defined terminology. Ontologies should also be language independent, which means independently motivated and not dictated by the linguistic patterns of a particular language. However, stumbling blocks appear in such cases as for example the concepts that are denoted by croup, croup syndrom, laryngeal spasm, laryngismus stridulus which are not the same for the French and for the American.

Coherence

This property requires that the defining axioms should be logically consistent. It means that the deduced information should not contradict a stored fact.

S21264 Facial pain
S68032 Facial pain: wrench type
S68061 Facial pain like burning
S68033 Facial pain like stab
S68030 Facial pain like bite
S68031 Facial pain like electric shock
S68020 Facial pain aggravated by swallowing
S68021 Facial pain aggravated by phonation
S68007 Facial pain calmed by massage of superficial temporal artery
S37630 Continuous facial pain
S37634 Continuous facial pain with paroxysms
S37639 Continuous facial pain with night paroxysms
S68014 Facial pain starting with phonation
S68015 Facial pain starting with tooth brushing
S15525 Diurnal facial pain
S37658 Shooting facial pain
S40715 Searing facial pain
S02217 Intense facial pain
S40346 Night facial pain
S37670 Facial pain that is not reduced by usual drugs
S37667 Paroxystic facial pain
S68013 Deep facial pain
S20719 Facial pain starting with swallowing
S37663 Rhythmical facial pain
S70977 Dull facial pain
S40714 Spontaneous facial pain

Fig. 18.3: Extract from ADM system enlisting facial pain

Following principles (axiomatic specification, Burgun et al. 2001) provides testing criteria for logical coherence as illustrated in Fig. 18.4:

1. Similarity Principle: child must share the meaning of a parent
2. Specificity Principle: child must differ from its parent in a distinctive way
3. Opposition Principle: distinguishable from and among its siblings
4. Unique Semantic Axis Principle: all subtypes must differ from their father on a common axis

Ambiguities

Liss et al. (2003) have discussed the term urinary tract infection (UTI) to show that a concept used widely within medical practice can be, and is described and defined in many different ways. Bodenreider and Burgun (2006) have cited some examples for abounding ambiguities in the medical definitions. For example, the ICD-9 code 'hematuria' is much more specific than the

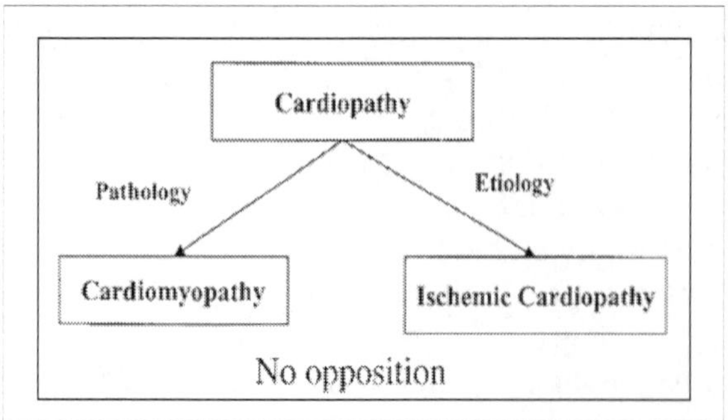

Fig. 18.4: Cardiopathy has two children which are cardiomyopathy and ischemic cardiopathy. With respect to the opposition principle, those siblings should not be compatible. But one cannot say that cardiomyopathy and ischemic cardiopathy are opposite since a cardiomyopathy can be caused by ischemy. Opposition of siblings exists when a unique principle for differentiation is applied (Burgun et al. 2001).

corresponding biomedical specialty 'urology'. Medical concepts are empirical rather than perfectly defined, leading to semantic and conceptual adaptation. Medicine, including research areas such as molecular biology or genetics, has historically used many terminological systems, i.e. classifications, thesauri, vocabularies, nomenclatures and various unstructured coding systems with diverse purposes.

As more biomedical ontologies are created, users might be tempted to integrate these sets of concepts and relations into a single system. However, the analysis of the differences in representation of blood (Fig. 18.5) illustrated the limitations of a naïve approach to merging ontologies, even when representations occur within a single theory of the domain (i.e. Western medicine). While difference in granularity is usually not a problem, different naming conventions, the lack of reliable textual definitions and the lack of explicit and consistently applied classificatory principles may result in merging difficulties. Additional difficulty is encountered when attempting to merge ontologies that convey different theories of the domain (e.g. Western and oriental medicine or modem medical knowledge and pre-scientific representations of the human body). In this case, the target system must be able to clearly identify the underlying theories and to represent them separately.

Developing Concept-Term Relation for Indian System

The modern, Western system of medicine reaches only a small group of people, it is understood that over half of the population of the world has no share in it. In India, the overwhelming majority of people receive medical service from traditional practitioners, who treat their patients according to the principles of Ayurveda. Also, in Sri Lanka, Bangladesh and Nepal a vast majority of the masses has been looking up to Ayurveda in its pure form or some of its variations

a. WordNet

Blood
- Liquid body substance
- • Body substance
- • • Substance
- • • • Entity

b. OpenGALEN

Blood
- Soft tissue
- • Tissue
- • • Body substance
- • • • Organic substance
- • • • • Substance
- • • • • • Generalised substance
- • • • • • • Phenomenon

c. UMLS

Blood
- Tissue
- • Fully-formed anatomical structure
- • • Anatomical structure
- • • • Physical object
- • • • • Entity

d. SNOMED CT

Blood
- Blood material
- • Body fluid
- • • Body substance
- • • • Substance

e. FMA

Blood
- Body substance
- • Material physical anatomical entity
- • • Physical anatomical entity
- • • • Anatomical entity

f. MENELAS

Blood
- Body fluid
- • Tissue
- • • Mass object
- • • • Real object
- • • • • Physical object
- • • • • • Abstract object
- • • • • • • Substratum
- • • • • • • • Entity

Fig. 18.5: Representation of blood in several biomedical ontologies (Bodenreider and Burgun 2006: 228)

in some form or other, for relief of various ailments. This is how Ayurveda has come to attract the attention of WHO.

The healing system of ancient cultures was inseparable from the cultures' religious beliefs and practices and had even some magic ingrained in it, as one find in ancient civilizations of India, Egypt and Mesopotamia. The *Rig Veda* refers to the notion of *tridaddu* in which the concept of *dhatu* (tissue) is one among the three most important clusters of ideas, the doctrine of *tri-doshas* (three humours) and *mala* (waste products) being the other two (Griffith 2009; Wujastyk 2001). Archeological evidences indicate the regular application of surgical practices in this pre-Aryan civilization. Meera Roy (1986) has traced the fact that Indo-Aryan (Vedic) medical practices facilitated the growth of certain concepts and theories relating to aetiology of diseases and three basic constituents of living organisms (*vata* or wind, *pitta* or bile and *kapha* or phlegm) which originated during pre-Aryan period. It may not be inapt to summarize the discussion on ontology for Indian traditional medicines by quoting the following extract from Microsoft Encarta (Sikorski and Peters 2008):

> The practices of ancient Hindu, or Vedantic, medicine (1500–1000 BC) are described in the works of two later physicians, Charaka (lived about AD second century) and Susruta (lived about AD fourth century). Susruta gave recognizable descriptions of malaria, tuberculosis, and diabetes. He also wrote about Indian hemp, or Cannabis, and henbane for inducing anesthesia, and included specific antidotes and highly skilled treatments

for bites of venomous snakes. An ancient Hindu drug derived from the root of the Indian plant *Rauwolfia serpentina* was the source of the first modern tranquilizer. In the field of surgery, the Hindus are acknowledged to have attained the highest skill in all antiquity. They were probably the first to perform successful skin grafting and plastic surgery for the nose.

With the rise of Buddhism, the study of anatomy was prohibited, and with the Muslim conquest of India, beginning around AD 1000, the field of medicine further declined and ultimately stagnated. Nevertheless, much valuable knowledge concerning hygiene, diet, and surgery was passed to the West through the writings of Indian physicians.

Ayurveda, as a science, deals with animal and vegetable medicines and enlists a comprehensive description of the chemical properties and medicinal worth of hundreds of species of flora. This enormous knowledge of time-tested scientific scrutiny and systematization inherited through generations of physicians could be mapped out as an apt starting point for ontological representation of the Indian and Western systems of medicine.

Terminological research and development have advanced significantly in the past 25 years or so, leading to creation of controlled biomedical ontologies. This work has had significant impact on the development of terminologies themselves, their acceptance and dissemination as standards, and their use in supporting biomedical information systems. Biomedical informatics involves a core set of methodologies that can provide a foundation for crossing the cultural barriers associated with the socio-political orientation of medicine. To this end, the fundamental aspects of biomedical informatics (e.g. bioinformatics, imaging informatics, clinical informatics, and public health informatics) may be essential in helping improve the ability to bring basic research findings to the bedside, evaluate the efficacy of interventions across communities, and enable the assessment of the eventual impact of complementary and alternative medicine practices on health policies.

One must be clear that mere collection of terminologies does not constitute ontology. Most existing controlled terminologies are collections of terms, wherein the terms are arranged in a simple list or organized in a hierarchy. These kinds of terminologies are considered useful for standardizing terms and encoding data and are currently used in many existing information systems. However, they suffer from a number of limitations that make data reuse difficult. Use of formal ontological methods was proposed relatively recently to overcome some of the problems of terminological design. Biomedical ontologies organize concepts (embodiments of knowledge about biomedical reality) whereas terminologies organize terms (what is used to code patient data at a certain point in time, based on the particular terminology version). However, the application of these methods to existing terminologies is not straightforward and incorporation of concepts from other medicine system might add to this problem. The use of these terminologies is firmly entrenched in many systems, and what might seem to be a simple option of replacing these terminologies is not possible.

Moreover, these terminologies evolve over time in order to suit the needs of users. Any methodology must therefore take these constraints into consideration, hence the need for formal methods of managing changes. One needs to work along these lines to develop a formal representation of the concept-term relation spanning a variety of medical practices.

Conclusion

Scholars working under Western medicine paradigm take it for granted that medicine is concerned with healing and problems of ill health. This constitutes a partial world view and one may infer that the way in which various medical systems define good health has not been adequately studied. Moreover, good health as such is usually regarded as a natural, normative state of being even by most medical anthropologists, who otherwise take a critical, relativist perspective on the subject of illness, pain, and disease. Ayurvedic medicine, on the other hand, has a very different way of looking at the question of how health is embodied. Ayurvedic perspective is proactive and concerned with overall fitness rather than reactivd and being primarily concerned with either illness or disease. A critical examination of the development of the philosophy of two different medicine systems is essential to highlight the contemporary arguments relating to scope of the discipline of medicine and the relation of the discipline to its cognate disciplines. Almost similar kind of research under the banner of 'philosophy of medicine' is being followed by a number of reputed scholars. Their works are often categorized as a general metaphysical world view, particular understandings of the cognate disciplines, and the perspective from which one asks the questions about the nature of the discipline is also required for creating a complete world view. If philosophy of medicine gains the due recognition, it may well combine the philosophical, sociological and historical studies in a mutually enriching way to form a fledgling steam of 'medicine studies'.

The process of designing the ontology begins after a language, a tool and standard terminology have been selected. The advantages of using ontology for knowledge representation are: standardization of medical terms, knowledge sharing, and support for automatic reasoning. It is also important to point out that any ontology is only a knowledge base and one should be aware about requirement for design and implement a decision support system so as to reason using the ontology. It can hardly be emphasized that there exist some regularities concerning the ontology classes, which the ontology creator should bear in mind. The concept from which a class is named should be known and already described in some terminology. The number of properties that a class possesses should always be kept as minimal as possible. In larger ontologies, it is usual that two or more classes use the same property.

Ontologies can help build more powerful and more interoperable information systems in health care. Ontologies can support the need of the health care process to transmit, re-use and share patient data. Ontologies can also provide semantic-based criteria to support different statistical aggregations for different purposes. Possibly the most significant benefit that ontologies may bring to health care systems is their ability to support the indispensible integration of knowledge and data. On the negative side, it may be mentioned that some remain skeptical about the impact that ontologies may have on the design and maintenance of real-world health care information systems. Thus, the creator of medical ontology must seek to go beyond the mere orientation of remedial health care and suggest a radical challenge to some of the most basic ontological assumptions in the cross-cultural comparative study of medical systems.

References

Baer, Hans, 'The American Dominative Medical System as a Reflection of Social Relations in the Larger Society', *Social Science and Medicine*, vol. 28, no. 11, 1989, pp. 1103–12.

Bodenreider, O. and O. Burgun, 'Biomedical Ontologies', in *Biomedical Informatics*, 2006, pp. 212–36.

Burgun, A., G. Botti, M. Fieschi and P. Le Beux, 'Issues in the Design of Medical Ontologies Used for Knowledge Sharing', *Journal of Medical Systems*, vol. 25, no. 2, 2001, pp 95–108.

Charles, M., Leslie and Allan Young, eds, 'Paths to Asian Medical Knowledge', University of California Press, pp. 129–208.

Baronov, David, *Biomedicine: An Ontological Dissection*, 2008, vol. 29, pp. 235–54.

Crnkovic Dodig Gordana and Stuart Susan, eds., 'Ontology as the Core Discipline of Biomedical Informatics: Legacies of the Past and Recommendations for the Future Direction of Research', in *Computing, Philosophy, and Cognitive Science*, Cambridge, 2006.

Eisenberg, Leon, 'Disease and Illness: Distinctions between Professional and Popular Ideas of Sickness', in *Culture, Medicine and Psychiatry*, vol. 1, 1977, pp. 9–23.

Gómez-Pérez, A., M. Fernández-López and O. Corcho, 'Ontological Engineering'. With examples from the areas of Knowledge Management, e-Commerce and the Semantic Web, Springer, 2004, London.

Gordon, D., 'Tenacious Assumptions in Western Medicine', in eds. *Biomedicine Reconsidered*, eds. Margaret Lock and Deborah Gordon, 1988, pp. 19–56 (Accessed: www.sanskritweb.net/rigveda/griffifth.pdf).

Griffith, R.T.H., *The Rig Veda* (English Translation), 2009.

Gruber, T.R., 'Toward Principles for the Design of Ontologies Used for Knowledge Sharing', *International Journal of Human-Computer Studies*, vol. 43, nos. 5–6, 1995, pp. 907–28.

Guarino, N. and C. Welty, 'A Formal Ontology of Properties', in EKA W-2000: The 12th International Conference on Knowledge Engineering and Knowledge Management, ed. R. Dieng and O. Corby, *Springer-Verlag*, 2000, pp. 97–112.

Hobsbawm, Eric, *The Age of Empire, 1875–1914*, New York, 1989.

Liss, P.-E., O. Aspevall, D. Karlsson and U. Forsum, 'Terms Used to Describe Urinary Tract Infections: The Importance of Conceptual Clarification', APMIS, 2003, pp. 291–9.

Payer, Lynn, *Medicine and Culture: Varieties of Treatment in the United States, England, West Germany and France*, New York, 1988.

Pisanelli, D.M., D. Zaccagnini, L. Capurso and M. Koch, 'An Ontological Approach to Evidence-based Medicine and Meta-analysis', in *Stud Health Technol Inform*, 95, pp. 543–8.

Porter, Roy, *The Greatest Benefit to Mankind: A Medical History of Mankind*, New York, 1997, p. 831.

Roy, Meera, 'Ayurveda', in *The Cultural Heritage of India*, vol. VI; *Science and Technology*, 2nd edn., ed. P. Ray, and S.N. Sen, Kolkata, 1986, pp. 152–76.

Sikorski, R. and R. Peters, 'Medicine. Microsoft ® Encarta [DVD]. Redmond, WA: Microsoft Corporation, 2007.

Smith, B., W. Ceusters and R. Temmerman, 'Wüsteria. Proc. of Medical Informatics Europe (MIE 2005)', *Studies in Health Technology and Informatics*, IOS Press, 2005, pp. 647–52.

Sowa, J.F., 'Knowledge Representation: Logical, Philosophical and Computational Foundations', 2000, pp. 594, xiv.

Wightman, W., *The Emergence of Scientific Medicine*, Edinburgh, 1971, p. 136.

Wujastyk, D., *The Roots of Ayurveda*, 2nd edn., New Delhi, 2001, p. 397.

Yach, D., C. Hawkes and C.L. Gould et al., *The Global Burden of Chronic Diseases: Overcoming Impediments to Prevention and Control.* JAMA, 2004, pp. 291, 2616–22.

Bibliography

AHIMA Foundation. Perspectives in Health Information Management. Available at http://www.ahima.org/perspectives/.

Pisanelli, D.M., ed., 'Ontologies in Medicine', vol. 102, Studies in Health Technology and Informatics, IOS Press.

Gruber, T.R., 'A Translation Approach to Portable Ontologies', *Knowledge Acquisition*, vol. 5, no. 2, 1993, pp. 199–220.

Stead, W.W. and H.S. Lin, eds., *Computational Technology for Effective Health Care: Immediate Steps and Strategic Directions*, Washington, Committee on Engaging the Computer Science Research Community in Health Care Informatics, National Research Council, 2009. Available at http://www.nlm.nih.gov/pubs/reports/comptech_prepub.pdf.

World Health Organization, *Manual of the International Classification of Diseases, Injuries, an Causes of Death*, Geneva, Switzerland, 1977.

IMIA Yearbook of Medical Informatics, 2006 (http://people.dbmi.Columbia.edu/cimino/Publications/2006 Meth Inf Med—The Practical Impact of Ontologies on Biomedical Informatics.pdf)

Hoehndorf, Robert et al., Thematic Series on Biomedical Ontologies in JBMS: Challenges and New Directions, *Journal of Biomedical Semantics*, vol. 5, no. 15, 2014 (Accessed http://........./content/pdf/2014-1480-5-15 pdf)

19

'Disease, Diet, Medicine'

Acharya Prafulla Chandra Ray's Writings on Food

Amrit Sen

> I assure you, my dear sister, that in serving my favourite science, I have only one idea in my mind, that through her I should serve my country. . . . God knows I have no other air in my life.
>
> —Acharya Prafulla Chandra Ray, in a letter to the wife of C.R. Das, December 1921, in *Life and Experience of a Bengali Chemist*, vol. 1, 1932, p. 233

Ray's contribution in the history of the nationalist project in science and industry has largely been documented in his writings on *Hindu Chemistry* and *Bengal Chemical.* It is worthwhile to note that a substantial body of Ray's writings discusses dietary practices as sources of preventive and curative medicine in the context of Bengali health in the early twentieth century. This essay explores Ray's *Khadya Bigyan* (*The Science of Food*, 1936) and attempts to locate within it Ray's nationalist project of devising ideal diets for the Bengali individual at this point in history.

It is important to note that the notion of health and masculinity had infiltrated the discourse of Indian, especially Bengali, nationalism during the period. The denigration of the Bengali middle class as effeminate and diseased had provoked a strong self-critical urge to create the alternative version of a Bengali manhood (imagined in Bankim Chandra for example) as healthy and active. The seamless integration of individual health and national health facilitated a serious rethink on the importance of dietary practices such as preventive practice in the cases of diseases like malaria, tuberculosis and dyspepsia. It is in this context that Prafulla Ray's writings need to be located.

It might be mentioned here that Ray's interest in food and its relation to disease can be traced to his early days of research at Presidency College. In his autobiography, he recollects:

> The adulteration of food-stuffs—a concomitant of modern 'civilized life'—was becoming a growing evil. Ghee and mustard oil are practically the only sources of fat which enter

into the diet of the people of Bengal. Articles in the ordinary markets that are sold as ghee and mustard oil are far from being pure. It is, however, by no means an easy task to detect by chemical analysis the adulterants used and their percentage. I undertook a searching examination of the food-stuffs of this description. I procured samples of these articles from the most reliable sources and also had them prepared under my personal supervision.[1]

Ray's use of Western scientific discourse also needs to be highlighted. While being situated within the paradigms of scientific rationality, Ray was also strongly arguing against critiques of India as a nation ever bereft of science. Dhruv Raina's analysis of *Hindu Chemistry* reveals Ray's documentation of a vibrant scientific tradition and its disruption by a rigid, monolithic Hindu superstition and submission to theoretical religion.[2] At the same time, he was conscious of the need to accept and utilize the benefits of modern scientific knowledge that the West had acquired:

Thus, for good or evil, the East has come in intimate contact with the West. The unchanging East had often in the past 'seen mighty legions pass and plunged in thought again'. This time, however, the impact is leaving behind a more permanent impress. To me personally, the civilization is a mosaic, the richer it is, the more diverse and picaresque are the elements that go to build it up. The world is in need of 'Karmayogins'—men of great purpose who delight in action, men of strong common sense, men who are constantly knocking at the locked door of Nature's secrets and are harnessing her forces to their own ends, men who in their communal and national life always try to play the game—and these typify Western culture at its best. The world—has equally the need for 'Jnanyogins'—men who love knowledge for its own sake, who renounce their all in contemplating the beauties of the universe, and in establishing direct contact between their own soul and the Universal spirit. The West, bereft of the spirit that suffered at the Cross, led to the world chaos of 1914 and its aftermath. In the East where the intellectuals withdrew from the world into the inner-self of spiritual life, ignorance and superstition, poverty and squalor have grown up as luxuriant tropical weeds and enveloped the lives of the masses. In their synthesis lies a new hope for the world; in their unmeaning clash—a wreckage of much that is of immense value in the scheme of life.[3]

Thus, with *Bengal Chemical*, Ray had used the resources of the kaviraji medical system but only after testing them scientifically in the laboratory:

Over and above that I began a regular campaign in favour of these and impressed upon the profession the fact that the efficacy of these drugs had been proved beyond doubt by their universal use in the households of Bengal. All that was needed was that their active principles should receive the *imprimatur* of the practicioners . . . slowly but surely they began to be favoured. It was the universal practice in those days to prescribe syrup of tolu as an expectorant; but it was found that syrup of vsaka acted more efficaciously. Our newly introduced indigenous drug preparations, thus, began to make headway on their own merits.[4]

Ray's self-critique was complimented by his trenchant critique of the colonial apparatus that was stripping India of its material resources and inculcating an education system designed to rob originality. He was also aware that colonialism had dealt a body blow to a nation that had known a healthier past, making an ironic contrast between the course charted out by the colonizer and the colonized:

> The facts and figures given by Sir George Newman show the 'amazing transformation', in the health of the British people which has taken place in the past 100 years. In India also, there has been 'amazing' transformation in the health of the people. But the transformation is such as to bring tears to the eyes of a man who has lived to be fifty or sixty and who remembers still the smiling villages which had not yet proved a prey to the epidemics of cholera due to scarcity of drinking water, or which had not yet felt the effects of the scourge of malaria.[5]

Khadya Bigyan embodies both a rigorous self-critique of the diet as well as a rejection of colonial diets to imagine a healthy Bengal.

The idea of a primer for familiarizing his countrymen to diet as preventive and curative medicine is defended in the conclusion to his text, 'In this book, researches into the science of food have been written in Bengali and I hope that the women of Bengal will choose the food she serves carefully so that she can preserve and cure health in the family and justify the title of mother.'[6]

Ray was aware of the need to introduce basic primers in science in the local languages to create awareness in the broader population:

> The medium of education is to be the vernacular languages of India, into which the best elementary treatises in English should be translated. Such translations are to be advertised for, and liberally rewarded by Government as the means of enriching vernacular literature. While, therefore, the vernacular languages are on no account to be neglected, the English language may be taught where there is a demand for it, but the English language is not to be substituted for the vernacular dialects of the country.[7]

Ray quotes Hopkins, the Nobel Prize winner, for his research on vitamins and proceeds to justify the importance of his primer on food:

> We now know that the satisfaction of appetites by mere bulk consumption is no final proof of a food supply as quantity; details are of the utmost significance; the absence of factors which add almost nothing to the bulk of a diet may make the whole entirely inadequate. . . . What is the relevance of research on food—we must look for the adequacy of food based on factors like place, time and person. We must learn how to supplement dietary inadequacies and choose our food accordingly.[8]

Accordingly, Ray defines the digestive system, types of food, vitamins and enzymes, food value, diets for various diseases and the reasons for the onset of diseases. Ray mentions diets for obesity, gout, diabetes, glycosma, nephritis, dyspepsia, constipation, pneumonia and typhoid. In many ways, this is a treatise that makes the reasons, indications and diets in a particular disease available to the population at large in a local language, thereby highlighting Ray's project of making scientific knowledge available to the masses. What does he reject? What is his ultimate project here?

Ray's initial proposition is that Bengali health had once been in pristine condition and various diseases had been given short shift. He locates this in three major presences in the Bengali diet—adequate milk, flesh, fruits, and vegetables. Looking at the presence of the flesh in the Bengali *shakta* tradition he regrets that this was disrupted by the turn towards the non-vegeterian diet. Ray refers to the Chandimangal as a source of recognition of meat in the diet and of Jagai Madhai as Brahmins who took meat: 'Unfortunately with Chaitanya that diet was rejected of course in Chaitanya's time there was a prevalence of milk products in the diet'.[9]

Interestingly Ray is here creating a social history of food much like his project of a social history of science in locating the fundamental shifts within dietary practices within the changing social movements in contemporary history.

In fact, Ray sees the drying up of milk as a major factor in the decline of health in Bengal:

> One potent reason is malnutrition, as the infants between age 0–5 and 5–10 get a very insufficient quantity of mother's or cow's milk; in short, they are fed on thin gruel of boiled rice, which neither contains nitrogenous (i.e. muscle-forming) stuff nor calcium (i.e. bone-forming) element. No wonder that the Census Report of 1931 points out that the Muslim population is to the Hindu as 55 to 45 (approx.); but if babies be left out of consideration, i.e. if adult population be taken into account, the ratio would be 51 to 48. In other words, the mortality of the babies among the Muslims is much more than among the Hindus, though the latter is appalling in all conscience.[10]

In his autobiography, he recollects the importance of the dairy products in the daily diet of Bengal: 'The tending of milch cows was a sort of religious duty with every Hindu. I still remember how my mother used to superintend personally the feeding of the cows of which there were various breeds. It was a rule with my parents that their children should be nourished chiefly on a milk diet till they were five years of age. Even ladies and gentlemen of rank did not disdain to cleanse the cowshed in the early morning.'[11]

He also locates within practices of the *prasad* and *suryapranam*, sources of vitamins and sunlight that can prevent diseases in India. Ray, thus, locates the sources of health within indigenous dietary practices. A key text in this analysis is his short essay 'Chira, Muri, Khai, Biscuit' where diets like *Chira, Muri* and *Khai* (varieties of beaten and puffed rice) are seen as rich sources of carbohydrates that are easily affordable to the Bengali individual.

Ray's point is that a return to and a respect of traditional dietary practices may prevent and cure numerous diseases. He urges against polished rice, urges the retaining of the decantation of boiled rice, retaining of the shin of potatoes in the increase of nutritive value. His advocaton of pulses and spinach or *sag* as rich sources of nutrition need special mention. Ray also looks at available fruits like the guava over imported fruits that are relatively difficult to obtain. In an ironic rejoiner he reminds us that a fractional investment in food might save a major expenditure in medicine and dietary supplements later: 'You had attempted to save money from expenses on food for six continuous months—more than five times that expense is now spent on buying medicines. I acknowledge that the poor are deprived of adequate food; but we are compounding the problem by an ignorant choice of diet and inviting disease'[12] (p. 433).

Ray's insistence on the diet for a healthy mother as a source of healthy children is a recurrent point within his writings.

An important trait of Ray's work is the constant reminder that rural health is a necessary aspect of the improvement of national health and there is a possibility of regenerating it: 'The health of our country can only be regenerated by the regeneration of its villages—in the prosperity of its ponds and rivers, agriculture and orchards, in its animal husbandry and poultry. I do not think there is a lack of food resources in our country. We have to turn to them.'[13]

Ray is, however, not insular in his adoption of elements of foreign diet, provided it suits the economic condition of the Bengali. Thus, he is in favour of soyabean as a cheap source of protein, while he is effusive about the benefits of tomato (bilati begun): 'Dr Nilratan Dhar used to say "A tomato a day keeps the doctor away" when it is impossible to cultivate apples, grapes and oranges in Bengal, we must irate the poor man's apple, the tomato with great respect'.[14]

Ray urges the Bengali to follow the ideal English breakfast and draws the comparative analysis of a Sikh diet versus a Bengali diet to highlight the importance of protein as a source of health: 'Indeed nothing could be more striking than the contrast between the manly, stalwart and resolute races of the North—the Pathans, Beluchis, Sikhs . . . and the poorly developed, toneless and supine people of the east and south; Bengalis, Madrassis, Kanarese . . . besides proteins, element of food vitamins and mineral elements are concerned in bringing about this result.'[15]

Ray's critique of adopting English food is intricately linked with the theme of colonial exploitation. The two sharpest targets are tea and biscuit. Ray's writings on tea draw upon tea as lacking food value and initiating disease like insomnia, dyspepsia and others. He, however, acknowledges that it is not an occasional cup of tea that he is against; it is the imagining of tea as an antidote to fatigue and disease that he protests. He locates the clever English projection of tea as a source of health in the English attempt to trap and economically exploit a huge population:

> The 'Educated' Bengali ever on the alert for imitating European ways, eagerly swallowed the bait. He has already become a confirmed tea-drinker and the habit is spreading like wild fire among the coolies, carters and labourers in general. The Tea Association, having captured Calcutta and emboldened by its phenomenal success, has begun propaganda on a large scale in the Provincial towns and big railway terminals with immense success.[16]

Ray is quick to count both the economic and the medical cost of such a replacement of the diet by tea:

As the vast majority of Indians are too poor to afford both their customary food and tea, it meant the substitution of their food by tea altogether . . . it possesses no dietetic value whatsoever . . . to strangle the salutary and universal dietetic custom of the country and undermine the health of the guileless people. He, momentarily, feels refreshed and goes on with his drudgery and again follows with another cup and in this way he often drinks half-a-dozen cups. He urges in support of this habit that it kills appetite and therefore he has no need for nourishing food. I am as much concerned here with the medical and physiological aspects of the question as with its economic bearing; 96 per cent of the tea produced in Bengal comes from the European Gardens and barely 4 per cent from the Indian. The tea-drinking habit is spreading fast among the masses and, if it goes on at this rate, in the course of the next 25 years the population of Bengal being taken at 50 millions, the European planters may safely count upon a yearly sale of 50 millions rupees worth of tea in Bengal alone. I have been appalled by the new fashions in diet in this age. We tend to imitate Europeans, but we forget that Europeans drink tea with plenty of food—we on the other hand drink it repeatedly without any food.[17]

The case of the biscuit replicates this process. Ray is at pain to point out the inferiority of biscuit as a source of energy. However, his sharpest critique is in the cultural perception of biscuit as replacing traditional Bengali food and an indicator of sophistication or civility:

In terms of food value and also in terms of price, the food articles that we make at home are far superior than biscuits that are largely imported. The Bengali woman can have far greater satisfaction in feeding her family members a diet of chira and muri rather than opening a shining new tin of biscuits.[18]

Ray also points to the fact how perceptions of food change culturally with colonialism so that perfectly nourishing food is seen as unacceptable in opposition to items without any significant food value, 'I would like to ask—what is the comparative price of chira, muri and biscuit. What I observe is that in servile imitation, we are moving towards a crisis in food habits. If a gentleman is offered muri he thinks he has not been shown respect!'[19]

In a way, Ray's analysis of food ties up with his project of decolonizing the mind through a rejection of certain underlying principles of a non-indigenous diet, 'In Bengal from time immemorial, every man, rich or poor, used to take his morning meal of Gur Chhola (molasses and gram) or phen bhat (rice with water) and milk, and as dietetic prescriptions they can hardly be improved upon either in general balance or in vitamin content.'[20]

Ray, thus, added:

We are afflicted with Malaria and other diseases. One of the major reasons is, thus, we shut off our houses (like chests) to light and winds—we use our ponds and water bodies as garbage disposal centers. We Hindus merely pay lip service to cleanliness. I am revolutionary—a rebel—not in politics but in the spite of health, education and social norms.[21]

Ray's analysis of the spread of malaria reflects an interesting response from the nationalist perspective. He traces the rise of malaria as an epidemic to the British project of laying railway lines across the breadth of the country:

> Choonakhally, Bhatpara, Cossimbazar, Kalkapore, Bamunghatta and Fureshdanga were situated on the curve of the river Hoogly until a straight cut was made some sixty years since forming the chord of the curve, thus changing the course of the river and throwing these places inland. This engineering operation was closely followed by the breaking out of an epidemic in all those places which, in the virulence and morality is unparalleled by any pestilential visitation in Bengal, saving perhaps that which depopulated Gour . . . not only the ravages of malaria but also the terrible calamity caused by the north Bengal flood would have been mitigated, if not altogether avoided if the railway authorities had taken the precaution to provide sufficient outlets for the passage of water. But they were more concerned to cheapen the cost of laying down the railroads. Earthworks had been thrown across partially silted up river-beds leaving narrow culverts for the flow of water. An engineer with only an elementary knowledge of the subject would have suggested the construction of bridges in such places. But the authorities were more anxious to consult the interest of the foreign capitalists and were thus utterly regardless of future consequences.[22]

Ray also accused the colonial government of importing quinine, therefore, pushing up the cost and thereby depriving the population of adequate medicine, 'There is a cinchona plantation at Mungpoo where quinine is manufactured at a government factory. But strange to say that the Indian public is supplied with Java Quinine at a higher price. It is, thus, evident that our benign government far from helping the malaria stricken peasants actually compel them to buy the drug at a dear price.'[23]

Interestingly knowledge about Ray sees pedagogy as a key tool in the overall enhancement of national health. Apart from education about diet as medicine, Ray sees the schoolteachers as imparting food to student. He also urges each school to monitor the weight of students and maintain charts of their growth so that children and their guardian are sensitized to the upkeep of their health. It is imperative that in the process of growth teachers accommodate and enthuse guardians in the health care of the ward.[24] Ray's vision is, thus, congruent with the mid-day meal project of the government where the school is seen as a source of holistic nourishment—both physical and intellectual.

Ray's writings on food as preventive and curative medicine, thus, dovetail nicely with his writings on *Hindu Chemistry* and *Bengal Chemical.* Using Bhaba's notion of third space as moving beyond imitation Ray borrows the discourse of Western science to establish the basis of his dietary logic. However, he locates this diet within indigenous food practices and in this location he underlines the rejection of colonial diets that exploit the economy and the population. Apart from its contribution as the first comprehensive manual of food as medicine, *Khadya Bigyan* needs to be placed and read alongside Ray's broader post-colonial outlook.

Notes

1. Prafulla Chandra Ray, *Life and Experiences of a Bengali Chemist*, vol. 1, Kolkata, 1932, p. 84.
2. Dhruv Raina, 'The Young P.C. Ray and the Inauguration of the Social History of Science in India 1885–1907', in *Science, Technology Society*, vol. 2, no. 1, pp. 2–40. Raina has identified the 'inauguration' of a 'social history of science' in Ray's identification of the cause of scientific decline in the consolidation of the caste system and social rigidities of medieval times. This is part of Raina's larger thesis of identifying Ray's project as a clear break from the orientalist paradigm, marking and initiating a new scientific discourse of colonial India. Raina argues that while orientalist literature on India tended to decontextualize Indian knowledge from its social matrix, Ray's analysis of the caste system located the problem both beyond the question of eastern and Western 'minds' as well as the nature of scientific practice in India. Moreover, through his unearthing of an Indian scientific past, Ray had articulated the logic of the universality of scientific and civilizational modes. Thus, a break from the fundamental postulate of Orientalism, which had proposed an ontological and epistemological divide between the Orient and the Occident was initiated (Raina 8).
3. Ray, *Life and Experiences*, vol. 2, p. 58.
4. Ibid., vol. 1, p. 104.
5. Ibid., vol. 2, p. 148.
6. Prafulla Chandra Ray, *Khadya Bigyan*, 1936, in *Acharya Prafulla Chandra Ray Rachana Sankalan*, ed. Anil Bhattacharya, vol. 1, Kolkata, 2008, pp. 310–503, see p. 318. All translations from this text are mine. Ray's text is the most comprehensive statement and analysis of food practices. He alludes to an earlier publication by Biresh Chandra Guha titled 'The Food Problem in India'. Ray also argues: 'Our lack of knowledge and interest about food is unfortunate. In our country the educated class increases the cost of motor fuel with an increase of earning, but they devote scant attention to their food habits.'
7. Ray, *Life and Experiences*, vol. 2, p. 56.
8. Ray, *Khadya Bigyan*, p. 479. Ray suggests that in the ideal diet of the middleclass household there should be (1) no monotony, (2) should contain fish, eggs, meat or paneer, (3) should contain fruits and salad, and (4) should contain milk.
9. Ibid., p. 399.
10. Ray, *Life and Experiences*, vol. 2, pp. 148–9.
11. Ibid., vol. 1, p. 396. Ray harps on milk as a diet which could revitalize the Bengali physique recurrently in his writings: 'Our lack of knowledge and interest about food is unfortunate. In our country, the educated class increase the cost of motor fuel with an increase of earning, but they devote scant attention to their food habits.'
12. Ray, *Khadya Bigyan*, p. 433.
13. Ibid., p. 493.
14. Ibid., p. 403. Ray also highlights the acute lack of proteins in the Bengali diet. 'Insufficiency of vitamins and of high-class protein, apart from racial factors, accounts for much of the short stature and proveners to disease observed in Bengal' (p. 361). Ray mentions—various pulses, *Kachu* (roots and stems), bringal and spinach as rich sources of protein (p. 357) which are, therefore, available to the impoverished Bengali individual. He also argues that the Prasad of the familiar pujas was a way of intake of fruits and vitamins: 'The prasad of our pujas is saturated with vitamins and we bow in respect to the far reaching vision of our saints.'
15. Ray, *Khadya Bigyan*, p. 402.
16. Ray, *Life and Experiences*, vol. 2, p. 334.

17. Ibid., p. 335.
18. Prafulla Chandra Ray, 'Chira Muri, Khoi, Biscuit', in *Shyamal Chakraborty*, ed. Acharya Prafullachandrer Prabandha, Kolkata: Aajkaal, 2001, pp. 69–75.
19. Ibid., p. 73.
20. Ray, *Khadya Bigyan*, p. 499.
21. Ibid.
22. Ray, *Life and Experiences*, vol. 2, pp. 137–8.
23. Ibid., p. 145.
24. Ray, *Khadya Bigyan*, p. 445. Ray's final words harp on the issue of food and exercise complementing each other: 'My advice for most Bengali gentlemen (1) Most of us dig our graves with our teeth. (2) Every mile you walk carries you a step away from the funeral pyre.'

Editors and Contributors

SYED EJAZ HUSSAIN is Professor in History at Visva-Bharati University, Santiniketan, West Bengal and has a deep interest in India's indigenous medicine. He specializes in medieval Indian history and numismatics as well as Islamic history and philosophy. His publications include *The Varied Facets of History: Essays in Honour of Aniruddha Ray* (co-edited with Ishrat Alam, 2011), *The Bengal Sultanate: Politics, Economy and Coins, AD 1205–1576* (2003) and *Mauji-i Sultani: A Memoir of the Mughal Prince Mirza Muhammad Zubairuddin Gorgani* (co-edited with Surendra Gopal, 2003).

MOHIT SAHA is Senior Medical Officer in Pearson Memorial Hospital, Visva-Bharati University, Santiniketan, West Bengal. He has participated in a number of conferences on medicine and is associated with several community services and public health initiatives. He is a votary of cross-medical practices.

ISHRAT ALAM is Professor at the Centre for Advanced Study, Department of History, Aligarh Muslim University, Aligarh. He has contributed research papers on ancient and medieval Indian technology, economy and society.

ANIS AHMAD ANSARI is Member, Executive Committee, Ibn-e-Sina Academy of Medieval Medicine & Science. He is Professor, at PG Department of Kulliyat, former Dean Faculty of Unani, Aligarh Muslim University, Aligarh and Principal Investigator, UGC Major Research Project A.K. Tibbiya College, Aligarh Muslim University, Aligarh.

NIRMALYA BANERJEE obtained his Ph.D. from University of Calcutta in Cytogenetics and Plant Biotechnology and worked as a Post-doctoral Fellow in Catholic University of Leuven, Belgium. He is Head, Department of Botany at Visva-Bharati. He has published about 80 research papers in reputed national and international journals. Vitro propagation and conservation of medicinal and ornamental plants and their cytogenetical and molecular analysis is presently his area of research.

ANIL BHARANI is a well-known cardiologist serving at Maharaja Yashwantrao Hospital, Indore. His area of expertise is clinical and drug trials. He has contributed several research articles on the subject in national and international journals of science and medicine.

JAYANTA BHATTACHARYA is a physician by training who obtained his doctorate in history of medicine from Medical College, Calcutta. He was awarded 'Honorable Mention for an Outstanding Essay' by the *Asian Society for the History of Medicine* in 2006. He has several reputed publications in renowned national and international journals like *Current Science*, *Historia Hospitalium* and *IESHR*.

DEBRAJ CHAKRABORTY teaches history at Rabindra Bharati University, Kolkata. He has received his doctoral degree in history from the Visva-Bharati University, Santiniketan. The areas of his research are history of environment, ecology, health, science and technology of pre-colonial India.

CHHANDA CHATTERJEE is Professor and Director, Centre for Guru Nanak Dev Studies and Programme Coordinator, UGC SAP DRS II of the Department of History at Visva-Bharati, Santiniketan, West Bengal.

NUPUR DASGUPTA has been teaching history at the Department of History, Jadavpur University since 1991. Her specialization is in ancient Indian history and the History of Science. She is currently working on the historical interfaces of chemistry, medicine and pharmacy in the Indian context. She has authored and edited a number of books and several of her research papers on her areas of specialization have been published in international and national journals and edited volumes.

ACHINTYA KUMAR DUTTA is Professor of History, The University of Burdwan. He is former postdoctoral Commonwealth Fellow at School of Oriental and African Studies, London, UK; and Visiting Fellow of The Wellcome Trust, London, UK; Foundation Maison des Sciences de l'Homme, Paris; Zakir Hussain Centre for Educational Studies, Jawaharlal Nehru University, New Delhi.

ARUNANGSHU GANGULY is a cardiologist of repute. He is Vice Chairman and Sr. Consultant at Mission Hospital, Durgapur, West Bengal. He also serves as Consultant, Interventional Cardiology at Suraksha Hospital, Kolkata. He has contributed several research papers on cardiology in reputed medical journals. Dr. Ganguly is also attached to several community services.

PARTHASARATHI GIRI is a well-known medical practitioner and worked for long in North Bengal. He has published a number of research papers in medical and scientific journals. He has recently developed his interests in ancient medicine and treatment systems.

DEEPAK KUMAR teaches history of science, medicine and education at the Zakir Husain Centre for Educational Studies, Jawaharlal Nehru University, New Delhi. He has been working in this area for almost four decades and is known for his book *Science and the Raj* (1995). In addition, he has edited separate volumes on medicine, technology, environment and education in the context of colonial India.

MADHUMITA MAJUMDAR completed her Ph.D. from Visva-Bharati University, Santiniketan and has published a number of research papers in scientific journals of national and international repute. She is now working as a Guest Faculty at Basirhat College, Basirhat, West Bengal.

SUJATA MUKHERJEE is Professor of History at Rabindra Bharati University, Kolkata. Her research interests include history of science, technology, medicine, environment, women's history, Gandhian studies, socio-cultural history of modern India. She has authored several books and articles and also edited monographs and journals.

S.N. OJHA completed his Ph.D. in the fledgling field of biophysics from Visva-Bharati and is Head of its Computer Center since 2002. Apart from his core research area, he has worked at the technology interfaces of humanities, languages, management and other social sciences. His publications also span the domains of ecology, higher education and philosophy of sciences.

ASHHAR QADEER is Head of the Department, Kulliyat (Fundamentals of Unani Medicine) at Jamia Hamdard University. He has published 9 books, 32 research papers and 133 articles to his name.

HABIBUR RAHAMAN is Associate Professor of Botany, Department of Botany, Visva-Bharati University, Santiniketan. He specializes in the area of phytoresources and has contributed 55 research papers in reputed national and international journals. Presently he concentrates his research on Applied Ethnobotany and Bioprospecting of Ethnomedicinal plants. His latest papers has come up in the *International Journal of Research in Ayurveda & Pharmacy* (2013).

ARABINDA SAMANTA is Professor of History at the University of Burdwan, West Bengal. He is also Visiting Professor, Zakir Husain Centre for Educational Studies, Jawaharlal Nehru University, New Delhi; Visiting Fellow, Wellcome Trust Centre for the History of Medicine at UCL, UK; and Visiting Fellow, Rockefeller Archive Center, New York, US. Professor Samanta has been working mainly on epidemics, medicine, and environment in colonial Bengal.

AMRIT SEN is Professor of English at Visva-Bharati University, Santiniketan. Interested in Eighteenth Century Studies, Travel Writing, Tagore Studies and the History of Science, he has won the outstanding research award for his doctoral dissertation, *The Narcissistic Mode: Metafiction as a Strategy in Moll Flanders, Tom Jones and Tristram Shandy*, published in 2007.

Index